T0309055

Recent Advances in
Predicting and Preventing
Epileptic Seizures

Recent Advances in Predicting and Preventing
Epileptic Seizures

edited by

Ronald Tetzlaff
Technische Universität Dresden, Germany

Christian E. Elger
Universitätsklinikum Bonn, Germany

Klaus Lehnertz
Universitätsklinikum Bonn, Germany

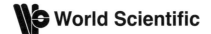

NEW JERSEY · LONDON · SINGAPORE · BEIJING · SHANGHAI · HONG KONG · TAIPEI · CHENNAI

Published by

World Scientific Publishing Co. Pte. Ltd.

5 Toh Tuck Link, Singapore 596224

USA office: 27 Warren Street, Suite 401-402, Hackensack, NJ 07601

UK office: 57 Shelton Street, Covent Garden, London WC2H 9HE

British Library Cataloguing-in-Publication Data
A catalogue record for this book is available from the British Library.

RECENT ADVANCES IN PREDICTING AND PREVENTING EPILEPTIC SEIZURES
Proceedings of the 5th International Workshop on Seizure Prediction

ISBN 978-981-4525-34-3

Printed in Singapore by World Scientific Printers.

Preface

This book comprises contributions delivered at the 5th International Workshop on Seizure Prediction held in Dresden, Germany in the September of 2011. This workshop followed a series of international meetings on seizure prediction, seizure dynamics, and seizure control hosted in Bonn in 2002, Bethesda in 2006, Freiburg in 2007, and Kansas City in 2009.

This series proved highly successful in bringing together specialists from a wide range of backgrounds - including epileptology, neurosurgery, neurosciences, physics, mathematics, computer science, and engineering - that are engaged in improving our understanding of mechanisms leading to seizures in humans and in developing new therapeutic options. The workshop covered topics such as recent approaches to seizure control, recent developments in signal processing of interest for seizure prediction, ictogenesis in complex epileptic brain networks, active probing of the pre-seizure state, non-EEG based approaches to the transition to seizures, microseizures and their role in the generation of clinical seizures, the impact of sleep and long-biological cycles on seizure prediction, as well as animal and computational models of seizures and epilepsy. Furthermore the workshop program covered recent developments of international databases and of parallel computing structures based on Cellular Nonlinear Networks that can play an important role for the realization of a portable seizure warning device.

In order to give an overview of recent advances in predicting and preventing epileptic seizures, the content of this book has been organized around three major themes. Theme 1 addresses the emerging concept of epileptic networks on different scales (from single neurons to the brain) and their role for seizure prediction and seizure control. Theme 2 summarizes recent computational models of seizures and epilepsy, and finally, Theme 3 conflates recent advances in EEG and network analyses as well as in measurement techniques. Multivariate signal processing and analysis methods that overcome the current limitiations of the univariate and bivariate techniques used in seizure prediction can be improved by gaining deeper insights from modeling dynamics on/of complex networks and from a data-driven characterization of their features. Especially, a signal processing platform based on Cellular Nonlinear Networks is proposed that implements a low-power sensor processor realization with stored programmability.

The workshop was sponsored by the German National Science Foundation (Deutsche Forschungsgemeinschaft), the Epilepsy Therapy Project (ETP), the American Epilepsy Society (AES), the Citizens United for Research in Epilepsy (CURE), Cyberonics, Inc., UCB Pharma GmbH, NeuroVista Corp., the Department of Epileptology of the University Hospital Bonn, and the Faculty of Electrical and Computer Engineering, Institute of Fundamentals of Electrical Engineering and Electronics, Technische Universität Dresden. We would like to express our appreciation and sincere thanks to the sponsoring organizations. Especially, we would like to thank Hitten Zaveri and Brian Litt for their valuable support in applying for grants from ETP, CURE, AES, and NeuroVista.

Finally, we would like to thank Mrs. Lempke who was in charge of the Conference Secretariat task, the members of the conference team (Gerrit Ansmann, Henning Dickten, Andreas Mögel, Jan Müller, Detlef Tolksdorf) for the invaluable job they have done, and Gerhard Thüner for designing the book cover.

Dresden and Bonn, March 2013

Ronald Tetzlaff, Christian E. Elger, Klaus Lehnertz

Contents

Epileptic networks and their role for seizure prediction and seizure control

TRANSITION INTO AND OUT OF A FOCAL SEIZURE

MARCO DE CURTIS

Unit of Experimental Neurophysiology and Epileptology
Fondazione Istituto Neurologico Carlo Besta, Milano, Italy

It is commonly assumed that seizure activity correlates with enhanced neuronal synchronization and increased excitation. Increasing evidence, based on both intracranial recordings in humans and data obtained in animal models, suggests that synchronization of inhibition is required to initiate a focal seizure and that synchronization among principal cells decreases at seizure onset and gradually recovers during late ictal phases. These findings are here reviewed and are discussed in the context of focal ictogenesis.

Key words: ictogenesis; Ictal discharges; interictal events; synchronization

The transition from the interictal state into a focal seizure and back to the interictal state is a highly dynamic phenomenon characterized by quite reproducible sequences of events/phases that develop in time and space. During different seizure phases, subpopulations of neurons may be selectively and transiently activated/inactivated and synchronized/decoupled; the relation between these largely unknown events shapes the rules of ictogenesis.

In spite of the extensive studies on the epileptic brain performed in animal models and in humans, we still have a very approximate understanding of how focal seizures initiate, develop and terminate. It is usually assumed that focal epileptiform discharges correlate with enhanced synchronization of neuronal activity and that both interictal and ictal events are due to a disturbed balance between excitation and inhibition, resulting in an increased excitation. Synchronization of excitation definitely occurs during the late phases of a seizure discharge, but seizure initiation and interictal epileptiform events are not always associated with synchronous enhancement of excitatory network interactions. The latter postulation is based on experimental evidence and is suggested by scalp or intracranial electroencephalographic (EEG) observations from patients with focal epilepsy.

I will revise the mechanism that promote and control the development of one of the most common neurophysiological pattern observed in focal seizures, characterized by the occurrence of low-voltage fast activity at onset, followed by irregular spiking ("tonic" phase) that progressively develops into periodic bursting intercalated by post-burst depressions ("clonic" phase: Figure 1). This pattern is habitually observed in human temporal lobe epilepsy (Lieb *et al.*, 1976; Allen et al., 1992; Fisher et al., 1992; Spencer et al., 1992; Gotman et al., 1995; Bartolomei et al., 1999; Bragin et al., 1999a) and in focal epilepsy of neocortical origin (Salanova et al., 1992; Lee et al., 2000; Tassi et al., 2002), as well as in experimental models of focal epilepsy (Bragin et al., 1999a; Bragin et al., 1999b; Karhunen et al., 2006; Kadam et al., 2010) and in acute models of focal seizures (Lopantsev and Avoli, 1998; Uva et al., 2005; Boido et al., 2012).

Low voltage fast activity that fragments and substitutes background rhythms (Allen et al., 1992; Fisher et al., 1992; de Curtis and Gnatkovsky, 2009), described as *EEG flattening*, is recognized since long time by clinical neurophysiologists and can be hardly interpreted as an event due to enhanced excitability. A major step forward in our understanding of focal ictogenesis (i.e., the processes that rule the transition from the interictal state into a seizure) was made when intracranial recordings started to be performed during pre-surgical diagnostic studies aimed at localizing the *epileptogenic zone* (EZ: the area involved in the generation of the epileptiform discharge) and the *seizure-onset zone* (SOZ: the area of initiation of the epileptiform discharge) in patients with focal epilepsies resistant to pharmacological treatment that could benefit of surgical removal of the epileptogenic region (Bancaud et al., 1970; Spencer et al., 1990; Engel, 1993; Munari et al., 1994). Interictal events of various amplitude, morphology and duration can be recorded between seizures with intracranial electrodes positioned within EZ and in the cortex around the EZ, defined as the *irritative zone* (IZ). Diverse patterns, such as spikes, sharp waves and brief spike bursts, as well as rhythmic sequences of activity in theta/delta frequency range and high frequency oscillations are included in the term "interictal event" (de Curtis and Avanzini, 2001; de Curtis and Gnatkovsky, 2009; Engel et al., 2009; de Curtis et al., 2012). Cortical surface recordings with grid and strip electrodes and intra-cerebral recordings performed with depth electrodes (stereo-EEG) in different cortical areas demonstrated that one of the most frequent and most localizing pattern of onset in focal epilepsies features a triad of electrographic traits (Gnatkovsky et al., 2011) that occur simultaneously: i) the abolition of the background activity, ii) the appearance of low-voltage fast activity in the beta-gamma range (20-100 Hz) that corresponds to the EEG flattening observed with scalp electrodes and iii) the activation of a very slow potential of high amplitude (Ikeda et al., 1996; Ikeda et al., 1999).

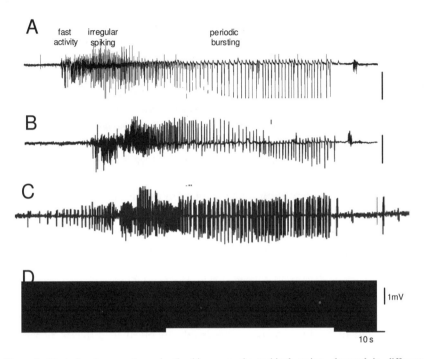

Figure 1. Typical seizure patterns in the hippocampal-entorhinal region observed in different experimental conditions and in patients. Seizure are always characterized by fast activity of low amplitude at onset followed by irregular spiking that gradually proceed into periodic bursting. The two seizures in the upper part of the figure were induced by acute application of either 2 mM bicuculline for 3 minutes (A; see Uva *et al.*, 2005) or 50 μM 4-aminopyridine (B; see Carriero *et al.*, 2010) in the *in vitro* isolated guinea pig brain preparation. The third trace reports a spontaneous seizure in a chronic model of temporal lobe epilepsy induced in the guinea pig by local hippocampal injection of kainic acid (C; Carriero *et al.*, 2012). The bottom trace (D) is the hippocampal recording of a seizure from a patient with temporal lobe epilepsy, performed during pre-surgical diagnostic intracranial recording to define the epileptogenic zone (courtesy of Stefano Francione and Laura Tassi, of the *Claudio Munari* Epilepsy Surgery Center, Milano, Italy).

The cellular correlates of interictal and ictal patterns in human epileptic brains showed that synchronization and enhanced excitation are not likely to occur in specific phases of ictogenesis. Unit recordings performed with micro-electrodes demonstrated that synchronous neuronal bursting suggestive of enhanced excitation is not observed during interictal spikes and during seizures (Babb et al., 1981; Wyler et al., 1982; Babb et al., 1987; Isokawa-Akesson et al., 1989; Colder et al., 1996). Recent intracranial human recordings performed during the early phase of a seizure demonstrated that neurons in the EZ and in the surrounding areas reduce their firing activity and synchronization, measured by spiking heterogeneity index (Truccolo *et al.*, 2011; Bower *et al.*, 2012). Microelectrode recordings also showed increased firing synchrony only several seconds after seizure onset, suggesting that action potential synchronization within the epileptogenic network is not required to initiate a seizure (Bower *et al.*, 2012; Schevon *et al.*, 2012). Non-linear correlation analysis between activities intracranially recorded during human focal seizures also demonstrated a desynchronization of the epileptogenic region during and just ahead seizure onset (Wendling *et al.*, 2003; Schindler *et al.*, 2007). These studies demonstrated that synchronization builds up and becomes prominent in the late phase of seizures close to seizure termination, characterized by large amplitude bursting patterns. Based on these human findings, the concept that transition into a seizure is due to a **synchronous enhancement of excitation** needs to be verified and perhaps revised.

A key concept to be discussed to understand transition in and out of seizure is the meaning of the term synchronization (Jiruska *et al.*, 2012). Synchronization can independently occur over time and/or over space. Moreover, synchronization may be promoted by enhanced activity in either excitatory or inhibitory neurons (or both) and may be mediated both by synaptic entrainment and via non-synaptic mechanisms. Synchronization of interneurons and/or excitatory neurons may be selectively involved in different phases of seizures and during the interictal state. Non-neuronal cells, such as astrocytes, also contribute to neuronal synchronization and their activation may be determinant to pace transition into seizure and to modify synchronization patterns during a focal seizure. These concepts will be discussed in the following paragraphs.

Space and time synchronization of neuronal activities during interictal phasic events, such as interictal spikes and sharp waves, is likely to happen. Large amplitude events recordable with extracellular or even extracerebral (scalp EEG) electrodes must be generated by the synchronous discharge of a considerable number of neurons. Spikes detected with scalp or intracranial EEG electrodes represent the integrate signal recorded over a wide cortical area (10 cm^2 and 5 mm^2 for scalp and intracranial electrodes, respectively; Buzsaki *et al.*, 2012). Simultaneous functional MRI and EEG recording in epilepsy patients demonstrated that interictal spikes can be detected by blood-oxygen-level-dependent signal changes; the cortical volume of tissue includes several voxels, over few mm^2 of tissue (Bagshaw *et al.*, 2006; Kobayashi *et al.*, 2006). Thus, in the case of spatial synchronization of interictal events, the spread and diffusion of a sharp, large-amplitude potential is measured, assuming that such potential originates from a "focus", i.e., a group of neurons that are simultaneously active for a brief time period. Incidentally, the term "epileptic focus" should be reconsidered and, in line with the new epilepsy classification proposal (Berg *et al.*, 2010; Berg and Scheffer, 2011), possibly replaced by the more neurobiologically appropriate concept of epileptogenic network.

Interictal spikes/sharp waves observed in different experimental and clinical conditions show similarities as grapho-elements, even though mechanisms and the type of synchronized networks underlying their generation can be considerably different, as revealed by studies performed on acute seizures induced by *in vitro* pharmacological manipulations. Interictal events with different time course are induced by 4-aminopyridine (4AP) applications on *in vitro* slices of rodent (Perreault and Avoli, 1989, 1992) and post-surgical human limbic and dysplastic cortices (Avoli *et al.*, 1991; Avoli *et al.*, 1995) and on the isolated guinea pig brain (Uva *et al.*, 2009). While fast spikes are sustained by glutamatergic synaptic potentials and are blocked by glutamate receptor antagonists, slow spikes are blocked by GABAa receptor blockers and, therefore, are sustained by inhibitory interneuronal networks.

Large amplitude spikes that may or may not be associated with high frequency oscillations are observed just ahead of the fast activity at seizure onset and are reproduced during consecutive seizures recorded from the same cortical region in the same patient (Lange, 1983; Bragin *et al.*, 2005; Wendling *et al.*, 2005) and in animal models of seizures (Avoli *et al.*, 1996b; Lopantsev and Avoli, 1998; Gnatkovsky *et al.*, 2008). These spikes have been termed "pre-ictal spikes", even though they should be considered as ictal events (as proposed by Jerome Jr. Engel during discussions at epilepsy meetings), since their occurrence is *always* associated with seizure onset. We demonstrated that in the transient dis-inhibition model of limbic seizure recorded in the *in vitro* isolated guinea pig brain preparation, pre-ictal spikes that lead to seizure onset correlate with a prominent activation of interneurons that generate large bursts of action potentials and are recorded as inhibitory potentials in principal neurons (Gnatkovsky *et al.*, 2008). In this model, epileptic spikes that occur between seizures (true **interictal** spikes) are sustained by glutamatergic transmission. Preliminary findings demonstrate that also when 4-AP is perfused in the *in vitro* isolated guinea pig brain, seizures in the entorhinal cortex are initiated by a large ictal spike possibly sustained by activation of inhibitory networks and coupled with depression of neuronal firing in principal excitatory neurons. In a different preparation, the *in vitro* slices containing the subiculum isolated from post-surgical specimens of patients with hippocampal sclerosis, interictal spikes are abolished by the GABAa receptor antagonist, bicuculline, while pre-ictal spikes are supported by glutamate-receptor mediated networks (Huberfeld *et al.*, 2007; Huberfeld *et al.*, 2011). These data demonstrate that in different cortical structures epileptic spikes can be sustained either by predominant excitatory or by inhibitory network activation.

Astrocytes are known to contribute to neuronal synchronization in a broad cortical region by enhancing excitation via the massive release of glutamate (and other neurotransmitters), probably mediated by waves of intracellular calcium rise that propagate via non-synaptic mechanisms in the astrocyte syncytium (Fellin and Carmignoto, 2004; Haydon and Carmignoto, 2006). One of the first studies on the role of astrocytes in epilepsy proposed that the activation of astrocytes was sufficient to promote seizures and interictal activities in different in vivo and in vitro preparations (Tian *et al.*, 2005). Subsequent experiments did not confirm these findings (Fellin *et al.*, 2006). Simultaneous imaging of calcium and patch recordings from both astrocytes and neurons demonstrated that astrocyte activation is not required for the generation of interictal spikes, whereas co-activation of astrocyte and neurons is needed to generate seizures (Gomez-Gonzalo *et al.*, 2010). In these in vitro experiments focal seizure-like activity induced in entorhinal cortex neurons by local application of NMDA was further reinforced and sustained by a reciprocal loop between astrocytes, revealing that neurons engage astrocytes in a recurrent excitation that promotes seizure ignition and sustains the ictal discharge.

High frequency oscillations (HFOs) have been reported to occur in isolation and in coincidence with an interictal spike in experimental models of temporal lobe epilepsy (Bragin *et al.*, 2004; Bragin *et al.*, 2007; Engel *et al.*, 2009; Jiruska *et al.*, 2010a) and in human pre-surgical recordings from patients with pharmaco-resistant focal epilepsies (Worrell *et al.*, 2004; Jirsch *et al.*, 2006; Urrestarazu *et al.*, 2006; Jacobs *et al.*, 2008; Engel *et al.*, 2009; Jacobs *et al.*, 2009). Under physiological conditions, HFOs at 100–200 Hz (ripples) implicated in memory consolidation are generated by population inhibitory postsynaptic potentials generated by synchronously active interneuron networks entrained via gap junctions with or without the contribution of glutamatergic networks (Buzsáki *et al.*, 1992; Csicsvari *et al.*, 1999; Jefferys *et al.*, 2012). HFOs with higher discharge rate (>250 Hz: fast ripples) are recorded exclusively from epileptic tissue in patients and in animal models during the interictal state (Khosravani *et al.*, 2005; Jacobs *et al.*, 2008; Engel *et al.*, 2009; Schevon *et al.*, 2009; Panuccio *et al.*, 2012) and during seizures (Jacobs *et al.*, 2008; Worrell *et al.*, 2008; Jacobs *et al.*, 2009). The mechanisms of generation of fast ripples are more controversial. Fast HFOs are due to synchronous burst firing of abnormally active principal neurons and are

9

independent on inhibitory neurotransmission. It has been proposed that epileptic HFOs are initiated and synchronized by excitatory interactions between pyramidal cells in the hippocampus (Dzhala and Staley, 2004; Jiruska *et al.*, 2010b). More recently, GABAergic mechanisms have been proposed as the source of epileptic HFOs (Lasztoczi *et al.*, 2009). The occurrence of spatial and time synchronization during HFO generation is still undetermined and the causal role of HFOs in the transition to seizure is debated (Worrell *et al.*, 2004; Jacob *et al.*, 2008; Engel *et al.*, 2009).

Spatial and temporal synchronization at the transition into seizure is an open issue and depends on what we consider as seizure onset and what is the pattern of seizure discharge we refer to. Substantial dissimilarities become obvious when seizure or seizure-like events are considered in different animal models and experimental preparations. As mentioned above, in most in vivo studies performed on animal models of focal epilepsy, such as posttraumatic epilepsy, temporal lobe epilepsy and post-ischemic epilepsy and in human intracranial recordings, the most common pattern observed at the beginning of a seizure is characterized by fast activity of low amplitude followed by large irregular spiking and rhythmic burst discharges (Figure 1). Fast activity at seizure onset is observed in limbic cortex slices in which connections between the hippocampus and parahippocampal cortices are preserved (Lopantsev and Avoli, 1998). Nevertheless, most experimental studies performed by exposing simplified brain tissue preparations, such as *in vitro* brain slices, to pro-epileptic conditions/drugs showed that these experimental conditions generate seizure-like patterns that are different form the pattern describe above and are often characterized by rhythmic bursting (also termed afterdischarges) from the very onset. Such a discharge is stereotyped, nonflexible and unchangeable over time and cannot be compared to the dynamic changes observed during seizure in more complex preparations and *in vivo* (see also de Curtis *et al.*, 2009). Network and tissue mechanisms during afterdischarges are obviously distinct and synchronization patterns should also expected to be different from those observed during seizures that initiate with low-voltage fast activity.

The measure of synchronization during low-voltage fast activity at seizure onset is based on different assumptions compared to spatial synchronization extent used to define activity spread observed during an interictal spike. Temporal synchrony, more than spatial synchronization, is evaluated during fast activity, on the basis of correlation between cycles of waves that form fast oscillations. Spatial synchrony is postulated to occur during low-voltage fast activity, but it is hardly measured or measurable. Desynchronization of neuronal firing during fast activity at seizure onset has been observed in human intracranial recordings (Le Van Quyen *et al.*, 2001; Schindler *et al.*, 2007) and was demonstrated in the hippocampus *in vitro* (Netoff and Schiff, 2002) and *in vivo* in models of temporal lobe epilepsy and seizures induced by chemoconvulsants (Cymerblit-Sabba and Schiller, 2010, 2012). In the transient dis-inhibition model of temporal lobe seizures induced in the *in vitro* isolated guinea pig brain, low-voltage fast activity at 20-30 Hz is associated to a block of action potential generation in principal neurons, coupled with enhanced firing of inhibitory neurons (Gnatkovsky *et al.*, 2008). Interestingly, also in slice models of seizures induced by 4AP a decrease in neuronal synchronization was observed at seizure onset (Ziburkus *et al.*, 2006). Large spatial and temporal synchronization occurs late during an epileptiform discharge, when rhythmic polyspike/bursting activity is recorded (Topolnik *et al.*, 2003; Ziburkus *et al.*, 2006; Cymerblit-Sabba and Schiller, 2012). Synchonization during late bursting is and can be correlated to the enhanced synchronization observed on *in vitro*-maintained slices during epileptiform afterdischarges.

Synchronization of neuronal activity can be mediated by synchronization of inhibition, through a mechanism of the post-anodal or post-inhibitory postsynaptic potential reset (Cobb *et al.*, 1995). Studies performed on *in vitro* slices of hippocampus, in the *in toto* hippocampal preparations, and on the isolated guinea pig brain confirmed that transition into seizures in different models of acute seizures (4AP, low-magnesium and tetanic stimulation) is associated with a prominent activation of interneurons (Kohling *et al.*, 2000; Fujiwara-Tsukamoto *et al.*, 2006; Ziburkus *et al.*, 2006; Derchansky *et al.*, 2008; Fujiwara-Tsukamoto *et al.*, 2010). Synchronous firing of inhibitory interneurons has also been proposed to mediate an "ictal penumbra" of inhibitory restraint to seizure propagation around the epileptogenic zone (Schevon *et al.*, 2012), in line with previous demonstration of a surround inhibition wavefront that control excitability around pharmacologically-induced cortical foci (Prince and Wilder, 1967).

Different mechanisms have been proposed to explain the development of seizure after an initial boosting of inhibitory networks. Depolarization block of interneuronal firing with consequent resurgence of activity in principal excitatory neurons was discussed (Ziburkus *et al.*, 2006). Depolarization block of GABAergic neurons does not explain, though, why excitatory neurons should increase their firing after inhibitory interneurons stop their activity. We proposed that the transition from prominent inhibition into recovery and further build-up of excitatory synchronization could be due to the direct excitatory action of extracellular potassium increase secondary to the intense firing of inhibitory interneurons (Avoli *et al.*, 1996b; Avoli *et al.*, 1996a; Gnatkovsky *et al.*, 2008; Trombin *et al.*, 2011). High potassium could promote generation of ectopic action potentials in principal cells (inhibited at soma by interneuronal firing) that gradually restore excitatory interaction within the epileptogenic network. This gradual transition from a prevalent activation of inhibitory networks to recovery of principal neuron firing could account for the activity pattern observed after low-voltage fast activity during a focal seizure, characterized by irregular extracellular spiking (Figure 1; de Curtis and Gnatkovsky, 2009; Trombin *et al.*, 2011). We hypothesized that when recurrent excitation reinforces via synaptic and non-synaptic mechanisms (gap junctions, field effects, K^+ increases), groups of spikes (bursts) are generated and the transition toward the last phase of a focal seizure progresses. A gradual increase in synchronization and intensity of neuronal excitation during population bursting is followed by synchronous and widespread increase in inhibition (or depression) of activity. This occurs through circuital interactions mediated by interneurons that have been shown to be preserved in several focal epileptic conditions. Alternative mechanisms of activity depression after increase in synchronous excitation may involve astrocytes release of inhibitory mediators, such as adenosine or ATP, progressive spatial and temporal synchronization of slow afterhyperpolarization due to Ca^{2+}-activated K^+ channels or extracellular changes in ion composition (see Lado and Moshe, 2008). Seizures stop when cycles of post-excitatory depression become too synchronous and too prolonged to allow re-excitation by synaptic activation.

In conclusion, experimental findings supported by intracranial human recordings suggest that desynchronization of excitation and enhanced inhibition may initiate a focal seizure. Concurrent and reciprocally nurtured synchronization of both excitation and inhibition develops during the course of a seizure and may promote an excessively synchronous depression/inhibition of the epileptic networks that brings the seizure to an end.

REFERENCES

1. P.J. Allen, D.R. Fish, S.J. Smith, *Electroencephalogr Clin Neurophysiol* **82**, 155 (1992).
2. M. Avoli, J. Louvel, C. Drapeau, R. Pumain, I. Kurcewicz, *J Neurophysiol* **73**, 468 (1995).
3. M. Avoli, T. Nagao, R. Köhling, A. Lücke, D. Mattia, *Brain Res* **735**, 188 (1996a).
4. M. Avoli, C. Drapeau, J. Louvel, R. Pumain, A. Olivier, J. G. Villemure, *Ann Neurol* **30**, 589 (1991).
5. M. Avoli, M. Barbarosie, A. Lücke, T. Nagao, V. Lopantsev, R. Köhling, *J Neurosci* **16**, 3912 (1996b).

6. T. L. Babb, C. L. Wilson, M. Isokawa-Akesson, *Electroencephalogr Clin Neurophysiol* **66**, 467 (1987).

7. T. L. Babb, E. Halgren, C. Wilson, J. Engel, P. Crandall, *Electroencephalogr Clin Neurophysiol* **51**, 104 (1981).

8. A. P. Bagshaw, E. Kobayashi, F. Dubeau, G. B. Pike, J. Gotman, *Neuroimage* **30**, 417 (2006).

9. J. Bancaud, R. Angelergues, C. Bernouilli, A. Bonis, M. Bordas-Ferrer, M. Bresson, P. Buser, L. Covello, P. Morel, G. Szikla, A. Takeda, J. Talairach, *Electroencephalogr Clin Neurophysiol* **28**, 85 (1970).

10. F. Bartolomei, F. Wendling, J. P. Vignal, S. Kochen, J. J. Bellanger, J. M. Badier, R. Le Bouquin-Jeannes, P. Chauvel, *Clin Neurophysiol* **110**, 1741 (1999).

11. A. T. Berg and I. E. Scheffer, *Epilepsia* **52**, 1058 (2011).

12. A. T. Berg, S. F. Berkovic, M. J. Brodie, J. Buchhalter, J. H. Cross, W. van Emde Boas, J. Engel, J. French, T. A. Glauser, G. W. Mathern, S. L. Moshe, D. Nordli, P. Plouin, I. E. Scheffer, *Epilepsia* **51**, 676 (2010).

13. D. Boido, N. Jesuthasan, M. de Curtis, L. Uva, *Cereb Cortex* **10**, 1093 (2012).

14. M. R. Bower, M. Stead, F. B. Meyer, W. R. Marsh, G. A. Worrell, *Epilepsia* **53**, 807 (2012).

15. A. Bragin, C. L. Wilson, J. J. Engel, *Epilepsia* **48 Suppl 5**, 35 (2007).

16. A. Bragin, J. J. Engel, C. L. Wilson, I. Fried, G. W. Mathern, *Epilepsia* **40**, 127 (1999a).

17. A. Bragin, J. J. Engel, C. L. Wilson, E. Vizentin, G. W. Mathern, (1999b) *Epilepsia* **40**, 1210 (1999a).

18. A. Bragin, C. L. Wilson, J. Almajano, I. Mody, J. J. Engel, *Epilepsia* **45**, 1017 (2004).

19. G. Buzsáki, Z. Horváth, R. Urioste, J. Hetke, K. Wise, *Science* **256**, 1025 (1992).

20. S. R. Cobb, E. H. Buhl, K. Halasy, O. Paulsen, P. Somogyi, *Nature* **378**, 75 (1995).

21. B. W. Colder, R. C. Frysinger, C. L. Wilson, R. M. Harper, J. J. Engel, *Epilepsia* **37**, 113 (1996).

22. J. Csicsvari, H. Hirase, A. Czurko, A. Mamiya, G. Buzsaki, *J Neurosci* **19**, RC20 (1999).

23. A. Cymerblit-Sabba and Y. Schiller, Network dynamics during development of pharmacologically induced epileptic seizures in rats in vivo. *J Neurosci* **30**, 1619 (2010).

24. A. Cymerblit-Sabba and Y. Schiller, *J Neurophysiol* **107**, 1718 (2012).

25. M. de Curtis and G. Avanzini, *Prog Neurobiol* **63**, 541 (2001).

26. M. de Curtis and V. Gnatkovsky, *Epilepsia* **50**, 2514 (2009).

27. M. de Curtis, J. G. R. Jefferys, M. Avoli, in: Jasper's Basic Mechanisms of the Epilepsies, 4th Edition (Noebels JL, Avoli M, Rogawski MA, Olsen RW, Delgado-Escueta AV, eds). Bethesda (MD) (2012).

28. M. Derchansky, S. S. Jahromi, M. Mamani, D. S. Shin, A. Sik, P. L. Carlen, *J Physiol* **586**, 477 (2008).

29. V. I. Dzhala and K. J. Staley, *J Neurosci* **24**, 8896 (2004).

30. J. J. Engel, *J Clin Neurophysiol* **10**, 90 (1993).

31. J. J. Engel, A. Bragin, R. Staba, I. Mody, *Epilepsia* **50**, 598 (2009).

32. T. Fellin and G. Carmignoto, *J Physiol* **559**, 3 (2004).

33. T. Fellin, M. Gomez-Gonzalo, S. Gobbo, G. Carmignoto, P. G. Haydon, *J Neurosci* **26**, 9312 (2006).

34. R. S. Fisher, W. R. Webber, R. P. Lesser, S. Arroyo, S. Uematsu, *J Clin Neurophysiol* **9**, 441 (1992).

35. Y. Fujiwara-Tsukamoto, Y. Isomura, M. Takada, *J Neurophysiol* **95**, 2013 (2006).

36. Y. Fujiwara-Tsukamoto, Y. Isomura, M. Imanishi, T. Ninomiya, M. Tsukada, Y. Yanagawa, T. Fukai, M. Takada, *J Neurosci* **30**, 13679 (2010).

37. V. Gnatkovsky, L. Librizzi, F. Trombin, M. de Curtis, *Ann Neurol* **64**, 674 (2008).

38. V. Gnatkovsky, S. Francione, F. Cardinale, R. Mai, L. Tassi, G. Lo Russo, M. de Curtis, *Epilepsia* **52**, 477 (2011).

39. M. Gomez-Gonzalo, G. Losi, A. Chiavegato, M. Zonta, M. Cammarota, M. Brondi, F. Vetri, L. Uva, T. Pozzan, M. de Curtis, G. M. Ratto, G. Carmignoto, *PLoS Biol* **8**, e1000352 (2010).

40. J. Gotman, V. Levtova, A. Olivier, *Epilepsia* **36**, 697 (1995).

41. P. G. Haydon and G. Carmignoto, *Physiol Rev* **86**, 1009 (2006).

42. G. Huberfeld, L. Wittner, S. Clemenceau, M. Baulac, K. Kaila, R. Miles, C. Rivera, *J Neurosci* **27**, 9866 (2007).

43. G. Huberfeld, L. Menendez de la Prida, J. Pallud, I. Cohen, M. Le Van Quyen, C. Adam, S. Clemenceau, M. Baulac, R. Miles, *Nat Neurosci* **14**, 627 (2011).

44. A. Ikeda, K. Terada, N. Mikuni, R. C. Burgess, Y. Comair, W. Taki, T. Hamano, J. Kimura, H. O. Luders, H. Shibasaki, *Epilepsia* **37**, 662 (1996).

45. A. Ikeda, W. Taki, T. Kunieda, K. Terada, N. Mikuni, T. Nagamine, S. Yazawa, S. Ohara, T. Hori, R. Kaji, J. Kimura, H. Shibasaki, *Brain* **122** (Pt 5), 827 (1999).

46. M. Isokawa-Akesson, C. L. Wilson, T. L. Babb, *Epilepsy Res* **3**, 236 (1989).

47. J. Jacobs, P. LeVan, R. Chander, J. Hall, F. Dubeau, J. Gotman, *Epilepsia* **49**, 1893 (2008).

48. J. Jacobs, R. Zelmann, J. Jirsch, R. Chander, C. E. Dubeau, J. Gotman, *Epilepsia* **50**, 1780 (2009).

49. J. G. R. Jefferys, P. Jiruska, M. de Curtis, M. Avoli, in: Jasper's Basic Mechanisms of the Epilepsies, 4th Edition (Noebels JL, Avoli M, Rogawski MA, Olsen RW, Delgado-Escueta AV, eds). Bethesda (MD) (2012).

50. J. D. Jirsch, E. Urrestarazu, P. LeVan, A. Olivier, F. Dubeau, J. Gotman, *Brain* **129**, 1593 (2006).

51. P. Jiruska, G. T. Finnerty, A. D. Powell, N. Lofti, R. Cmejla, J. G. Jefferys, *Brain* **133**, 1380 (2010a).

52. Jiruska P, de Curtis M, Jefferys JG, Schevon CA, Schiff SJ, Schindler K (2012) Synchronization and Desynchronization in Epilepsy: Controversies and Hypotheses. J Physiol.

14

53. P. Jiruska, J. Csicsvari, A. D. Powell, J. E. Fox, W. C. Chang, M. Vreugdenhil, X. Li, M. Palus, A. F. Bujan, R. W. Dearden, J. G. Jefferys, *J Neurosci* **30**, 5690 (2010b).
54. S. D. Kadam, A. M. White, K. J. Staley, F. E. Dudek, *J Neurosci* **30**, 404 (2010).
55. H. Karhunen, J. Nissinen, J. Sivenius, J. Jolkkonen, A. Pitkanen, *Epilepsy Res* **72**, 25 (2006).
56. H. Khosravani, C. R. Pinnegar, J. R. Mitchell, B. L. Bardakjian, P. Federico, P. L.Carlen, *Epilepsia* **46**, 1188 (2005).
57. E. Kobayashi, A. P. Bagshaw, C. G. Benar, Y. Aghakhani, F. Andermann, F. Dubeau, J. Gotman, *Epilepsia* **47**, 343 (2006).
58. R. Kohling, M. Vreugdenhil, E. Bracci, J. G. Jefferys, *J Neurosci* **20**, 6820 (2000).
59. F. A. Lado and S. L. Moshe, *Epilepsia* **49**, 1651 (2008).
60. H.. Lange, *EEG ClinNeurophysiol* **56**, 543 (1983).
61. B. Lasztoczi, G. Nyitrai, L. Heja, J. Kardos, *J Neurophysiol* **102**, 2538 (2009).
62. M. Le Van Quyen, J. Martinerie, V. Navarro, M. Baulac, F. J. Varela, *J Clin Neurophysiol* **18**, 191 (2001).
63. S. A. Lee, D. D. Spencer, S. S. Spencer, *Epilepsia* **41**, 297 (2000).
64. J. P. Lieb, G. O. Walsh, T. L. Babb, *Epilepsia* **17**, 137 (1976).
65. V. Lopantsev and M. Avoli, *Journal of neurophysiology* **79**, 352 (1998).
66. C. Munari, D. Hoffmann, S. Francione, P. Kahane, L. Tassi, G. Lo Russo, A. L. Benabid, *Acta Neurol Scand Suppl* **152**, 56, discussion 68 (1994).
67. T. L. Netoff and S. J. Schiff, *The J Neurosci* **22**, 7297 (2002).
68. G. Panuccio, G. Sanchez, M. Levesque, P. Salami, M. de Curtis, M. Avoli, *Epilepsia* **53**, 459 (2012).
69. P. Perreault and M. Avoli, *J Neurophysiol* **61**, 953 (1989).
70. P. Perreault and M. Avoli, *J Neurosci* **12**, 104 (1992).
71. D. A. Prince and B. J. Wilder,) *Arch Neurol* **16**, 194 (1967.
72. V. Salanova, F. Andermann, A.Olivier, T. Rasmussen, *Brain* **115**, 1655 (1992).
73. C. A. Schevon, A. J. Trevelyan, C. E. Schroeder, R. R. Goodman, G. McKhann Jr., R. G. Emerson, *Brain* **132**, 3047 (2009).
74. C. A. Schevon, S. A. Weiss, G. McKhann Jr., R. R. Goodman, R. Yuste, R. G. Emerson, A. J. Trevelyan, *Nat Commun* **3**, 1060 (2012).
75. K. Schindler, H. Leung, C. E. Elger, K. Lehnertz, *Brain* **130**, 65 (2007).
76. S. S. Spencer, D. D. Spencer, P. D. Williamson, R. Mattson, *Neurology* **40,** 74 (1990).
77. S. S. Spencer, P. Guimaraes, A. Katz, J. Ki, D. Spencer, *Epilepsia* **33**, 537 (1992).
78. L. Tassi, N. Colombo, R. Garbelli, S. Francione, G. Lo Russo, R. Mai, F. Cardinale, M. Cossu, A. Ferrario, C. Gall, M. Bramerio, A. Citterio, R. Spreafico, *Brain* **125**, 1719 (2002).
79. G. F. Tian, H. Azmi, T. Takano, Q. Xu, W. Peng, J. Lin, N. Oberheim, N. Lou, X. Wang, H. R. Zielke, J. Kang, M. Nedergaard, *Nat Med* **11**, 973 (2005).
80. L.Topolnik, M. Steriade, I. Timofeev, *Cereb Cortex* **13**, 883 (2003).

81. F. Trombin, V. Gnatkovsky, M. de Curtis, *J Neurophysiol* **106**, 1411 (2011).
82. W. Truccolo, J. A. Donoghue, L. R. Hochberg, E. N. Eskandar, J. R. Madsen, W. S. Anderson, E. N. Brown, E. Halgren, S. S. Cash, *Nat Neurosci* **14**, 635 (2011).
83. E. Urrestarazu, J. D. Jirsch, P. LeVan, J. Hall, *Epilepsia* **47**, 1465 (2006).
84. L. Uva, M. Avoli, M. de Curtis, *Eur J Neurosci* **29**, 911 (2009).
85. L. Uva, L. Librizzi, F. Wendling, M. de Curtis, *Epilepsia* **46**, 1914 (2005).
86. F. Wendling, F. Bartolomei, J. J. Bellanger, J. Bourien, P. Chauvel, *Brain* **126**, 1449 (2003).
87. F. Wendling, A. Hernandez, J. J. Bellanger, P. Chauvel, F. Bartolomei, *J Clin Neurophysiol* **22**, 343 (2005).
88. G. A. Worrell, L. Paris, S. D. Cranstoun, R. Jonas, G. Baltuch, B. Litt, *Brain* **127**, 1496 (2004).
89. G. A. Worrell, A. B. Gardner, S. M. Stead, S. Hu, S. Goerss, G. J. Cascino, F. B. Meyer, R. Marsh, B. Litt, *Brain* **131**, 928 (2008).
90. A. R. Wyler, G. A. Ojemann, A. A. J. Ward, *Ann Neurol* **11**, 301 (1982).
91. J. Ziburkus, J. R. Cressman, E. Barreto, S. J. Schiff, *J Neurophysiol* **95**, 3948 (2006).

NEURONAL AND NETWORK DYNAMICS PRECEDING EXPERIMENTAL SEIZURES

P. JIRUSKA[1,2,3], F. MORMANN [4] and J.G.R. JEFFERYS[2]

[1] Department of Developmental Epileptology, Institute of Physiology, Academy of Sciences of Czech Republic,
Prague, CZ-14220, Czech Republic
* E-mail: jiruskapremysl@gmail.com

[2] Neuronal Networks Group, School of Clinical and Experimental Medicine, University of Birmingham,
Birmingham B15 2TT, United Kingdom

[3] Department of Neurology, Charles University, 2nd School of Medicine, University Hospital Motol,
Prague, CZ-15006, Czech Republic

[4] Department of Epileptology, University of Bonn,
53105 Bonn, Germany

How seizures are initiated remains far from clear. Understanding the dynamics of neuronal networks, which lead to transition to seizure, and identifying reliable markers for this process remains an area of active research. Recent studies demonstrated that seizures can be preceded by detectable changes in cellular and network dynamics. These dynamical features resemble a process of critical slowing which is characterized by an increase variance in time series, shift to lower frequencies, increased skewness etc. Additionally, it is accompanied by a progressive decrease of neuronal network resilience, which manifests as enhanced sensitivity to external or internal perturbations. Transition to seizure occurs during a very unstable state of network dynamics when even very weak perturbations are capable of tipping the dynamical regime of the network to seizure. Demonstrating that the dynamics of epileptic neuronal networks are governed by similar principles to other dynamical systems opens new ways to design better methods to examine network dynamical state and to control and/or reverse the transition to seizure.

Keywords: seizures, preictal dynamics, critical transition, tipping point, complex systems, in vitro

1. Introduction

Epileptic seizures used to be viewed as a sudden alteration of brain function, which occurs randomly and unpredictably. This view dramatically changed during the last two decades when several studies indicated that seizures can be preceded by detectable changes in brain dynamics.[1,2] The presumed existence of preictal changes stimulated attempts to develop seizure warning algorithms and provided new ideas on how to treat epilepsy. However, despite extensive research and the application of a range of sophisticated mathematical techniques to analyse human and experimental data, we are still not able to reliably predict seizures above chance level, or even to determine when seizures are most likely to occur.[3–5] Currently seizure prediction research focuses on two main areas which can advance this research field. The first area relates to the application of mathematical tools developed in previous studies on data obtained from multichannel recordings using macro- and microelectrodes which could provide more precise insights into the spatial dynamics of transition to seizures at various spatial scales. New recording techniques enable the evaluation of established seizure prediction algorithms on wide band data, particularly on the preictal dynamics of brain activities beyond traditional EEG frequencies (> 80 Hz).[6,7] The second area is neurobiologically oriented research, which focuses on identification of changes in cellular and network behaviour which precede the onset of seizure and on understanding of mechanism how seizures are generated.[2] Contemporary epilepsy research, and particularly seizure prediction research, substantially overlaps with mathematical and physical disciplines studying complex systems. This multidisciplinary approach is mutually beneficial: epilepsy research gains new ideas on transition to, and generation of, seizures; fundamental research on complex systems benefits from analysing the complexity of the pathophysiological brain dynamics. There is growing evidence that preictal changes in the behaviour of single neurons and neuronal populations can be identified experimentally.[8–10] It is proving more difficult to identify robust preictal changes at the single neuron level in clinical cases[11,12] but this may be because it is remarkably difficult to find the specific site of seizure initiation.[13] Dynamical features of experimental observations, particularly of *in vitro* experiments, demonstrate striking similarities with process of critical transition in complex systems.[14,15] From this perspective seizures can be viewed as a transition to a different dynamic regime (state) of the brain. Such regime shifts occur in various processes including climate change, market collapse, changes in ecosystems etc.[14,16–19] Intense research in these fields identified several early warning indicators which discern that the system is heading towards the critical transition and that these various phenomena are governed by common principles and rules.

2. Critical transition and early warning indicators

Abrupt changes in dynamics of a system and the shift to a different regime can be caused by an unpredictable external perturbation, usually in the form of a strong stochastic event (weather extremes, fire outbreaks etc.)[15] Alternatively, regime shift may be a gradual process during which the probability of transition to alternative state may progressively increase as a system approaches the tipping point or catastrophic bifurcation. When the system reaches a tipping point, it becomes very unstable so that even minor perturbations may result in self-propagating shift to the different state (Figure 1). Using stability landscape the systems state can be visualized as a basin of attraction (or potential well), which provides information on several aspects of the systems dynamical state and vulnerability.[18,19] Valleys in the basin correspond to stable (equilibrium) states. Peaks in the basin of attraction are tipping, or bifurcation, points and represent highly unstable states. If the basin of attraction is large, then displacing the system from one basin of attraction to another (hence to a different state) requires a large perturbation to push the system over the tipping point. Such a system is described as having high resilience. Resilience can be also understood as the maximum perturbation which can be accepted by the system without causing a shift to an alternative stable state. Thus, the probability of transition between two states is dependent on the shape and size of the basin and on the perturbing force. The impact of stochastic perturbations on systems characterized by the existence of multiple stable states does not necessarily impact directly on the systems state by causing regime switches. But these perturbations may lead to changes in the size and shape of the basin of attraction, which may gradually shrink, which in turn will manifest as decreased resilience so that the system becomes more fragile and may switch with small perturbations (Fig. 1).

Perturbations usually are stochastic and can be external, but also internal, events resulting from the systems own dynamics. All systems are permanently exposed to natural perturbations, and the impact of perturbation on the system can be used passively to obtain information to determine the systems dynamical state. Increased sensitivity to perturbations represents one of the early warning indicators of gradually approaching the critical transition. Slowing down of recovery from the perturbation represents a

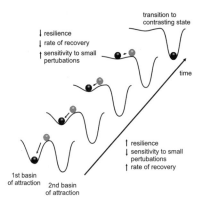

Fig. 1. Stability of the system can be depicted as a landscape map with basins of attraction (potential wells). Valleys in the basin of attraction represent regions of stable equilibrium, while the hill represents an unstable state. If the basin becomes narrower and shallower, the system has low resilience and becomes sensitive to weaker perturbations which can shift the system to an alternative basin of attraction. Shallow basins of attraction slow down the recovery rate from perturbations.

second feature of a system that is becoming unstable.[14,20] This is called critical slowing down which causes decreases in intrinsic rates of change in a system. Future states of the system become more like its past state. This increase in systems memory can be measured, for instance, when time-series data becomes more correlated with itself, which manifests as an increase in autocorrelation.[21] In the frequency domain critical slowing down will manifest by shift of the power spectra from higher to lower frequencies. Due to low resilience, such a system exposed to perturbations will move further from the basin of attraction, resulting in increased variance of the time series. Additionally, as the system approaches the tipping point it may demonstrate asymmetric deviations in amplitude, which are in the direction of the state to which it is shifting (in our case seizure). This may manifest as increased skewness.[14] Signs of critical slowing can be used to provide early warnings of system vulnerability to switching state. Testing methods using controlled external perturbations can be designed to examine vulnerability. These experimental perturbations should not be too strong, to avoid shifting the system to the different dynamic regime, but should be strong enough to measure the recovery rate and system fragility. A list of early warning measures associated with critical slowing down is summarized in Tab. 1.

Table 1. Early warning indicators of
critical transition.

EARLY WARNING INDICATORS
increase in autocorrelation
increased variance
shift to lower frequencies
increased skewness
increased sensitivity to perturbations
decreased recovery rate
small signal amplification
changes in spatial patterns
spatial expansion

3. Preictal dynamics in *in vitro* models of seizures

Can early warning indicators be observed preceding seizures? Recent data
from several studies of *in vitro* models of seizures suggests that similar types
of behaviour can be observed at cellular and network levels, and that some
of them may share similarities with critical slowing down.

Perfusion of hippocampal slice with low-calcium artificial cerebrospinal
fluid is an *in vitro* model of seizures. They originate in CA1 of the hippocampus and are generated by mainly non-synaptic mechanisms (Fig. 2
A). We recently showed that seizures in this model are preceded by a progressive build-up of activity at ~180 Hz (Fig. 2 B, E).[9] The temporal profile
of the build-up was characterized by a combination of linear and quadratic
increases in summated power in the frequency band 80–250 Hz (Fig. 2 E).
The increase in summated power was caused by increased incidence of high-
frequency activity combined with a progressive increase in the amplitude of
the individual cycles.[9] The progressive increase in amplitude manifests as
an increase in the standard deviation of the recorded signal (i.e. square root
variance) (Fig. 2 D). The frequency composition, particularly the median
frequency, of power spectra was not stable: as the seizure approached the
median frequency gradual shifted towards lower frequencies (from 229 to
158 Hz) (Fig. 2 F).

We also examined whether similar changes can be observed in another
seizure model with intact synaptic activity, the isolated CA1 area perfused
with high (8 mM) potassium cerebrospinal fluid. This second model revealed
similar warning indicators of approaching seizures, i.e. increasing summated

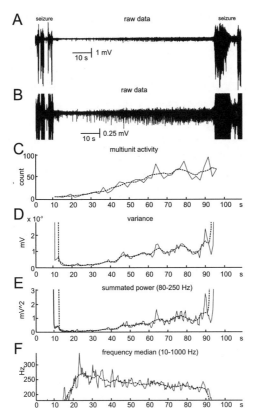

Fig. 2. Low-calcium seizures are preceded by detectable preictal changes in network dynamics. A: Single electrode recording from the CA1 area of hippocampal slice perfused with low-calcium artificial cerebrospinal fluid. B: Period between seizures with higher-amplitude resolutions shows low-amplitude field potentials with superimposed multiunit activity. C: Multiunit activity progressively increases preceding the onset of seizure (dashed line represents smoothed data). D: Variance and its square root (standard deviation) accompany increase in multiunit activity. E: Summated power in the 80-250 Hz band represents another early warning indicator of critical slowing down. F: Median frequency, derived from power spectra, shows the shift towards lower frequencies with an approaching seizure.

power of high-frequency activity and progressive shifting towards lower frequencies.[9] Preictal increases in the power of high-frequency activity were observed by other groups using *in vitro* models: low-magnesium[10] and high-potassium in intact hippocampal slices.[8] Furthermore, studies in humans also suggest that a build-up in high-frequency activity may precede the onset of seizures.[6] To identify the underlying cellular mechanisms of high-frequency activity build-up, and to interpret the observations described above, we used tetrode recordings to study the behaviour of multiple single neurons simultaneously. We found that changes in high-frequency activity are accompanied by progressive increases in overall neuronal activity (multiunit activity) (Figure 2 C). At the level of individual cells, these changes included both increased frequencies of neurons that were already firing, and the recruitment of new cells, which could then either increase their firing frequency or fire at constant rate.[9] However, individual cells did not necessarily demonstrate preictal changes, rather it was the overall neuronal activity which increased progressively. These tetrode recordings also revealed that individual cycles of high-frequency activity are generated by co-firing of small numbers of principal cells. Increases in the amplitude and the slowing of frequency of the high-frequency activity before seizure onset reflect increases in the numbers of principal cells firing together. We hypothesize that between seizures the underlying neuronal network is organized into small functional clusters of principal cells. These clusters are distributed along the CA1 area and generate high-frequency activity. As a seizure approaches, the size of these clusters increases, manifesting as a build-up in summated high-frequency power.[9] The nature of the driving force and/or mechanism responsible for recruiting more cells, and driving the network towards transition to seizure, is not entirely clear. One candidate mechanism is an alteration of potassium homeostasis. Failure of potassium clearance can play an important role in seizure genesis. Several studies demonstrated that seizures can be preceded by tonic increases in extracellular potassium with superimposed short-term fluctuations (Fig. 3).[22–24] This reflects a failure of glial cells to buffer extracellular potassium. Potassium accumulation in extracellular space depolarizes neurons, increases their excitability and/or results in spontaneous neuronal firing. It creates a positive feedback loop in which these phenomena reinforce each other, causing further increase in cellular activity (excitability) and extracellular potassium load, and leading to cell swelling and shrinkage of extracellular space which will further amplify these processes. As the seizure approaches, these mechanisms become more intense and their consequences are more pronounced. In the low-calcium model increased cellular firing may result in 1) higher incidence of high frequency activity (HFA), 2) formation of larger bursts of HFA and 3) pre-seizure bursts. It has been shown that pharmacological manipulation targeting extracellular potassium transients, and limiting the neuronal firing rate by applying electric fields, may be effective in suppressing the transition to seizure.[25]

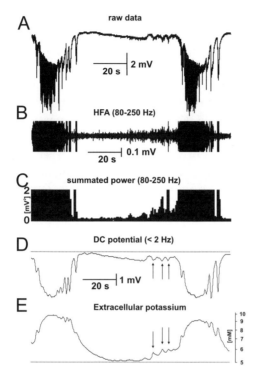

Fig. 3. Preictal changes in extracellular potassium. A: Period between seizures in the low-calcium model of seizures. B: Band-pass filtered signal (80–250 Hz) demonstrates the presence of high-frequency activity. C: Summated power in 80–250 Hz band shows progressive increase before the seizure, with phasic fluctuations in the summated power. D: DC potentials show a negative trend, with superimposed low frequency negative fluctuations, which are accompanied by tonic and phasic increases in extracellular potassium (E).

All the above described changes have features of early warning indicators of critical slowing down which mark progressive shifts of network dynamics towards seizure generation. These observations predict that the neuronal network becomes more vulnerable to stochastic perturbations, and recovers from them more slowly. Stability landscape diagrams of approaching seizures should show the basin of attraction becoming progressively shallower.

4. Active probing of the network dynamics

Active probing of the state dynamics is one of the very promising research direction in epilepsy research and seizure prediction.[26-28] External perturbation can be delivered by electrical stimulation of the neuronal network. In our study we perturbed and tested CA1 network by antidromic stimulation of neuronal axons. With approaching seizures we observed prolongation of epileptiform antidromic responses (Fig. 4). The prolongation of the response can be converted into a recovery rate, which gradually decreased. These experiments confirm that the CA1 neuronal network undergoes a process of critical slowing down. Supporting information was obtained by testing the network with application of uniform electrical fields.[9,29] Application of brief DC fields of varying intensity demonstrated that the CA1 network becomes progressively more sensitive to applied fields as the seizure approaches. Close to the seizure even very week depolarizing fields were able to tip the dynamics of the network to an ictal regime.[9] Application of brief electrical fields revealed an increased sensitivity to external stimuli. Weak electrical fields with strength of 2–4 V/m were capable to trigger seizures. In the normal hippocampus, in which the dynamical state is very stable, such field intensities are harmless. To evoke seizures in normal brain requires field intensities 20–40 times stronger.[29] Epileptic activity, however, does not persist beyond the duration of the applied field, and neuronal networks quickly shift back to the original state. The progressive increase in sensitivity of electric fields and slowing of recovery rates from antidromic stimulations demonstrates decreased resilience and increased excitability of the network.

5. Critical transition and seizure onset

Decreased resilience and increased excitability designate that the neuronal network is approaching the tipping point. One of the main questions in complex system dynamics is what determines the properties of the systems tipping point and what determines its response to perturbations.[15] Two network properties were identified to be the most critical: heterogeneity and connectivity between network components. In certain subtypes of networks the probability of the network occupying a particular state is promoted by having neighbouring components in similar state. Homogenous networks in which individual components are similar and highly interconnected initially provide high resistance to change. But if the state of the homogeneous network reaches the tipping point for critical transition, then a small and local perturbation may shift all components in synchrony into the alternative state through a so-called domino effect.[15,30]

The switch to seizure in the low-calcium model is characterized by a rapid expansion of synchronization, which reflects the expansion and coa-

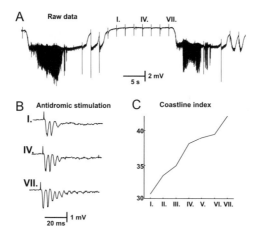

Fig. 4. Active probing of the network dynamics before seizure onset. A: Antidromic stimulation. Recording electrode was positioned in stratum pyramidale of the CA1 area of hippocampus perfused with low-calcium artificial cerebrospinal fluid. The stimulating electrode was located in the alveus to stimulate axons of CA1 pyramidal cells antidromically. B: As a seizure approaches, the antidromic response increases in duration, due to increased numbers of cycles. Antidromic stimulation can be viewed as an external perturbation, and prolongation of the response as a delayed recovery from the perturbation. Antidromic stimulation can be also used to test the CA1 network excitability. C: Prolonged response is characterized by increased signal line length of the response and quantified as coastline index.

lescence of small neuronal populations generating preictal high-frequency activity.[9,31,32] Multichannel recording demonstrated that the gradual pre-ictal increase in neuronal excitability is widespread (global) and can be monitored by the global build-up of high-frequency activity, which appears across the entire CA1 region.[9] Immediately preceding the onset of seizure, the whole CA1 area is in a very unstable state with globally low resilience and "high preparedness" to seize — the population is homogeneous. These properties mean that any area of CA1 can initiate transition to seizure and that adjacent areas being in the same state can promote this transition. What determines which area will initiate the transition and where the seizure will exactly start may be less predictable and may depend on the stochastic nature of small internal and local perturbations. The concept of functional cluster organization of seizure onset area and neuronal cluster expansion at the beginning of seizure was demonstrated in other studies.[32–35] Stead et al. showed in humans that the areas from which seizures initiate can be organized into functional clusters (microdomains).[35] Each cluster generates not only high-frequency activity, but also local ictal activity called microseizures.[35,36] Expansion of areas generating microseizures and coalescence with adjacent clusters results in macroseizures.[35] Expansion of clusters generating high-frequency activity was also described in animal models of chronic temporal lobe epilepsy.[34]

6. Mechanisms of transition to seizure – small stochastic perturbations

What are the cellular mechanisms of endogenous perturbations that can tip the balance towards the seizure? There is a myriad of pathophysiological processes which have been identified as playing roles in transition to seizure. Each could have a very small effect on normal networks, but in an unstable epileptic network their impact on network dynamics can be critical. These processes can have features of stochastic perturbation, but they would be expected to be seizure promoting, i.e. they should have depolarizing and/or synchronizing effects. One candidate mechanism is a sudden and excessive release of potassium. Several studies demonstrated intense interneuronal activity immediately before and during the seizure onset. In the low-calcium model interneurons become very active, firing series of action potentials which may convert to continuous firing immediately before seizure.[9] Such intense firing may cause substantial release of potassium and trigger the seizure. In models with intact synaptic activity, transition to seizure can be caused by abnormalities of inhibition. Intense interneuronal activity may result in a depolarisation block followed by failure to provide inhibitory inputs to principal cells.[37] Interneuronal firing and resulting GABAergic postsynaptic currents may lead to increases in extracellular potassium, probably due to the activity of transporters reuptaking GABA and extruding chloride from the cells. Additionally, excessive inhibitory currents can overload the ability of the adult neuronal chloride transporter (KCC2) to maintain a low intracellular chloride concentration and allow HCO_3- to dominate the postsynaptic current.[38–41] Both mechanisms result in shifting inhibitory synapses from hyperpolarizing to depolarizing, and can contribute to transition to seizures. There are other mechanisms implicated in seizure initiation, including modulation of glutamatergic synaptic transmission,[42–44] activation of presynaptic receptors, decreased probability of GABA release due to activation of presynaptic GABAB receptors, depletion of the available pool of stored GABA due to intense interneuronal activity; desensitization of GABA receptors, loss of inhibitory surround,[13,45] sudden withdrawal of inhibition[46] etc.

7. Conclusions and therapeutic implications

Seizures can be preceded by detectable changes which express features similar to early warning indicators of critical transition. These changes may reflect changes that enhance pro-ictogenic and/or weaken anti-ictogenic processes, shifting the dynamics and excitability of epileptic networks towards the ictal state. The majority of the observations described above were obtained in simplified brain preparations which comprise only limited parts of the epileptic network. In the intact brain the epileptic network is usually much more extensive and often includes several structures. The dynamics of such larger networks will be much more complex and will also involve other non-ictal regimes depending on the brain state (for example circadian and infradian rhythms) which will substantially modify transition to seizure. New and challenging results from patients and from *in vivo* models of epilepsy are starting to emerge, and hopefully will advance our understanding of the preictal dynamics.[11–13] Utilization of methods from the theory of complex systems may also provide better understanding of transition to seizure, and crucially may suggest more effective therapeutic interventions. Studies of complex systems already have demonstrated that rather than controlling or preventing perturbations and system fluctuations, therapy should focus on stabilizing the systems state and strengthening the systems resilience.[18,19] Seizures can be initiated by various processes which perturb the epileptic network. Treating only one of them will most likely mean it will be replaced by perturbations by other processes. That may explain why certain epilepsies can be difficult to control with drugs targeting only one mechanism. It may be more effective to treat epilepsy by focusing on preictal phenomena and factors which drive the system dynamics towards the catastrophic point of transition to the alternative state of the seizure.

Acknowledgments

Supported by Czech Ministry of Health Grant IGA NT/11460-4, Epilepsy Research UK grant P1102 and MRC Grant G0802162.

References

1. B. Litt and K. Lehnertz, *Curr Opin Neurol* **15**, 173 (2002).
2. F. Mormann, R. G. Andrzejak, C. E. Elger and K. Lehnertz, *Brain* **130**, 314 (2007).
3. F. E. Dudek and K. J. Staley, *Neurosci Lett* **497**, 240 (2011).

28

4. P. A. Williams, J. L. Hellier, A. M. White, K. J. Staley and E. F. Dudek, *Epilepsia* **48 Suppl 5**, 157 (2007).
5. W. Stacey, M. L. V. Quyen, F. Mormann and A. Schulze-Bonhage, *Epilepsy Res* **97**, 243 (2011).
6. G. A. Worrell, L. Parish, S. D. Cranstoun, R. Jonas, G. Baltuch and B. Litt, *Brain* **127**, 1496 (2004).
7. J. Jacobs, R. Zelmann, J. Jirsch, R. Chander, C. E. Dubeau and J. Gotman, *Epilepsia* **50**, 1780 (2009).
8. V. I. Dzhala and K. J. Staley, *J Neurosci* **23**, 7873 (2003).
9. P. Jiruska, J. Csicsvari, A. D. Powell, J. E. Fox, W. C. Chang, M. Vreugdenhil, X. Li, M. Palus, A. F. Bujan, R. W. Dearden and J. G. R. Jefferys.
10. H. Khosravani, C. R. Pinnegar, J. R. Mitchell, B. L. Bardakjian, P. Federico and P. L. Carlen, *Epilepsia* **46**, 1188 (2005).
11. W. Truccolo, J. A. Donoghue, L. R. Hochberg, E. N. Eskandar, J. R. Madsen, W. S. Anderson, E. N. Brown, E. Halgren and S. S. Cash, *Nat Neurosci* **14**, 635 (2011).
12. M. R. Bower, M. Stead, F. B. Meyer, W. R. Marsh and G. A. Worrell, *Epilepsia* **53**, 807 (2012).
13. C. A. Schevon, S. A. Weiss, G. M. Jr., R. R. Goodman, R. Yuste, R. G. Emerson and A. J. Trevelyan, *Nat Commun* **3**, p. 1060 (2012).
14. M. Scheffer, J. Bascompte, W. A. Brock, V. Brovkin, S. R. Carpenter, V. Dakos, H. Held, E. H. van Nes, M. Rietkerk and G. Sugihara, *Nature* **2009**, 53 (461).
15. M. Scheffer, S. R. Carpenter, T. M. Lenton, J. Bascompte, W. Brock, V. Dakos, J. van de Koppel, I. A. van de Leemput, I, S. A. Levin, E. H. van Nes, M. Pascual and J. Vandermeer, *Science* **338**, 344 (2012).
16. L. Chen, R. Liu, Z. P. Liu, M. Li and K. Aihara, *Sci Rep* **2**, p. 342 (2012).
17. V. Dakos, S. Kefi, M. Rietkerk, E. H. van Nes and M. Scheffer, *Am Nat* **177**, E153 (2011).
18. M. Scheffer, S. Carpenter, J. A. Foley, C. Folke and B. Walker, *Nature* **413**, 591 (2001).
19. T. M. Lenton, *Nature Climate Change* **1**, 201 (2011).
20. A. J. Veraart, E. J. Faassen, V. Dakos, E. H. van Nes, M. Lurling and M. Scheffer, *Nature* **481**, 357 (2012).
21. V. Dakos, M. Scheffer, E. H. van Nes, V. Brovkin, V. Petoukhov and H. Held, *Proc Natl Acad Sci USA* **105**, 14308 (2008).
22. A. Konnerth, U. Heinemann and Y. Yaari, *Nature* **307**, 69 (1984).
23. A. Konnerth, U. Heinemann and Y. Yaari, *J Neurophysiol* **56**, 409 (1986).
24. S. F. Traynelis and R. Dingledine, *J Neurophysiol* **59**, 259 (1988).
25. M. Bikson, B. R. Id, M. Vreugdenhil, R. Kohling, J. E. Fox and J. G. R. Jefferys, *Neuroscience* **115**, 251 (2002).
26. D. R. Freestone, L. Kuhlmann, D. B. Grayden, A. N. Burkitt, A. Lai, T. S. Nelson, S. Vogrin, M. Murphy, W. D'Souza, R. Badawy, D. Nesic and M. J. Cook, *Epilepsy Behav* **22 Suppl 1**, S110 (2011).
27. S. Kalitzin, D. Velis, P. Suffczynski, J. Parra and F. L. da Silva, *Clin Neurophysiol* **116**, 718 (2005).

28. P. Suffczynski, S. Kalitzin, F. L. da Silva, J. Parra, D. Velis and F. Wendling, *Phys Rev E Stat Nonlin Soft Matter Phys* **78**, p. 051917 (2008).
29. M. Bikson, M. Inoue, H. Akiyama, J. K. Deans, J. E. Fox, H. Miyakawa and J. G. R. Jefferys, *J Physiol* **557**, 175 (2004).
30. E. H. van Nes and M. Scheffer, *Ecology* **86**, 1797 (2005).
31. X. Li, D. Cui, P. Jiruska, J. E. Fox, X. Yao and J. G. R. Jefferys, *J Neurophysiol* **98**, 3341 (2007).
32. M. Bikson, J. E. Fox and J. G. R. Jefferys, *J Neurophysiol* **89**, 2330 (2003).
33. A. Bragin, C. L. Wilson and J. E. Jr., *Epilepsia* **41 Suppl 6**, S144 (2000).
34. A. Bragin, I. Mody, C. L. Wilson and J. E. Jr., *J Neurosci* **22**, 2012 (2002).
35. M. Stead, M. Bower, B. H. Brinkmann, K. Lee, W. R. Marsh, F. B. Meyer, B. Litt, J. V. Gompel and G. A. Worrell, *Brain* **133**, 2789 (2010).
36. C. A. Schevon, S. K. Ng, J. Cappell, R. R. Goodman, G. M. Jr., A. Waziri, A. Branner, A. Sosunov, C. E. Schroeder and R. G. Emerson, *J Clin Neurophysiol* **25**, 321 (2008).
37. J. Ziburkus, J. R. Cressman, E. Barreto and S. J. Schiff, *J Neurophysiol* **95**, 3948 (2006).
38. M. Avoli, M. Barbarosie, A. Lucke, T. Nagao, V. Lopantsev and R. Kohling, *J Neurosci* **16**, 3912 (1996).
39. M. Avoli, M. D'Antuono, J. Louvel, R. Kohling, G. Biagini, R. Pumain, G. D'Arcangelo and V. Tancredi, *Prog Neurobiol* **68**, 167 (2002).
40. V. Lopantsev and M. Avoli, *J Neurophysiol* **79**, 352 (1998).
41. I. Pavlov, K. Kaila, D. M. Kullmann and R. Miles, *J Physiol* (2012).
42. R. D. Traub, R. Miles and J. G. R. Jefferys, *J Physio* **461**, 525 (1993).
43. R. D. Traub, J. G. R. Jefferys and M. A. Whittington, *J Physiol* **478**, 379 (1994).
44. G. Huberfeld, L. M. de la Prida, J. Pallud, I. Cohen, M. L. V. Quyen, C. Adam, S. Clemenceau, M. Baulac and R. Miles, *Nat Neurosci* **14**, 627 (2011).
45. D. A. Prince and B. J. Wilder, *Arch Neurol* **16**, 194 (1967).
46. A. Klaassen, J. Glykys, J. Maguire, C. Labarca, I. Mody and J. Boulter, *Proc Natl Acad Sci USA* **103**, 19152 (2006).

INTERICTAL EEG AND ITS RELEVANCE
FOR SEIZURE PREDICTION*

ANDREAS SCHULZE-BONHAGE

Epilepsy Center, University Hospital Freiburg, Germany

The variability of interictal EEG dynamics has attracted attention due to increasing evidence that the performance of seizure prediction methods critically depends on the duration and continuity of interictal time periods on which training and assessment of algorithms is performed [1]. Here an overview on physiological and pathological EEG patterns during the interictal period is given with an emphasis on aspects relevant to seizure prediction. In particular, similarities in interictal patterns with ictal and preictal discharges are highlighted, including bursts of fast activity, repetitive spike patterns and subclinical electrographic ictal events. The manifestation of clinical seizures and its relation to these interictal discharges is discussed in terms of dynamical interactions of epileptic focus and network.

1. Introduction

Electroencephalography permits to assess the bioelectric activities of extended brain areas at various levels, from lobar information obtained from conventional scalp recordings to intracranial recordings of single neuronal units [2]. For seizure prediction, either scalp recordings or recordings using subdural and intracerebral macroelectrodes have been used so far [3-10]. Both during seizures and in the interictal period, a variety of activity patterns may occur which so far pose relevant problems to automated EEG analysis. Here, an overview of morphological EEG patterns occurring in the interictal period of epilepsy patients is given. In particular, pathological epileptic activity is discussed which may have relevance for the performance of prediction algorithms in that their electrographic patterns and suspected pathophysiology resembles activities at the transition to or onset of epileptic seizures. The discussion is targeted to focal epilepsy as only in epilepsies with focal generation seizures are regarded as potentially predictable [11].

* This work was supported by the EU (grant 211713).

2. Interictal versus ictal activity: general properties and physiological activity

Ictal epileptic activity in focal epilepsy is characterized by rhythmic activities in various frequency bands, rhythmic spiking or "electrodecremental" patterns with low amplitude high frequency discharges which show an evolution in terms of the degree and extent of synchronization, reflected by amplitude, steepness and field extension of the patterns over time [12,13]. In clinical practice, these ictal patterns are mostly defined as the EEG-correlate during the manifestation of clinical signs of seizures, like abnormal motor behavior, impairments in cognition or vegetative signs like tachycardia. These ictal patterns are presumed to cause the ictal phenomenology.

Interictal EEG activity consists of various physiological rhythms like alpha- and beta-activity expressed differentially depending on the topography of the brain. Alpha-rhythms are considered as indicative of an "idling state" which show higher amplitude and regularity when the respective brain areas have little working load [14]. Accordingly, rhythmic alpha activity arises over the visual cortex (occipital) when eyes are closed, over the auditory cortex (temporal "τ-rhythm") during silence, and over the motor cortex ("μ-rhythm", Fig 1) when the contralateral extremity is relaxed. These rhythms are blocked as soon as adequate stimuli occur, with imagination of the respective quality, with motor activity, or unspecifically during problem solving (a famous example being alpha blockade when performing complex multiplications as shown by Berger [15]). Frequent physiological fluctuations in the power of rhythmic alpha activity render the detection of seizures with either new appearance or suppression of rhythmic alpha activity difficult and prone to false classifications particularly if only single channels are analyzed and the topography of seizure patterns and their spread is not taken into account [16].

With changes in vigilance, a variety of new patterns arise; this includes not only a shift of power to lower frequencies but also the occurrence of sharp potentials (e.g. vertex waves, rhythmic "saw tooth" patterns, posterior sharp transients of sleep, benign epileptiform transients of sleep) which differ from epileptic sharp waves based on topographical distribution, field, width, morphology and repetitive occurrence. Whereas these potentials pose problems mainly for spike and seizure detection algorithms, some seizure prediction algorithms are sensitive to the dynamical changes associated with transition from wakefulness to sleep; capturing these dynamics may statistically perform better than chance in predicting seizures in patients with nocturnal seizures without addressing the specific dynamical alterations leading to ictal discharges (Fig. 2). On the other hand, adaptations of algorithms relating analyses to differing EEG dynamics during wakefulness and sleep may improve the performance of seizure prediction, e.g. when moving time windows are compared to fixed interictal time intervals [17].

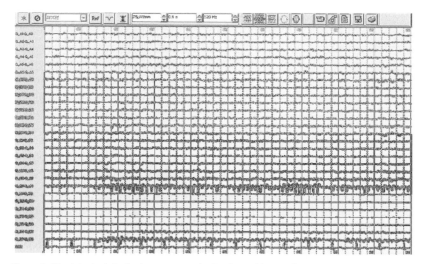

Figure 1. Physiological rhythmic patterns: μ rhythm in a grid recording covering the motor cortex

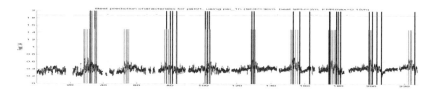

Figure 2. Prediction performance of an algorithm sensitive to circadian alterations in EEG dynamics. Despite correct prediction of most nocturnal seizures, false predictions arise when a patient only falls asleep. Green bars: correct predictions in a subsequent time window (seizure occurrence period), orange bars: false predictions, black bars: seizure time points.

3. Interictal abnormal activity: unspecific changes vs. epileptic patterns

In patients with focal epilepsy, electrophysiological abnormalities are frequently visible also in the interictal period; the presence of these interictal discharges constitutes the value of widespread clinical EEG use in confirming a suspected diagnosis of epilepsy. EEG alterations in patients with focal epilepsy are in part unspecifically related to a structural brain lesion (like focal slowing consisting of continuous intrusions of polymorphic theta and delta waves). In contrast, interictal spikes / sharp waves, repetitive spikes (polyspikes, spike-runs) and other steep field potentials representing abnormal synchronization of pyramidal cell discharges, and rhythmic theta or delta activities representing the slow waves following a spike (related to GABA-ergic inhibition of synaptically coupled areas, Fig. 3) occur almost exclusively in patients with manifest epilepsy and are therefore termed interictal epileptic discharges. Sharp waves and rhythmic activities also occur during seizures, and morphological differences may only consist of a higher degree of rhythmicity or a longer duration during seizures [18].

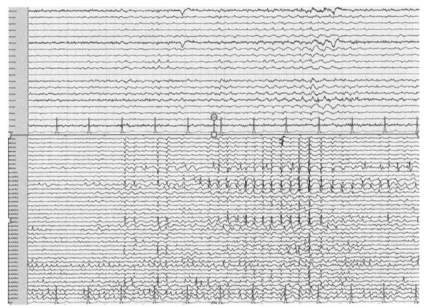

Figure 3. Simultaneous scalp (upper part) and intracranial (lower part) EEG recordings during an interictal period. Rhythmic slowing in the interictal EEG as seen on the surface EEG corresponds to the slow wave part of ongoing interictal spiking as recorded epicortically.

4. Fast interictal discharges

Interictal epileptic activities also includes high frequency discharges ("low amplitude high frequency activity", "lafa") of variable duration and spatial extension, which is much better visible in intracranial EEG recordings. Depending on the etiology of the epilepsy, such lafa activity and spiking can occur not only as identifiable single events on a more or less normal background but may dominate the activity over brain areas of variable extent. In particular, developmental disorders ("cortical dysplasia"), characterized by altered cortical layering, abnormal cell types and connectivity [19,20] In these patients, only the degree of confluence of such fast discharges may distinguish ictal periods from

34

the interictal state which may pose particular problems to algorithms based on the analyses of high frequency power content (Fig. 4).

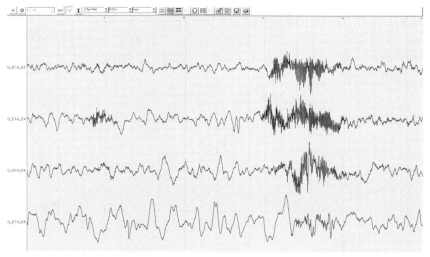

Figure 4. Detail from an interictal subdural intracranial recording showing low amplitude fast activities (lafa) with variable spread and duration. More extended and prolonged lafa activity is found during a clinically manifest seizure.

5. High frequency oscillations

Local oscillatory activity at frequencies of >80 Hz are termed high frequency oscillations (HFO). They occur in the interictal period particularly in the seizure onset zone, and may be a better marker of the "epileptogenic zone" than interictal spikes [21]. So far no clear long-term trends in the preictal phase have been convincingly shown [22], but HFO appear to increase with antiepileptic drug tapering [23] and during the interictal-ictal transition [24]. Analyses of more extended time periods with automated detection algorithms [25] will be required to better assess the relationship of HFO with seizure propensity.

6. Preictal spiking

In some brain areas, rhythmic spiking may regularly precede a seizure [26]. This is particularly well known in patients with hippocampal sclerosis, where rhythmic repetitive spiking has been a matter of debate regarding their attribution as an interictal or already ictal discharge pattern. They may thus constitute a rare example of a visible "preictal" discharge, not yet being accompanied by clinical correlates but regularly preceding high frequency discharges which then give rise to clinical phenomena. Whereas such repetitive spikes may consistently precede an ictal pattern, spiking of similar morphology and variable repetitiveness may also occur without transition to a subsequent high frequency ictal discharge. Algorithms focusing on the detecting of rhythmic spiking of a given topography for seizure detection or prediction may not be able to distinguish preictal from interictal spiking, i.e. apparently identical EEG dynamics will only at times transform into an ictal discharge (Fig. 5a,b).

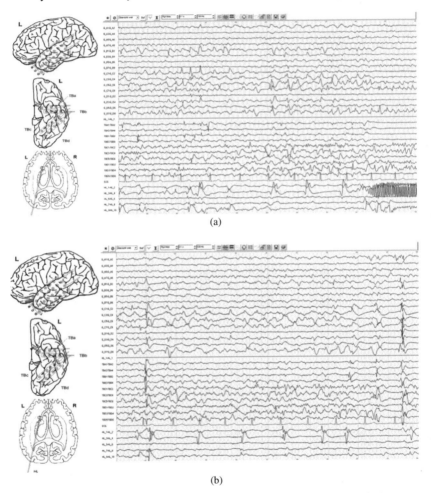

(a)

(b)

Fig. 5a,b. a) Interictal-ictal transition in the hippocampus. Note repetitive high amplitude sharp waves in hippocampal contacts H3-H4 before high frequency spike runs occur, indicating the ictal onset (combined subdural grid recording from temporal neocortex and hippocampal depth recording from a longitudinal approach). b) similar repetitive spiking without subsequent transition to a seizure.

7. Subclinical electrographic seizure patterns

In a given patient, seizures are typically accompanied by a remarkably stereotyped ictal EEG pattern, particularly if the epilepsy is unifocal and has more or less constant patterns of spread. Many of these patients show similar discharges also during the interictal period which are not accompanied by phenomena to which the patient or an observer become aware of. These discharges which fulfill the criteria for ictal patterns given above (rhythmicity, evolution in frequency, amplitude, steepness and topographical extension) are thus called "subclinical electrographic events". It is highly probable that these events do impair the computational capacity of the areas involved but remain unnoticed as the areas involved are quite limited, as there is no spread to "eloquent" brain regions and as observation of a patient is not sufficiently elaborated to discover associated minor or selective performance deficits.

Such subclinical electrographic ictal discharges have by definition similarities in appearance with ictal patterns during a clinically manifest seizure, posing a major problem for detection algorithms, particularly if they are tuned to early detection. They can occur much more frequently than clinically manifest seizures (Fig. 6). Without appropriate EEG monitoring (often requiring intracranial recordings), such events remain unnoticed and are not be reflected in seizure diaries.

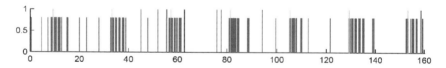

Fig. 7: Continuous long-term recording in a patient from the European Epilepsy Database [27]. Subclinical electrographic patterns (short bars) may occur much more frequently than more prolonged ictal discharges associated with clinical symptomatology (long bars). The clinical appearance thus is not explained by dynamical changes in the seizure onset zone (focus) alone.

Beyond seizure detection, such electrographic ictal discharges (like preictal repetitive spiking) pose a key problem also to seizure prediction. Whereas the occurrence of these epileptic discharges assumedly depends on the dynamics in the epileptic focus (or, more precisely, the seizure onset zone from which they arise), the evolution of repetitive spiking into an ictal discharge and even more the extension of an ictal discharge in time and space critically depend on interactions of the focus and surrounding brain areas (Fig. 7).

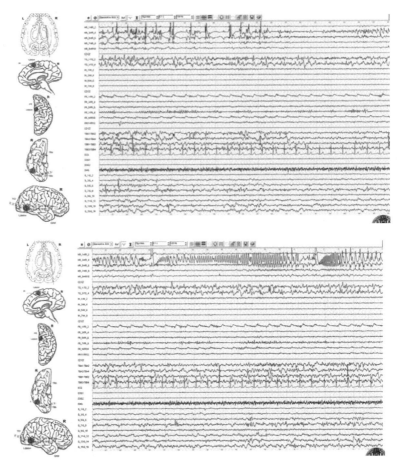

Fig. 7: Intracranial recording of a subclinical event. Upper part: Onset of a low frequency discharge showing a typical evolution (slowing of frequency, increase in amplitude) but limited spatial extension to the right hippocampus. Clinically manifest seizures occurred only when this activity spread to the neocortex.

Taking into account subclinical events may thus influence the evaluation of sensitivity and specificity of a seizure prediction algorithm [28]. Beyond this, capturing different dynamics (generation of electrographic events versus propensity of surrounding brain networks to limit such discharges) may not be possible using only a single type of EEG analysis. The propensity of a spatially limited ictal discharge may thus depend on "proictal" dynamics in the focus surround which determines the probability of an ictal discharge to spread and thus transform a subclinical ictal patterns into a pattern accompanied by a clinically signs. This dynamic property of the focus surround may, however, not be critical to the propensity for the primary generation of an ictal discharge in the seizure onset zone. Given the distinct factors relevant to focal and extrafocal dynamics, analysis of either alone may not be able to perform sufficiently well to achieve seizure prediction performances to a degree which fulfills clinical requirements in terms of sensitivity and specificity [29,30]. Even if the individual algorithm would capture the respective dynamics perfectly well, periods under false warning may occur when proictal changes in the dynamics in either the focus or in the surround occur in isolation.

8. Conclusions

Interictal periods in epilepsy patients show a diversity of phenomena which are relevant to seizure prediction. Physiological changes (either depending on the variations in information processing or on circadian alterations in brain dynamics) affect the performance of many algorithms and may in fact influence seizure propensity (as more or less specific triggers). In patients with reflex seizures or seizures with circadian propensities, it has to be analyzed if a prediction algorithm captures changes specifically related to seizure occurrence or only to changes in the background on which seizures arise. Interictal epileptic discharges may show a more or less well-defined border to ictal discharges, particularly in the case of fast activities and of repetitive spikes. Finally, generation of ictal electrographic discharges and generation of clinically manifest seizure have to be accounted for when terminological aspects of "preictal" or "proictal" are discussed, when seizure prediction performances are analyzed, and when concepts are discussed which may lead to improvements in prediction performance, e.g. by combining algorithms capturing dynamics in the primary generator and in the surrounding network. The latter critically determine if ictal electrographic discharges persist in time and spread in space thus resulting in the clinical seizure count on which seizure prediction is assessed. On the other hand, consideration of the independent dynamics in the seizure onset zone and in network hubs critical for limitation of spread of discharges may open up new windows for differential topical intervention approaches and contribute to an improved approach to seizure prediction in the future [31].

Acknowledgments

The writing of this paper was supported by Funding by the BMBF (Bernstein Center for Neurotechnology) and by the Excellence Cluster BrainLinks-BrainTools.

References

1. Schulze-Bonhage A, Feldwisch-Drentrup H, Ihle M: The role of high-quality EEG databases in the improvement and assessment of seizure prediction methods. Epilepsy Behav 2011; 22 Suppl. 1: S88-S93.

2. Schulze-Bonhage A. Human single unit recording as an approach to understand the neurophysiology of seizure generation. In: I. Fried, U. Rutishauser, M. Cerf and G. Kreiman (eds.): Single Neuron Studies of the Human Brain. MIT Press, Cambridge, 2013, in press

3. Mormann F, Andrzejak RG, Elger CE, Lehnertz K: Seizure prediction: the long and winding road. Brain 2007; 130:314-33.

4. Le Van Quyen M, Adam C, Baulac M, Martinerie J, Varela FJ. Nonlinear interdependencies of EEG signals in human intracranially recorded temporal lobe seizures. Brain Res 1998; 792:24-40.

5. Litt B, Lehnertz K. Seizure prediction and the preseizure period. Curr Opin Neurol 2002;15:173-177.

6. Aschenbrenner-Scheibe R, Maiwald T, Winterhalder M, Voss HU, Timmer J, Schulze-Bonhage A: How well can epileptic seizures be predicted? An evaluation of a nonlinear method. Brain 2003; 126: 2616-2626.

7. Maiwald T, Winterhalder M, Aschenbrenner-Scheibe R, Voss HU, Schulze-Bonhage A, Timmer J: Comparison of three non-linear seizure prediction algorithms by means of the seizure prediction characteristic Physica D 2004; 194: 357-368.

8. Winterhalder M, Schelter B, Kurths J, Schulze-Bonhage A, Timmer J: Sensitivity and specificity of coherence and phase synchronization analysis Phys Lett A, 2006; 356: 26-34.

9. Winterhalder M, Schelter B, Maiwald T, Brandt A, Schad A, Schulze-Bonhage A, Timmer J: Spatio-temporal patient-individual assessment of synchronization changes for epileptic seizure prediction. Clin Neurophysiol, 2006; 117: 2399-2413.

10. Schad A, Schindler K, Schelter B, Maiwald T, Brandt A, Timmer J, Schulze-Bonhage A: Application of a multivariate seizure detection and prediction method to non-invasive and intracranial long-term EEG recordings Clin Neurophysiol, 2008; 119: 197-211.

11. Suffczynski P, Lopes da Silva FH, Parra J, Velis DN, Bouwman BM, van Rijn CM, van Hese P, Boon P, Khosravani H, Derchansky M, Carlen P, Kalitzin S. Dynamics of epileptic phenomena determined from statistics of ictal transitions. IEEE Trans Biomed Eng. 2006; 53:524-32.

12. Geiger LR, Harner RN. EEG patterns at the time of focal seizure onset. Arch Neurol. 1978; 35:276-86.

13. Schulze-Bonhage A. An Introduction to Epileptiform Activities and Seizure Patterns Obtained by Scalp and Invasive EEG Recordings. In: I. Osorio et al. (eds.) Epilepsy. Ther Intersection of Neurosciences, Biology, Mathematics, Engineering, and Physics. CRC Press, Boca Raton, 2011, pp. 51-64

14. Buzsáki G. Rhythms of the Brain. Oxford Univ. Press, New York, 2006, pp. 212 ff

15. Berger H: Über das Electrenkephalogramm des Menschen. Archiv für Psychiatrie und Neverkrankheiten 1929; 23:527 – 570.

16. Meier R, Dittrich H, Schulze-Bonhage A, Aertsen A. Detecting epileptic seizures in long-term human EEG: a new approach to automatic online and real-time detection and classification of polymorphic seizure patterns. J Clin Neurophysiol 2008; 25: 119-131

17. Schelter B, Winterhalder M, Maiwald T, Brandt A, Schad A, Timmer J, Schulze-Bonhage A: Do false predictions of seizures depend on the state of vigilance? A report from two seizure-prediction methods and proposed remedies. Epilepsia 2006; 47: 2058-2070.

18. Chang BS, Schomer DL, Niedermeyer E. Epilepsy in adults and the elderly. In: D.L. Schomer, F.H. Lopes da Silva: Niedermeyer´s Electroencephalography. Lippincott Williams & Wilkins, Philadelphia, 2011, p. 541.

19. Palmini A, Gambardella A, Andermann F, Dubeau F, da Costa JC, Olivier A, Tampieri D, Gloor P, Quesney F, Andermann E et al. : Intrinsic epileptogen-icity of human dysplastic cortex as suggested by corticography and surgical results. Ann Neurol 1995; 37:476-487.

20. Fauser S, Schulze-Bonhage A: Epileptogenicity of cortical dysplasia in temporal lobe dual pathology: an electrophysiological study with invasive recordings. Brain 2006; 129: 82-95.

21. Jacobs J., Zijlmans M., Zelmann R, Chatillon CE, Hall J, Olivier A, Dubeau F, Gotman J: High-frequency electroencephalographic oscillations correlate with outcome of epilepsy surgery. Annals of Neurology 2010; 67: 209–220.

22. Jacobs J, Zelmann R, Jirsch J, Chander R, Dubeau CE, Gotman J: High frequency oscillations (80–500 Hz) in the preictal period in patients with focal seizures. Epilepsia 2009; 50,:1780–1792.

23. Zijlmans M, Jacobs J, Zelmann R, Dubeau F, Gotman J: High-frequency oscillations mirror disease activity in patients with epilepsy. Neurology 2009; 72:,979–986.

24. Khosravani H, Mehrotra N, Rigby M, Hader WJ, Pinnegar CR, Pillay N, Wiebe S, Federico P: Spatial localization and time-dependant changes of electrographic high frequency oscillations in human temporal lobe epilepsy. Epilepsia 2009; 50: 605–616.

25. Dümpelmann M, Jacobs J, Kerber K, Schulze-Bonhage A: Automatic 80-250Hz "ripple" high frequency oscillation detection in invasive subdural grid and strip recordings in epilepsy by a radial basis function neural network. Clin Neurophysiol 2012; 123: 1721-1731.

26. Wendling F, Hernandez A, Bellanger JJ, Chauvel P, Bartolomei F: Interictal to ictal transition in human temporal lobe epilepsy: insights from a computational model of intracerebral EEG. J Clin Neurophysiol 2005; 22:343–356.

27. Klatt J, Feldwisch-Drentrup H, Ihle M, Navarro V, Neufang M, Teixeira C, Adam C, Valderrama M, Alvarado-Rojas C, Witon A, Le Van Quyen M, Sales F, Dourado A, Timmer J, Schulze-Bonhage A, Schelter B: The EPILEPSIAE database-An extensive electroencephalography database of epilepsy patients. Epilepsia 2012; 53: 1669-1676.

28. Feldwisch-Drentrup H, Ihle M, Quyen Mle V, Teixeira C, Dourado A, Timmer J, Sales F, Navarro V, Schulze-Bonhage A, Schelter B: Anticipating the unobserved: prediction of subclinical seizures. Epilepsy Behav 2011; 22 Suppl 1: S119-S126.

29. Schulze-Bonhage A, Sales F, Wagner K, Teotonio R, Carius A, Schelle A, Ihle M. Views of patients with epilepsy on seizure prediction devices. Epilepsy Behav 2010; 18: 388-396.

30. Stacey W, Le Van Quyen M, Mormann F, Schulze-Bonhage A: What is the present-day EEG evidence for a preictal state? Epilepsy Res 2011; 79: 243-251.

31. Feldwisch-Drentrup H, Schelter B, Jachan M, Nawrath J, Timmer J, Schulze-Bonhage A: Joining the benefits: Combining epileptic seizure prediction methods. Epilepsia 2010; 51: 1598-1606.

INVASIVE BRAIN STIMULATION IN THE TREATMENT OF EPILEPSY

MATHIEU SPRENGERS*, ROBRECHT RAEDT*, ALFRED MEURS*, EVELIEN CARRETTE*, DIRK VAN ROOST§, PAUL BOON*, KRISTL VONCK*

*Department of Neurology, Ghent University Hospital, De Pintelaan 185
9000 Ghent, Belgium

§ Department of Neurosurgery, Ghent University Hospital, De Pintelaan 185
9000 Ghent, Belgium

Invasive brain stimulation has emerged as an alternative treatment for refractory epilepsy patients and an increasing number of trials evaluating its efficacy and safety have been published. Various brain structures have been targeted, including the cerebellum, the anterior and centromedian thalamic nucleus, the hippocampus, the ictal onset zone and the subthalamic and caudate nucleus. The rationale for each of these targets and the results obtained in open-label and randomized controlled trials (RCTs) are discussed, with particular emphasis on two large RCTs that investigated open-loop anterior thalamic deep brain stimulation and responsive stimulation of the ictal onset zone. We conclude that promising results have been published for most targets, mainly in open-label trials, and that more RCTs are needed.

1. Introduction

1.1. General Introduction

Epilepsy and epileptic seizures are characterized by both electrical and chemical abnormalities. Research on the treatment of epilepsy patients has mainly focused on the neurochemical part, leading to the development of many antiepileptic drugs (AEDs). Over the past decades, interest in neurostimulation as an alternative treatment for refractory epilepsy patients has grown. Neurostimulation can be defined as the administration of electrical or magnetic pulses to neural tissue in order to modulate neuronal activity. A distinction should be made between invasive and noninvasive neurostimulation strategies. Invasive neurostimulation modalities can be subdivided in extracranial, today still being synonymous to vagus nerve stimulation (VNS), and intracranial stimulation. Whereas VNS is nowadays the only neurostimulation treatment which has become routinely available in clinical practice and has received FDA approval, this review focuses on the experience gained with invasive intracranial stimulation.

1.2. *Historical Background*

The concept of stimulating the brain to treat epilepsy patients is not new. Already in the 19th century Brown-Séquard,[1] Jackson[2] and Gowers[3] suggested 'counter-irritation' as a potential strategy to abate epileptic activity.[4] In the mid-20th century animal studies and preliminary acute human experiments provided further evidence to support this hypothesis.[5,6] The first chronic trials in humans were initiated in the seventies.[7,8] Promising results in these and various other open-label trials[7,9-12] led to the initiation of three randomized-controlled trials[13-15] (RCTs) but these failed to confirm the optimistic outcomes reported in the initial pilot trials. However, given the vast progress in biotechnology along with the experience with brain stimulation in movement disorders and other neuropsychiatric diseases,[16,17] interest in intracranial stimulation for the management of medically intractable epilepsy has been renewed over the past 10-15 years and has resulted into an exponential growth of publications on this topic.

1.3. *Classification of Intracranial Neurostimulation*

There are several ways to categorize intracranial neurostimulation. One way is to focus on the anatomical location of the targeted structure: intracranial electrodes may be inserted into deep subcortical targets for deep brain stimulation (DBS) or be placed over the cortical convexity for cortical stimulation. Another possibility is to classify intracranial stimulation treatments according to the presumed pathophysiological function of the targeted structure, being either the ictal onset zone (e.g. the neocortex, the hippocampus in medial temporal lobe epilepsy,...) or a more remote structure thought to be involved in the epileptic network (e.g. anterior thalamic nucleus, centromedian thalamic nucleus, cerebellar stimulation, caudate nucleus, subthalamic nucleus,...). Finally, with regards to the timing of stimulation, a distinction should be made between open- and closed-loop stimulation paradigms. In open-loop or scheduled stimulation, stimulation is administered at certain prespecified given time points, either continuously or intermittently (following a specific duty cycle). On the contrary, in closed-loop or responsive stimulation, electrical stimuli are only delivered upon seizure detection.

2. Overview of the Different Targets

2.1. *Cerebellar Stimulation*

The rationale behind cerebellar stimulation is that inhibitory Purkinje cells are activated and thus intensify the inhibitory cerebellar output to the ventrolateral thalamus which results into a decreased excitation of thalamocortical projections and ultimately into diffuse cortical inhibition.[18,19] Although a decreased number of Purkinje cells in epilepsy patients[7,11,13] and a further reduction with cerebellar stimulation[20] as well as a decreased activity[21,22] of Purkinje cells in response to cerebellar stimulation have been used as arguments against this theory,[18,23] it should be noticed that none of these truly discard the hypothesis of increased efferent[24] output.

After animal studies[6,18,22,25,26] had shown variable but at the same time hopeful results, Cooper and colleagues conducted a first chronic cerebellar cortical stimulation trial in humans and reported at least 50% seizure reduction in 18 of their 32 patients (56%) suffering from various forms of medically intractable epilepsy.[7] Various open-label trials followed and demonstrated a significant improvement in the majority (up to > 90%) of patients, who often even achieved seizure freedom.[11,12,18,20,27] Inspired by these promising results, Van Buren *et al.*[13] and Wright *et al.*[14] recruited five and twelve patients respectively with focal and/or generalized seizures for two randomized controlled cross-over trials. Although family members of all the subjects in Van Buren's trial and 11 out of 12 patients of Wright's trial felt better for cerebellar stimulation, this probably reflected a placebo effect as statistically significant seizure frequency reductions could not be demonstrated. Looking at the individual patient data, there was no more than one patient who clearly did benefit from the stimulation (97% seizure reduction) in the Wright's trial.[14] On the contrary, although Van Buren *et al.*[13] reported increased seizure frequency with regard to the baseline period in 4/5 patients (with as well as without stimulation), directly comparing seizure frequency of (only) 2 weeks with and without stimulation leads to somehow more favourable – albeit still heterogeneous – results: blinded evaluations during hospital admissions in the first 10 months after electrode implantation revealed unknown, -69%, -73%, unknown and +102% changes in seizure frequency (not enough data in 2/5 patients), whereas late blinded evaluations during hospital admissions 10-21 months after electrode implantation showed -53%, -12%, -7%, -19% and +131% differences in seizure frequency. The most recent RCT was performed in 2005 by Velasco and coworkers and included five patients with intractable motor seizures (generalized epilepsy (n=3) or (multi)focal epilepsy from frontal origin (n=2)).[28] During the 3-month randomized blinded phase of the trial, generalized tonic-clonic seizures (GTCS) (n=5) decreased with 67% in the stimulated group (n=3) compared to 7% in the control group (n=2) (p=0.023). Seizure rate reductions for tonic seizures (TS) (n=4) and drop attacks (DA) (n=2) were comparable for both groups and not statistically significantly different. After the randomized period, stimulators were turned on in all patients. This resulted in a 59% GTCS reduction (n=5), a 48% TS reduction (n=4), a 74% DA reduction (n=2) and a 84% reduction in myoclonic seizures with atypical absences (n=1). Cerebellar stimulation was well-tolerated across the different studies,[13,14,18,28] but electrode migration necessitating repeated surgery constitutes a non-negligible complication that needs to be resolved.[14,28]

As conflicting results have been published, considerable interest in cerebellar stimulation remains and further investigation is warranted. Identifying optimal stimulation protocols will be an important step in this process, e.g. both animal and human studies have suggested that stimulation of the superomedial surface of the cerebellum (as in all RCTs) may be most efficacious.[18, 25, 27]

2.2. Anterior Thalamic Nucleus Stimulation

Being part of the circuit described by Papez, the anterior thalamic nucleus (ATN) has widespread projections to the limbic structures and ultimately also to the – mainly frontal and temporal – neocortex.[29] Besides these anatomical connections, its relatively small size,[19,30] its involvement in seizure propagation,[31] the improved seizure control in lesional studies in animals[32-35] and humans,[36] and the promising results in some acute[34,35,37,38] (but not chronic[39]) animal models, have made the ATN an appealing target for DBS in epilepsy.

Cooper and Upton[9] were the first to explore chronic ATN stimulation in humans and reported an over 60% seizure reduction in 5/6 patients suffering from refractory (multi)focal epilepsy (2-6 years of follow-up). Many other open-label trials have followed and have reported variable results with mean seizure reductions of 14-76% and 50% responder rates of 25-100%[9,40-46] (see Table 1). Except for 2 (or 3) patients with symptomatic generalized epilepsy in Hodaie's[42] and Andrade's[44] patient series (same patients but different follow-up), all patients included so far suffered from (multi)focal epilepsy. Although seizure reductions reported by Hodaie et al.[40] were more pronounced in (multi)focal (75 and 89% reduction) compared to symptomatic generalized (23 and 34% reduction) epilepsy patients, conclusions on this topic are too premature to draw. Most favourable results were reported by Osorio et al.[44] in 4 patients with

Table 1. Overview of open-label trials evaluating anterior thalamic nucleus stimulation

Study	Number of Patients	Follow-Up (months)	Mean Seizure Reduction	Responder Rate
Cooper et al. 1985[9]	6	24-72	> 60% reduction in 83%	
Hodaie et al. 2002[40, 41]	5	12-21	54%	60%
Kerrigan et al. 2004[41]	5	6-36	14%	20%
Andrade et al. 2006[42]	6	48-84	64%	83%
Lee et al. 2006[43]	3	?	75%	100%
Osorio et al. 2007[44]	4	36	76%	100%
Lim et al. 2007[45]	4	24	49%	25%
Lee et al. 2012[46]	15	27	70%	?

inoperable al.[44] in 4 patients with inoperable medial temporal lobe epilepsy. Stimulation of the ATN in idiopathic generalized epilepsy has not been evaluated yet. Despite the encouraging results published in literature, doubt about the efficacy of ATN stimulation as such remained, as 1) Lim et al.[42] and Hodaie et al.[47] reported a significant postoperative seizure reduction, but no further improvement after initiation of stimulation (suggestion of lesional or implantation effect), and 2) turning stimulation off for 2 months in a single-blind manoeuvre and unblindedly for months or years thereafter did not increase seizure frequency in Hodaie's and Andrade's patient series.[40,42] In contrast, Osorio et al.[44] did not observe an important and immediate postoperative prestimulation seizure reduction and Kerrigan et al.[41] did report an increased seizure frequency after switching stimulation off (as also in one of Osorio's patients[44]).

Ultimate evidence with regards to the efficacy and safety of ATN stimulation has been provided by the SANTE trial.[47] This multicenter double-blind, parallel-design RCT recruited 110 adults (18-65 years, IQ $\geq$ 70) suffering from refractory partial-onset epilepsy (failure of $\geq$ 3 AEDs and $\geq$ 6 seizures per month). About half of the patients had prior VNS and/or resective surgery. In the first postoperative month seizure frequency decreased by 22% and this was before any stimulation took place (just as had been reported in some of the open-label trials). However, in the ensuing 3-month randomized period, median percentage seizure frequency change increased from 33.9 to 40.4% in the stimulation group and decreased from 25.3 to 14.5% in the control group, resulting in a net treatment effect of -17% over the entire blinded period (p=0.04). This net stimulation effect became statistically significant only in the third month of the randomized phase (-29%, p=0.002; month 1: -10%, month 2: -11%). Differences in seizure freedom and the 50% responder rate were not statistically significant. With further follow-up (AEDs kept constant for another 9 months) median percentage seizure reduction increased to 41% at 13 months (n=99) and 56% (n=81) at 25 months. The same trend for increasing efficacy over time was observed for the 50% responder rate, being 43% and 54% respectively, and 6/81 patients were seizure-free in the 3-month period preceding the 25-month follow-up visit. However, this moderately improved seizure control was not without any cost. Over the entire study period, five – albeit asymptomatic – haemorrhages were detected incidentally by neuroimaging and 14 participants (13%) developed implant site infections (but no parenchymal brain infections). Moreover, there were more subjects with self-reported depression (14.8 versus (vs) 1.8%, p=0.02) and subjective memory impairment (13.0 vs 1.8%, p=0.03) in the stimulated group compared to the control group, and one subject experienced a dramatic (but reversible) seizure frequency increase linked to the stimulation. On the contrary, there were less epilepsy-related injuries (7.4 vs 25.5%, p=0.01).

In conclusion, good evidence exists that ATN stimulation can reduce seizure frequency in highly refractory focal epilepsy patients. However, benefits in double-blind and controlled conditions were less substantial than what could have been expected based on open-label trials.

2.3. *Hippocampal Stimulation*

As outlined in the introductory part, targeting the area of presumed ictal onset instead of more remote network structures is another strategic DBS approach in epilepsy. In medial temporal lobe epilepsy (MTLE), the hippocampus plays a crucial role in the ictal onset, as has been demonstrated by various (invasive) electrophysiological and other studies in humans.[48-51] Significant seizure reductions observed after selective amygdalohippocampectomy are in line with this presumed key function of the hippocampus in MTLE.[52-54]

Velasco *et al.*[55] were the first to use diagnostic depth electrodes in humans to deliver electrical pulses to medial temporal lobe structures for 2-3 weeks prior to resective surgery. In 7/10 patients whose stimulation contacts were placed within the hippocampal formation and gyrus, one week of stimulation completely abolished seizures and significantly decreased the number of interictal spikes. At Ghent University Hospital, we were able to confirm these preliminary results in a chronic pilot trial in 2002.[56] After 3-6 months of hippocampal and amygdalar stimulation, a 50-95% seizure reduction in three patients was found. Since then more patients were included in this open-label trial.[57,58] After 6-10 years of stimulation, 3/11 patients are now seizure-free for > 3 years, 3/11 achieved a

> 90% seizure reduction, 3/11 responded moderately with a 40-70% seizure reduction and two patients are considered non-responders.[58] Interestingly, in some of the unilateral MTLE patients maximum seizure frequency reduction was only achieved after initiation of bilateral hippocampal stimulation (further reduction compared to unilateral stimulation in 3/5 patients). These results are comparable to those in two other open-label trials with long-term follow-up and a similar number of patients[58-60] (see Table 2). However, although in one RCT reported seizure frequency reductions reached statistical significance,[61] patients in two (albeit small) RCTs did not improve to the same extent.[61,62]

Table 2. Overview of trials evaluating hippocampal stimulation in MTLE

Study	Number of Patients	Follow-Up (months)	% Seizure Reduction	Responder Rate	Seizure Freedom
Velasco et al. 2007[60]	9	18-84	84%	100%	44%
Boëx et al. 2011[59]	8	12-74	67%	75%	25%
Vonck et al. 2013[58]	11	66-120	67%	73%	27%
Tellez-Zenteno et al. 2006[62]*	4	3x 1	26%[#]	25%	0%
McLachlan et al. 2007[61]*	2	3	33%[¶]	0%	0%

* Randomized controlled trial; [#] and [¶]: 15 and 29% respectively when comparing ON and OFF periods (no responders)

Velasco and colleagues[60] reported a slower (after 6-8 months vs 1-2 months) and less pronounced seizure reduction (50-70% vs 95-100%) in 4 patients with hippocampal sclerosis (HS) on magnetic resonance imaging (MRI). This discrepancy was not distinctly observed in other open-label trials with however slightly smaller numbers of HS patients.[58,59] Boëx et al.[59] hypothesized that the reduced efficacy reported by Velasco and coworkers in their HS patients[60] could result from suboptimal stimulation parameter settings, as Boëx and colleagues did report the need for stronger stimulation (higher stimulus amplitudes or/and multipolar configuration) in HS patients.[59] Because 5/6 patients in the RCTs[61,62] showed typical findings of HS on their MRI, it is difficult to draw any conclusions with regards to this issue from these studies.

With long-term seizure freedom of 50-75%, resective surgery remains the treatment of choice for pharmacologically refractory MTLE patients.[63-65] However, hippocampal DBS seems a valuable alternative for those patients who are unsuitable surgical candidates (independent bitemporal foci, high risk of memory decline,...) or who are reluctant to undergo resective brain surgery. In this context, it is worthwhile mentioning that with appropriate stimulation parameter settings neither uni- nor bilateral hippocampal stimulation resulted in neuropsychological deterioration and has actually been associated with enhanced emotional well-being.[58-60,62,66] Future research and optimization of the stimulation protocol could further improve outcome of hippocampal DBS.

2.4. *Centromedian Thalamic Stimulation*

The centromedian thalamic nucleus (CMTN) is part of the reticulo-ascending system with diffuse projections from the brain stem to the cerebral cortex and is thought to mediate cortical excitability and desynchronisation and thus having seizure modulating potential.[67-70]

Velasco and colleagues were the first to explore CMTN stimulation during 2 hours/day (h/d) for 3 months in five patients, with significant reductions in GTCS (80-100% reductions, 3/5 seizure-free) and complex partial seizures (CPS) (4/5 seizure-free).[10] Further experience with this technique in larger patient series (n=23,[71] n=5[72]) confirmed the efficacy for GTCS but could not reproduce the beneficial effects on CPS. In addition, > 90% seizure reductions in 3 patients with partial motor seizures were found[71]. Results in Lennox-Gastaut type patients were more inconclusive,[71,72] but more recent trials (n=8,[73] n=13;[74] stimulation 24 h/d) showed very favourable seizure outcomes especially in this difficult-to-treat patient group (mean seizure frequency reduction of 81% compared to 57% in five patients with (multi)focal epilepsy). Subgroup analysis of patients with optimal (*i.e.* in the ventrolateral or parvocellular region of the CMTN) stereotactic electrode placement yielded even higher seizure reductions. Surprisingly, turning stimulators off for 3 months in a double-blind protocol did not increase seizure frequency.[73] Authors attributed this phenomenon to residual stimulation effects. This effect, however, may not be present in every single patient and could only be temporary, as could be derived from – in some cases delayed – seizure frequency increases after mainly unblinded discontinuations in five other patients due to battery depletion, pulse generator removal or lead rupture.[73,74]

After the hopeful initial results of Velasco *et al.*,[10] Fisher and coworkers conducted a RCT in seven patients.[15] One patient had CPS only, another had CPS and secondarily GTCS and five suffered from primarily generalized seizures (2/5 with Lennox-Gastaut syndrome (LGS)). There were no significant differences between stimulation ON (2 h/d) and OFF periods in this cross-over trial with a 3-month washout period, even after exclusion of one patient with only CPS who reported a seizure increase during the trial (ON -30% versus OFF -8%, p=ns). In fact, only one LGS patient seemed to benefit from CTMN stimulation (-89% reduction with stimulation ON but then dropped from the blinded protocol due to a seizure increase in the washout period). However, during the unblinded open-label phase of the study (stimulation 24 h/d) 3/6 patients showed a > 50% response.

In line with the negative findings in the randomized period of the RCT, two other research groups[42,75] failed to demonstrate important seizure reductions with CMTN stimulation in very small open-label trials (n=1 with generalized epilepsy, n=2 with multifocal epilepsy). In contrast, Cukiert et al.[76] revealed a 65-98% improvement and increased attention level after 1-2 years of CMTN stimulation in 4 patients with generalized epilepsy who had previously been submitted to callosotomy.

In conclusion, Velasco and colleagues have demonstrated marked seizure frequency reductions after initiation of CMTN stimulation, especially in patients suffering from GTCS, atypical absences and LGS. Nevertheless, apart from Cukiert et al.,[76] other smaller trials including one RCT failed to confirm these results. In future, large RCTs in homogeneous patient populations and with 24 hours of stimulation per day are needed before making unambiguous statements with regards to the efficacy of CMTN stimulation.

2.5. Subthalamic Nucleus Stimulation

Inhibition of the excitatory output of the subthalamic nucleus (STN) to the reticular part of the substantia nigra reduces inhibitory output of the substantia nigra to the dorsal midbrain anticonvulsant zone and in this way ultimately leads to decreased inhibition of the GABAergic tectocortical projections.[77] Besides this mechanistic rationale, supporting animal studies[78-80] coupled with ample experience with STN DBS in Parkinson's disease[16] have resulted into various pilot trials in epilepsy patients.

Not surprisingly, STN DBS was first explored by Benabid's group, who reported a significant seizure frequency reduction (67-80%) in three patients with focal epilepsy originating from the central region.[81] Improvement was less pronounced in a patient with Dravet syndrome (-42%) and no effect could be observed in a patient with autosomal dominant nocturnal frontal lobe epilepsy with hypermotor seizures (left insulofrontal focus). Other open-label trials reported similar results with significant improvements in about half of the patients: Loddenkemper et al.[77] showed a 60-80% reduction in 2/5 patients suffering from focal intractable epilepsy and 33 to 50% reductions were observed by Handforth et al.[82] in 2 patients with unifrontal and bitemporal epilepsy respectively.

In addition to these focal epilepsy patients, STN DBS has also been investigated in generalized epilepsy. In a case report published in 2001, STN DBS completely abolished GTCS and diminished myoclonic and absence seizures with > 75% in one LGS patient.[83] More recently Wille et al.[84] reported on five patients with progressive myoclonic epilepsy who had been treated with STN DBS. In all patients a reduction of myoclonic seizures was observed and ranged between 30 and 100%. Temporary discontinuation of stimulation was associated with an almost immediate deterioration in 3/3 patients. Stimulation of the ventral intermediate thalamic nucleus in the same study failed to achieve acute therapeutic effects and therefore was interrupted, so no long-term data are available.

2.6. Caudate Nucleus Stimulation

Sramka, Chkhenkeli and their coworkers have published several reports on stimulation of the caudate nucleus,[75, 85-87] activation of which has been correlated with hyperpolarization of cortical neurons via the 'caudate loop'.[75,85,88] After having demonstrated a decrease in interparoxysmal activity and focal discharges in neocortical and mesial temporal lobe foci as well as abrupt cessation of spreading and generalized discharges,[87] Chkhenkeli et al.[75] published their results of chronic low-frequency stimulation of the ventral part of the head of the caudate nucleus. Patients suffered from epilepsy with various and not well-described seizure origins, but the majority had temporal lobe epilepsy. An impressive 53% of participants achieved seizure-freedom and an additional 29% experienced a 'worthwhile' improvement. Comparable figures were obtained in 21 patients after combined DBS and ablation (total cryoamygdalohippocampectomy or anterior temporal lobectomy) of the dominant epileptic focus. However, as these results were those of 25 years of follow-up, they should be interpreted with caution because significant medication-related improvements cannot be excluded. In addition, in 1980 Sramka et al.[86] reported good early therapeutic effects in only 2 out of 10 patients.

2.7. Various Targets

Electrical stimulation of the epileptogenic region may be an alternative in focal epilepsy patients with seizures originating from a well-circumscribed focus in the motor cortex which cannot be resected for obvious reasons. Elisevich et al.[89] (n=1) and Velasco et al.[90] (n=2) observed > 90% seizure reductions in all patients with elimination of spreading and Todd's phenomenon. One patient even became seizure-free.[90] There were no adverse events, including preserved motor function.

Franzini et al.[91] employed DBS for stimulating two unconventional targets. Posteriomedial hypothalamic DBS led to 75-80% reductions in 2 patients with multifocal epilepsy and stimulation of the caudal zona inserta in focal motor epilepsy was associated with a 85% seizure reduction in one patient and focal motor status disappearance in another.

Various research groups have evaluated the potential of DBS to treat intractable seizures related to hypothalamic hamartomas.[92-95] Khan et al.[92] found significant improvements of gelastic and CPS in 2 patients after initiation of mamillothalamic tract stimulation, with no seizures for the last 10 months in one patient. In another trial (n=1) direct stimulation of the hamartoma resulted into complete abatement of gelastic seizures, a significant reduction of CPS and had no effect on drop attacks.[93] In contrast, two other case reports could not observe any beneficial effect.[94,95]

Two older publications report on stimulation of the locus coeroleus (LC)[96] and the corpus callosum (CC).[97] Unilateral LC stimulation in 2 epilepsy patients appeared to reduce both incidence and severity of seizures, but Feinstein and coworkers[96] warned at the same time this was not 'rigorously established' yet. Finally, Marino Junior et al.[97] planned to evaluate chronic CC stimulation in several patients, but disappointing results in their first patient along with negative experimental findings in cats[98] made them focus on stereotactic anterior callosotomy.

2.8. Closed-loop Stimulation

In studies investigating closed-loop stimulation, implanted intracranial electrodes serve a dual function: continuous monitoring of electro-encephalographic activity and delivery of electrical pulses. In concept, electrical stimuli are only administered after epileptiform electro-encephalographic activity has been detected, aiming to disrupt ongoing seizure activity. Potential advantages of this responsive strategy include minimization of adverse effects, temporary use of higher stimulation settings, lower daily doses, prolonged battery life and higher efficacy.[99] An additional challenge compared to open-loop stimulation is that, apart from an effective stimulation paradigm, the applicability and success of closed-loop stimulation is highly dependent on the implementation of a sensitive, specific and fast seizure detection or prediction algorithm. Finally, one could hypothesize that possible but still controversial long-term neuromodulatory effects of intracranial stimulation are less likely to occur with – inherently less frequent – closed-loop stimulation.

Early proof-of-concept trials provided initial evidence that responsive stimulation is feasible, safe and has seizure reducing potential in focal epilepsy.[4,100-102] Six to 24 months of stimulation resulted in a > 45% reduction in seizure frequency in 7/8 patients[102] and 50-75% reductions after 2 years of follow-up were reported by Anderson and coworkers (n=4).[101] These trials selected the seizure focus as stimulation target but in a short-term trial (4-12 days) Osorio et al.[4] demonstrated that responsive stimulation of the ATN may be efficacious too.

The results of a multi-institutional parallel-group RCT of a cranially implanted responsive neurostimulator (RNS® System, NeuroPace, Mountain View, CA) were published in 2011.[103] All subjects (n=191) were adults (18-70 years) who had ≥ 3 disabling seizures per month (mean 1.2 seizures/day) which had been localized to 1 or 2 epileptogenic regions. Prior VNS (34%) or epilepsy surgery (32%) did not exclude patients from participation. As in the SANTE trial[47] an important postoperative prestimulation seizure reduction was observed, with subsequent further improvement from -34.2% (month 1) to -41.5% (month 3) after responsive stimulation of the ictal onset zone had been initiated but in contrast a gradual return towards baseline in the control group (from -25.2% in month 1 to -9.4% in month 3). Differences were statistically significant from the second month on as well as for the entire blinded evaluation period as a whole (-37.9% vs -17.3%, p=0.012). Two subjects in the treatment group were seizure-free, compared to none in the sham group. Responder rates were very similar in both groups (29% vs 27%). Seizure reductions were sustained and even improved over time with responder rates of 43 and 46% after 1 and 2 years of open-label follow-up. Seven per cent of subjects had no seizures in the 3 months preceding their most recent visit. There were no significant differences in mild or serious adverse events in the blinded phase of the trial. Nine subjects had an intracranial haemorrhage (6/9 postoperative, 7/9 serious), but none of them had permanent neurologic sequelae. Implant or incision site soft tissue infections occurred in 5.2% of patients (no brain infections). Most commonly reported adverse events were related to the cranial implantation of the pulse generator and include implant site pain (15.7% in year 1), headache (10.5%) and dysesthesia (6.3%).

3. Conclusions and Future Perspectives

After pioneering work of Cooper and later Velasco and colleagues, many trials evaluating invasive brain stimulation have followed and different structures have been targeted often showing promising results. However, notwithstanding that at least some RCTs have demonstrated significant improvements with cerebellar, ATN, hippocampal and responsive ictal onset zone stimulation, results in those trials were in general quite moderate compared to the often very favourable outcomes reported in open-label trials. Besides the placebo effect, some other issues may have overestimated efficacy of stimulation *an sich* in open-label trials. These include an implantation effect,[40,45,47,97,103] microlesions resulting from electrode insertion[59,104,105] and medication-induced and spontaneous improvements.[106,107] However, as a trend for increasing efficacy over time,[44,47,60,91,92,103] results consistent with a possible outlasting effect after stimulation[42,45,58,61,73] and further improvement due to optimization of stimulation parameter settings[58,59,84] have been reported, efficacy may at the same time have been underestimated in RCTs due to their short duration, cross-over design and fixed stimulation protocol.

Apart from two large RCTs providing good evidence for ATN[47] and responsive ictal onset zone stimulation,[103] a drawback of most trials is the small number of patients they included. More and large RCTs are certainly needed to fully appreciate efficacy and safety of intracranial stimulation and to define optimal stimulation targets and parameters. Furthermore, substantiating still poor but increasing knowledge about the mechanism of action of invasive brain stimulation in epilepsy may rationalize study designs in future.

Acknowledgments

Dr. M. Sprengers is supported by an FWO-aspirant grant. Prof. Dr. P. Boon is supported by grants from FWO-Flanders, grants from BOF and by the Clinical Epilepsy Grant from Ghent University Hospital. Prof. Dr. K. Vonck is supported by a BOF-ZAP grant from Ghent University Hospital.

References

1. C.E. Brown-Séquard, *Boston Medical and Surgical Journal,* **55-57** (1856-1857).
2. H. Jackson, *Lancet* **91**, 618 (1868).
3. W.R. Gowers, *Epilepsy and Other Chronic Convulsive Diseases: Their Causes, Symptoms and Treatment,* 235 (1885).
4. I. Osorio, M. G. Frei, S. Sunderam, J. Giftakis, N. C. Bhavaraju, S. F. Schaffner and S. B. Wilkinson, *Ann. Neurol.* **57**, 258 (2005).
5. R. G. Heath, 'Electrical Self-Stimulation of Brain in Man', *Am. J. Psychiatry* **120**, 571 (1963).
6. P. M. Cooke and R. S. Snider, *Epilepsia* **4**, 19 (1955).

7. I. S. Cooper, I. Amin and S. Gilman, *Trans. Am. Neurol. Assoc.* **98**, 192 (1973).

8. R. Davis and S. E. Emmonds, *Stereotact. Funct. Neurosurg.* **58**, 200 (1992).

9. I. S. Cooper and A. R. Upton, *Biol. Psychiatry* **20**, 811 (1985).

10. F. Velasco, M. Velasco, C. Ogarrio and G. Fanghanel, *Epilepsia* **28**, 421 (1987).

11. S. Gilman, G. Dauth, V.M. Tennyson, L.T. Kremzner, R. Defendini and J.W. Correll, *Functional Electrical Stimulation: Applications in Neural Prosthesis*, 191 (1977).

12. L. F. Levy and W. C. Auchterlonie, *Epilepsia* **20**, 235 (1979).

13. J. M. Van Buren, J. H. Wood, J. Oakley and F. Hambrecht, *J. Neurosurg.* **48**, 407 (1978).

14. G. D. Wright, D. L. McLellan and J. G. Brice, *J. Neurol. Neurosurg. Psychiatry* **47**, 769 (1984).

15. R. S. Fisher, S. Uematsu, G. L. Krauss, B. J. Cysyk, R. McPherson, R. P. Lesser, B. Gordon, P. Schwerdt and M. Rise, *Epilepsia* **33**, 841 (1992).

16. M. S. Okun, *N. Engl. J. Med.* **367**, 1529 (2012).

17. R. S. Shah, S. Y. Chang, H. K. Min, Z. H. Cho, C. D. Blaha and K. H. Lee, *J. Clin. Neurol.* **6**, 167 (2010).

18. K. N. Fountas, E. Kapsalaki and G. Hadjigeorgiou, *Neurosurg. Focus.* **29**, E8 (2010).

19. C. H. Halpern, U. Samadani, B. Litt, J. L. Jaggi and G. H. Baltuch, *Neurotherapeutics* **5**, 59 (2008).

20. G. L. Krauss and M. Z. Koubeissi, *Acta. Neurochir. Suppl.* **97**, 347 (2007).

21. R. Mutani, L. Bergamini and T. Doriguzzi, *Epilepsia* **10**, 351 (1969).

22. R. S. Dow, A. Fernandez-Guardiola and E. Manni, *Electroencephalogr. Clin. Neurophysiol.* **14**, 383 (1962).

23. J. Fridley, J. G. Thomas, J. C. Navarro and D. Yoshor, *Neurosurg. Focus* **32**, E13 (2012).

24. C. C. McIntyre, M. Savasta, L. Kerkerian-Le Goff and J. L. Vitek, *Clin. Neurophysiol.* **115**, 1239 (2004).

25. K. D. Laxer, L. T. Robertson, R. M. Julien and R. S. Dow, *Adv. Neurol.* **27**, 415 (1980).

26. R. Mutani and R. Fariello, *Brain Res.* **14**, 749 (1969).

27. R. Davis, *Arch. Med. Res.* **31**, 290 (2000).

28. F. Velasco, J. D. Carrillo-Ruiz, F. Brito, M. Velasco, A. L. Velasco, I. Marquez and R. Davis, *Epilepsia* **46**, 1071 (2005).

29. J.W. Papez, *Arch. Neur. Pscyh.* **38**, 725 (1937).

30. C. Hamani, D. Andrade, M. Hodaie, R. Wennberg and A. Lozano, *Int. J. Neural. Syst.* **19**, 213 (2009).

31. M. A. Mirski and J. A. Ferrendelli, *Epilepsia* **27**, 194 (1986).

32. M. A. Mirski and J. A. Ferrendelli, *Science* **226**, 72 (1984).

33. J. A. Kusske, G. A. Ojemann and A. A. Ward, Jr., *Exp. Neurol.* **34**, 279 (1972).

34. S. Takebayashi, K. Hashizume, T. Tanaka and A. Hodozuka, *Epilepsia* **48**, 348 (2007).

35. C. Hamani, F. I. Ewerton, S. M. Bonilha, G. Ballester, L. E. Mello and A. M. Lozano, *Neurosurgery* **54**, 191 (2004).

36. S. Mullan, G. Vailati, J. Karasick and M. Mailis, *Arch. Neurol.* **16**, 277 (1967).

37. M. A. Mirski, L. A. Rossell, J. B. Terry and R. S. Fisher, *Epilepsy Res.* **28**, 89 (1997).

38. C. Hamani, M. Hodaie, J. Chiang, M. del Campo, D. M. Andrade, D. Sherman, M. Mirski, L. E. Mello and A. M. Lozano, *Epilepsy Res.* **78**, 117 (2008).

39. F. A. Lado, *Epilepsia* **47**, 27 (2006).

40. M. Hodaie, R. A. Wennberg, J. O. Dostrovsky and A. M. Lozano, *Epilepsia* **43**, 603 (2002).

41. J. F. Kerrigan, B. Litt, R. S. Fisher, S. Cranstoun, J. A. French, D. E. Blum, M. Dichter, A. Shetter, G. Baltuch, J. Jaggi, S. Krone, M. Brodie, M. Rise and N. Graves, *Epilepsia* **45**, 346 (2004).

42. D. M. Andrade, D. Zumsteg, C. Hamani, M. Hodaie, S. Sarkissian, A. M. Lozano and R. A. Wennberg, *Neurology* **66**, 1571 (2006).

43. K. J. Lee, K. S. Jang and Y. M. Shon, *Acta Neurochir. Suppl.* **99**, 87 (2006).

44. I. Osorio, J. Overman, J. Giftakis and S. B. Wilkinson, *Epilepsia* **48**, 1561 (2007).

45. S. N. Lim, S. T. Lee, Y. T. Tsai, I. A. Chen, P. H. Tu, J. L. Chen, H. W. Chang, Y. C. Su and T. Wu, *Epilepsia* **48**, 342 (2007).

46. K. J. Lee, Y. M. Shon and C. B. Cho, *Stereotact. Funct. Neurosurg.* **90**, 379 (2012).

47. R. Fisher, V. Salanova, T. Witt, R. Worth, T. Henry, R. Gross, K. Oommen, I. Osorio, J. Nazzaro, D. Labar, M. Kaplitt, M. Sperling, E. Sandok, J. Neal, A. Handforth, J. Stern, A. DeSalles, S. Chung, A. Shetter, D. Bergen, R. Bakay, J. Henderson, J. French, G. Baltuch, W. Rosenfeld, A. Youkilis, W. Marks, P. Garcia, N. Barbaro, N. Fountain, C. Bazil, R. Goodman, G. McKhann, K. B. Krishnamurthy, S. Papavassiliou, C. Epstein, J. Pollard, L. Tonder, J. Grebin, R. Coffey, N. Graves and SANTE Study Group, *Epilepsia* **51**, 899 (2010).

48. T. H. Swanson, *J. Clin. Neurophysiol.* **12**, 2 (1995).

49. D. King and S. Spencer, *J. Clin. Neurophysiol.* **12**, 32 (1995).

50. S. S. Spencer, P. Guimaraes, A. Katz, J. Kim and D. Spencer, *Epilepsia* **33**, 537 (1992).

51. C. L. Wilson and J. Engel Jr., *Adv. Neurol.* **63**, 103 (1993).

52. D. Spencer and K. Burchiel, *Epilepsy Res. Treat.* **2012**, 382095 (2012).

53. A. S. Wendling, E. Hirsch, I. Wisniewski, C. Davanture, I. Ofer, J. Zentner, S. Bilic, J. Scholly, A. M. Staack, M. P. Valenti, A. Schulze-Bonhage,

P. Kehrli and B. J. Steinhoff, *Epilepsy Res.* http://www.sciencedirect.com/science/article/pii/S0920121112002744 (2012).
54. T. Tanriverdi, A. Olivier, N. Poulin, F. Andermann and F. Dubeau, *J. Neurosurg.* **108**, 517 (2008).
55. A. L. Velasco, M. Velasco, F. Velasco, D. Menes, F. Gordon, L. Rocha, M. Briones and I. Marquez, *Arch. Med. Res.* **31**, 316 (2000).
56. K. Vonck, P. Boon, E. Achten, J. De Reuck and J. Caemaert, *Ann. Neurol.* **52**, 556 (2002).
57. P. Boon, K. Vonck, V. De Herdt, A. Van Dycke, M. Goethals, L. Goossens, M. Van Zandijcke, T. De Smedt, I. Dewaele, R. Achten, W. Wadman, F. Dewaele, J. Caemaert and D. Van Roost, *Epilepsia* **48**, 1551 (2007).
58. K. Vonck, M. Sprengers, E. Carrette, I. Dauwe, M. Miatton, A. Meurs, L. Goossens, V. De Herdt, R. Achten, E. Thiery, R. Raedt, D. Van Roost and P. Boon, *Int. J. Neural. Syst.* **23**, 1250034 (2013).
59. C. Boex, M. Seeck, S. Vulliemoz, A. O. Rossetti, C. Staedler, L. Spinelli, A. J. Pegna, E. Pralong, J. G. Villemure, G. Foletti and C. Pollo, *Seizure* **20**, 485 (2011).
60. A. L. Velasco, F. Velasco, M. Velasco, D. Trejo, G. Castro and J. D. Carrillo-Ruiz, *Epilepsia* **48**, 1895 (2007).
61. R. S. McLachlan, S. Pigott, J. F. Tellez-Zenteno, S. Wiebe and A. Parrent, *Epilepsia* **51**, 304 (2010).
62. J. F. Tellez-Zenteno, R. S. McLachlan, A. Parrent, C. S. Kubu and S. Wiebe, *Neurology* **66**, 1490 (2006).
63. S. Wiebe, W. T. Blume, J. P. Girvin, M. Eliasziw and Effectiveness and Efficiency of Surgery for Temporal Lobe Epilepsy Study Group, *N. Engl. J. Med.* **345**, 311 (2001).
64. J. Engel, S. Wiebe, J. French, M. Sperling, P. Williamson, D. Spencer, R. Gumnit, C. Zahn, E. Westbrook and B. Enos, *Neurology* **60**, 538 (2003).
65. J. de Tisi, G. S. Bell, J. L. Peacock, A. W. McEvoy, W. F. Harkness, J. W. Sander and J. S. Duncan, *Lancet* **378**, 1388 (2011).
66. M. Miatton, D. Van Roost, E. Thiery, E. Carrette, A. Van Dycke, K. Vonck, A. Meurs, G. Vingerhoets and P. Boon, *Epilepsy Behav.* **22**, 759 (2011).
67. W. Penfield, *Arch. Neurol. Psychiatr.* **40**, 417 (1938).
68. M. Velasco, F. Velasco, A. L. Velasco, F. Jimenez, F. Brito and I. Marquez, *Arch. Med. Res.* **31**, 304 (2000).
69. G. Moruzzi and H. W. Magoun, *Electroencephalogr. Clin. Neurophysiol.* **1**, 455 (1949).
70. J. W. Miller and J. A. Ferrendelli, *Brain Res.* **508**, 297 (1990).
71. F. Velasco, M. Velasco, A. L. Velasco and F. Jimenez, *Epilepsia* **34**, 1052 (1993).
72. F. Velasco, M. Velasco, A. L. Velasco, F. Jimenez, I. Marquez and M. Rise, *Epilepsia* **36**, 63 (1995).

73. Velasco, M. Velasco, F. Jimenez, A. L. Velasco, F. Brito, M. Rise and J. D. Carrillo-Ruiz, *Neurosurgery* **47**, 295 (2000).

74. A. L. Velasco, F. Velasco, F. Jimenez, M. Velasco, G. Castro, J. D. Carrillo-Ruiz, G. Fanghanel and B. Boleaga, *Epilepsia* **47**, 1203 (2006).

75. S. A. Chkhenkeli, M. Sramka, G. S. Lortkipanidze, T. N. Rakviashvili, ESh Bregvadze, G. E. Magalashvili, TSh Gagoshidze and I. S. Chkhenkeli, *Clin. Neurol. Neurosurg.* **106**, 318 (2004).

76. A. Cukiert, J. A. Burattini, C. M. Cukiert, M. Argentoni-Baldochi, C. Baise-Zung, C. R. Forster and V. A. Mello, *Seizure* **18**, 588 (2009).

77. T. Loddenkemper, A. Pan, S. Neme, K. B. Baker, A. R. Rezai, D. S. Dinner, E. B. Montgomery Jr. and H. O. Luders, *J. Clin. Neurophysiol.* **18**, 514 (2001).

78. F. A. Lado, L. Velisek and S. L. Moshe, *Epilepsia* **44**, 157 (2003).

79. L. Vercueil, A. Benazzouz, C. Deransart, K. Bressand, C. Marescaux, A. Depaulis and A. L. Benabid, *Epilepsy Res.* **31**, 39 (1998).

80. N. Usui, S. Maesawa, Y. Kajita, O. Endo, S. Takebayashi and J. Yoshida, *J. Neurosurg.* **102**, 1122 (2005).

81. S. Chabardes, P. Kahane, L. Minotti, A. Koudsie, E. Hirsch and A. L. Benabid, *Epileptic. Disord.* **4**, S83 (2002).

82. A. Handforth, A. A. DeSalles and S. E. Krahl, *Epilepsia* **47**, 1239 (2006).

83. A. Alaraj, Y. Comair, M. Mikati, J. Wakim, E. Louak and S. Atweh, *Presented as a poster at Neuromodulation: defining the future. Cleveland, OH.* (June 8-10, 2001).

84. C. Wille, B. J. Steinhoff, D. M. Altenmuller, A. M. Staack, S. Bilic, G. Nikkhah and J. Vesper, *Epilepsia* **52**, 489 (2011).

85. M. Sramka, G. Fritz, M. Galanda and P. Nadvornik, *Acta Neurochir. Suppl. (Wien)* **23**, 257 (1976).

86. M. Sramka, G. Fritz, D. Gajdosova and P. Nadvornik, *Acta Neurochir. Suppl. (Wien)* **30**, 183 (1980).

87. S. A. Chkhenkeli and I. S. Chkhenkeli, *Stereotact. Funct. Neurosurg.* **69**, 221 (1997).

88. M.R. Klee and H.D. Lux, *Arch. Psychiatr. Nervenkr.* **203**, 667 (1962).

89. K. Elisevich, K. Jenrow, L. Schuh and B. Smith, *J. Neurosurg.* **105**, 894 (2006).

90. A. L. Velasco, F. Velasco, M. Velasco, J. Maria Nunez, D. Trejo and I. Garcia, *Int. J. Neural. Syst.* **19**, 139 (2009).

91. A. Franzini, G. Messina, C. Marras, F. Villani, R. Cordella and G. Broggi, *Stereotact. Funct. Neurosurg.* **86**, 373 (2008).

92. S. Khan, I. Wright, S. Javed, P. Sharples, P. Jardine, M. Carter and S. S. Gill, *Epilepsia* **50**, 1608 (2009).

93. G. Savard, N. H. Bhanji, F. Dubeau, F. Andermann and A. Sadikot, *Epileptic Disord.* **5**, 229 (2003).

59

94. C. E. Marras, M. Rizzi, F. Villani, G. Messina, F. Deleo, R. Cordella and A. Franzini, *Neurosurg. Focus* **30**, E4 (2011).
95. P. Kahane, P. Ryvlin, D. Hoffmann, L. Minotti and A. L. Benabid, *Epileptic. Disord.* **5**, 205 (2003).
96. B. Feinstein, C. A. Gleason and B. Libet, *Stereotact. Funct. Neurosurg.* **52**, 26 (1989).
97. R. Marino Junior and G. Gronich, *Arq. Neuropsiquiatr.* **47**, 320 (1989).
98. A. Cukiert, S. W. Baumel, M. Andreolli and R. Marino, *Stereotact. Funct. Neurosurg.* **52**, 18 (1989).
99. I. Osorio, M. G. Frei, B. F. Manly, S. Sunderam, N. C. Bhavaraju and S. B. Wilkinson, *J. Clin. Neurophysiol.* **18**, 533 (2001).
100. E. H. Kossoff, E. K. Ritzl, J. M. Politsky, A. M. Murro, J. R. Smith, R. B. Duckrow, D. D. Spencer and G. K. Bergey, *Epilepsia* **45**, 1560 (2004).
101. W. S. Anderson, E. H. Kossoff, G. K. Bergey and G. I. Jallo, *Neurosurg. Focus* **25**, E12 (2008).
102. K. N. Fountas, J. R. Smith, A. M. Murro, J. Politsky, Y. D. Park and P. D. Jenkins, *Stereotact. Funct. Neurosurg.* **83**, 153 (2005).
103. M. J. Morrell and RNS Syst Epilepsy Study Group, *Neurology* **77**, 1295 (2011).
104. A. Schulze-Bonhage, D. Dennig, K. Wagner, J. Cordeiro, A. Carius, S. Fauser and M. Trippel, *J. Neurol. Neurosurg. Psychiatry* **81**, 352 (2010).
105. N. M. Katariwala, R. A. Bakay, P. B. Pennell, L. D. Olson, T. R. Henry and C. M. Epstein, *Neurology* **57**, 1505 (2001).
106. A. Neligan, G. S. Bell, M. Elsayed, J. W. Sander and S. D. Shorvon, *J. Neurol. Neurosurg. Psychiatry* **83**, 810 (2012).
107. L. M. Selwa, S. L. Schmidt, B. A. Malow and A. Beydoun, *Epilepsia* **44**, 1568 (2003).

Computational Models of Seizures and Epilepsy

PATIENT-SPECIFIC NEURAL MASS MODELING - STOCHASTIC AND DETERMINISTIC METHODS

D.R. FREESTONE, L. KUHLMANN, M.S. CHONG, D. NEŠIĆ and D.B. GRAYDEN

NeuroEngineering Laboratory, Department of Electrical and Electronic Engineering, and The Center for Neural Engineering, The University of Melbourne, Parkville, VIC, 3010, Australia, and The Bionics Institute, 384-388 Albert St. East Melbourne, VIC, 3002, Australia
E-mail: {deanrf,levink,chongms,dnesic,grayden}@unimelb.edu.au, @unimelb.edu.au

P. ARAM

Department of Automatic Control and Systems Engineering, The University of Sheffield, Mappin Street, Sheffield, S1 3JD, United Kingdom
E-mail: p.aram@sheffield.ac.uk

R. POSTOYAN

Université de Lorraine, CRAN, UMR 7039 and CNRS, CRAN, UMR 7039, France
E-mail: romain.postoyan@univ-lorraine.fr

M.J. COOK

The University of Melbourne, Department of Neurology, St. Vincent's Hospital Melbourne, Fitzroy VIC 3065, Australia
E-mail: markcook@unimelb.edu.au

Deterministic and stochastic methods for online state and parameter estimation for neural mass models are presented and applied to synthetic and real seizure electrocorticographic signals in order to determine underlying brain changes that cannot easily be measured. The first ever online estimation of neural mass model parameters from real seizure data is presented. It is shown that parameter changes occur that are consistent with expected brain changes underlying seizures, such as increases in postsynaptic potential amplitudes, increases in the inhibitory postsynaptic time-constant and decreases in the firing threshold at seizure onset, as well as increases in the firing threshold as the seizure progresses towards termination. In addition, the deterministic and stochastic estimation methods are compared and contrasted. This work represents an important foundation for the development of biologically-inspired methods to image underlying brain changes and to develop improved methods for neurological monitoring, control and treatment.

Keywords: Estimation; Neural Mass Model; EEG; Epilepsy

1. Introduction

This chapter describes two methods for forming patient-specific mesoscopic neural mass models: a stochastic method and a deterministic method. The aim of these methods is to form a bridge between clinical and computational neuroscience that will facilitate the application of control engineering tools[1] to develop new therapies for neurological conditions, such as epilepsy.

The human brain is arguably the most complicated system known to man. The development of a complete theory of its function is one of the greatest challenges faced by researchers today. To address this challenge, researchers have used both theoretical and experimental frameworks to develop and test hypotheses. Experimental frameworks are typically designed to uncover causal relationships between the system's properties or parameters and its function (reverse engineering the brain). Theoretical studies are typically used in one of two ways. The first is to explain data acquired in an experiment and the second is to predict system behaviour. This work is aimed at developing two more applications for theoretical studies and computational models. The first is to use the models as filters, providing insight into the physiology of the brain by estimating the states (i.e. neural activity) and the parameters (e.g. synaptic strength) of the modelled physiology. The second is to use the model as a tool for developing new therapies, where they can be used to provide feedback to a system that can systematically deliver an intervention (e.g. electrical stimulation) in a robust, controlled manner.

Presently, it is almost half a century since Hodgkin and Huxley shared the Nobel prize (in 1963 with Eccles for Physiology and Medicine) for their influential model that helped to establish the field of theoretical neuroscience. Over this time period, both experimental and theoretical methods have developed considerably. Experimental approaches have been able to isolate neural function using various forms of manipulation in greater detail. In parallel, theoretical and computational models have been able to explain and provide new hypotheses for an ever increasing assortment of neural phenomena. Through the development of these models, a fundamental set of parametric equations has been established that explain neuronal responses to sensory input at varying spatiotemporal scales, from small patches of membrane to networks of neural ensembles.

Although the predictive explanatory power of the theoretical models is rather vast when they are tuned to mimic experimental conditions, a major limitation has been in establishing a rigorous method for choosing model parameters in more general situations. For example, over the last decade, it has come to light that there is significant variability in neural systems across subjects despite seemingly similar network activity.[2] We expect an analogous situation in disease states and pathological activity such as epileptic seizures. Therefore, for models to be clinically useful, they must be subject-specific.

By assimilating experimental or clinical measurements with mathematical models, one can infer unmeasured or latent system properties or parameters from standard clinical (electrophysiological) recordings. Inference of patient-specific parameters has the potential to revolutionise the treatment of disease. Typically, one can measure the blood-oxygen level dependent signal through functional magnetic resonance imaging (fMRI) or the electromagnetic fields of the brain through electroencephalography (EEG) or magnetoencephalography (MEG). In clinical neurology, these measurement modalities give a 'where and when' indication of the presence of a pathology, but provide little information on the causative mechanisms for disease. A classic example of this is in epilepsy management, where the disease is diagnosed using EEG by identifying electrographic seizures. If electrical seizures are recorded with EEG, a medication plan is prescribed. The choice of medication is not based on the data acquired with the EEG, but based upon the clinician's experience and the patient's circumstance, then the treatment plan is often modified based on trial and error. This process of searching for the best drug combination is often required since similar electrographic seizures can have fundamentally different mechanisms of initiation.[3] This means that epilepsy is difficult to treat. Ideally, in epilepsy monitoring we would like to image the concentration of ions, the synaptic dynamics, the connectivity strength and structure, or other parameters to better inform a treatment plan by understanding physiological changes that lead to seizures. This is also highly desirable for epileptic seizure prediction which has shown limited progress to date.[4,5]

The signal processing and control theory literature generally provides two approaches to state and parameter estimation of models using measured data (otherwise known in engineering as 'system identification'): stochastic and deterministic. In deterministic approaches,[6,7] there is no universal technique that can be applied to a given general nonlinear system. Rather, the synthesis of deterministic approaches is often more specific to the form of the system being estimated and the convergence of the estimates toward the true values is analytically guaranteed. Often deterministic assumptions are initially quite strict when first devising an estimator; however, these assumptions can usually be relaxed in order to deal with noise issues. Stochastic approaches[1,8,9] on the other hand can be applied more easily to arbitrary systems; however, these approaches depend on initialization. Moreover, the convergence of the estimates to the true values is not guaranteed for every trajectory.

In this chapter, we first describe the basic structure of neural mass models and give specific reference to the formulation of Jansen and Rit with which we will perform estimation.[10] Then we show how two different estimation methods, one stochastic and one deterministic, can perform state and parameter estimation to illustrate their usefulness in inferring underlying and unmeasured physiological variables using only limited physiological measurements. Specifically, we apply a deterministic approach, referred to as an adaptive observer,[7,11] to estimation of the states and parameters using simulated data. Then we apply a stochastic approach based on the unscented Kalman filter (UKF)[12,13] to estimation of the states and parameters using both simulated data and real electrocorticography (ECoG) data of a seizure. Finally, we contrast and compare the stochastic and deterministic approaches in the discussion.

2. Neural Mass Model

To define a standard neural mass model, we begin by defining the post-synaptic potential of population n as a result of an input firing rate from population m as their convolution

$$v_n(t) = v_{r,n} + \frac{\alpha_{mn}}{\tau_{mn}} \int_{-\infty}^{t} h_{mn}(t - t')g_m(v_m(t')) \, dt' \qquad (1)$$

$$v_n(t) - v_{r,n} = \frac{\alpha_{mn}}{\tau_{mn}} \int_{-\infty}^{t} h_{mn}(t - t')g_m(v_m(t')) \, dt' \qquad (2)$$

$$\tilde{v}_n(t) = \frac{\alpha_{mn}}{\tau_{mn}} \int_{-\infty}^{t} h_{mn}(t - t')g_m(v_m(t')) \, dt', \qquad (3)$$

where α_{mn} is the gain for the post-synaptic response kernel, denoted by $h_{mn}(t)$, from neural population m to n, and τ_{mn} is the membrane time constant. Typically, α_{mn} and τ_{mn} are constants (particularly for current based synapses), but later in this chapter we will consider them as time varying quantities. Also, $g_m(v_m(t))$ describes the input firing rate as a function of the pre-synaptic membrane potential. The resting membrane potential of the post-synaptic population is denoted by $v_{r,n}$, $v_n(t)$ is the post-synaptic membrane potential and $\tilde{v}_n(t)$ is the deviation of the membrane from the resting potential. For the network of neural masses that we are considering in the chapter, the index n (post-synaptic) may represent either the pyramidal (p), excitatory interneuron (spiny stellate) (e), external (x) or inhibitory interneuron (i) populations.

The post-synaptic response kernel, $h_{mn}(t)$, typically takes one of three different forms: one first-order and two second-order. The first-order form has an instantaneous rise time and a decay defined by a single time constant.[14] The second-order kernels have finite rise and decay times, with the difference being with one form having separate time constants[15] (bi-exponential) for the rise (synaptic time constant) and decay (membrane time constant), whereas, the other form is defined using a single time constant variable by[16]

$$h_{mn}(t) = \eta(t)t \exp\left(-\frac{t}{\tau_{mn}}\right), \tag{4}$$

where $\eta(t)$ is the Heaviside step function. This is the form that we shall use; however the framework holds for other forms.

This convolution can conveniently be written as

$$\mathrm{D}\tilde{v}_n(t) = \frac{\alpha_{mn}}{\tau_{mn}} g_m(v_m(t)), \tag{5}$$

where the linear differential operator is

$$\mathrm{D} = \frac{\mathrm{d}^2}{\mathrm{d}t^2} + \frac{2}{\tau_{mn}} \frac{\mathrm{d}}{\mathrm{d}t} + \frac{1}{\tau_{mn}^2}. \tag{6}$$

This allows the dynamics of the neural mass to be described by the differential equation

$$\frac{\mathrm{d}^2\tilde{v}_n(t)}{\mathrm{d}t^2} + \frac{2}{\tau_{mn}} \frac{\mathrm{d}\tilde{v}_n(t)}{\mathrm{d}t} + \frac{1}{\tau_{mn}^2}\tilde{v}_n(t) = \frac{\alpha_{mn}}{\tau_{mn}} g_m(v_m(t)). \tag{7}$$

This second-order ODE can be written as two coupled first-order ODEs by defining

$$z_n(t) = \frac{\mathrm{d}\tilde{v}_n(t)}{\mathrm{d}t}. \tag{8}$$

Recasting the system in this way allows formation of a state-space model in a canonical format. This gives the system:

$$\frac{\mathrm{d}\tilde{v}_n(t)}{\mathrm{d}t} = z_n(t) \tag{9}$$

$$\frac{\mathrm{d}z_n(t)}{\mathrm{d}t} = \frac{\alpha_{mn}}{\tau_{mn}} g_m(v_m(t)) - \frac{2}{\tau_{mn}} z_n(t) - \frac{1}{\tau_{mn}^2}\tilde{v}_n(t). \tag{10}$$

68

There is a sigmoidal relationship between the mean membrane potential and firing rate of each of the populations. This sigmoid nonlinearity may take different forms, for example the cumulative density function (error function) or the logistic / hyperbolic tangent. Typically, the logistic function form is used, which is defined by

$$g\left(\tilde{v}_n(t)\right) = \frac{1}{1 + \exp\left(\varsigma_n\left(v_{0n} - \tilde{v}_n(t)\right)\right)} \tag{11}$$

$$g\left(\tilde{v}_n(t)\right) = \frac{1}{1 + \exp\left(\varsigma_n\left(v_{0n} + v_{rn} - v_n(t)\right)\right)} \tag{12}$$

$$g\left(v_n(t)\right) = \frac{1}{1 + \exp\left(\varsigma_n\left(\tilde{v}_{0n} - v_n(t)\right)\right)}, \tag{13}$$

where $\tilde{v}_{0n} = v_{0n} + v_{rn}$. Note that in this formulation, we are absorbing the maximal firing rate, which is typically a linear coefficient on the sigmoid, into the PSP gain (α_{mn}). This removes a redundant parameter that can not be recovered by estimation methods. The quantities ς_n and v_{0n} describe the slope of the sigmoid (variance of firing thresholds within the populations) and the mean firing threshold, respectively. These quantities are usually considered as constants, but again later in this chapter they will be treated as time varying. The parameter $\tilde{v}_{0n}$ describes the deviation from the resting membrane potential, which becomes our lumped threshold parameter. For ease of notation we can drop the *tilde* remembering the resting membrane potential resides within this term. Figure 1 depicts a standard neural mass.

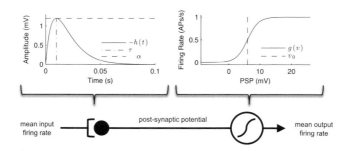

Fig. 1. **Graphical Representation of the Neural Mass Model.** The neural mass model converts an input firing rate to a mean post-synaptic potential by a convolution with the post-synaptic response kernel. The membrane potential is converted to output firing rate, given in action potentials per second (APs/s), by the sigmoidal activation function.

This neural mass maps from a mean pre-synaptic firing rate to a post-synaptic mean membrane potential, which in turn determines the output firing rate of the post-synaptic population. The terms that are usually considered parameters of the model include τ, α, v_0, and ς. These can be set to model different neural populations, such as pyramidal neurons, spiny stellate cells, and fast and slow inhibitory interneurons ($GABA_a$ and $GABA_b$). The neural populations can then be configured to represent the circuitry of a cortical column and networks of cortical columns. Various kinds of neural mass models have been developed.[10,17–19]

The parameters of the neural masses not only define the population type, but also the behaviour the model exhibits. For example, for certain parameter combinations we get a model of a cortical column that will generate alpha type activity and for another set of parameters we get another model that will exhibit epileptic behaviour.[20] Therefore, we consider this neural mass as a family of models, which we define as

$$\dot{\mathbf{x}}(t) = f_\theta\left(\mathbf{x}(t), \mathbf{u}(t)\right) \tag{14}$$

$$y(t) = \mathbf{C}\mathbf{x}(t) + e(t), \tag{15}$$

where $\mathbf{x}(t) \in \mathbb{R}^{n_x}$ is a state vector representing the postsynaptic membrane potentials, generated by each population synapse, and their time derivatives, n_x is the number of states, $\mathbf{u}(t)$ represents the system input, which may be from afferent connections, other brain regions or electrical stimulation or other model inaccuracies. The function $f_\theta(\cdot)$ describes the dynamics, where $\theta \in \mathbb{R}^{n_\theta}$ determines the model type and the behaviour it exhibits. The EEG is denoted by $y(t)$, $\mathbf{C}$ is the observation matrix, and $e(t)$ is the observation noise.

The model focused on in the following estimation sections is the formulation by Jansen and Rit.[10] Given space limitations we refer the reader to the article by Jansen and Rit[10] where the original state-space equations are presented. The parameters that were described in this section are related to the Jansen and Rit paper by

$$A = \frac{\alpha_{pe}}{2e_0 c_1} = \frac{\alpha_{pi}}{2e_0 c_3} = \frac{\alpha_{ep}}{2e_0 c_2} = \frac{\alpha_{xp}}{2e_0} \tag{16}$$

$$B = \frac{\alpha_{ip}}{2e_0 c_4} \tag{17}$$

$$a = \frac{1}{\tau_{pe}} = \frac{1}{\tau_{pi}} = \frac{1}{\tau_{ep}} = \frac{1}{\tau_{xp}} \tag{18}$$

$$b = \frac{1}{\tau_{ip}}, \tag{19}$$

where e_0 is a parameter that scales the maximum firing rate, A and B are synaptic gains for excitation and inhibition respectively, and a and b are the reciprocals of the synaptic time constants for excitation and inhibition, respectively, and the subscripts p, e, x, and i denote pyramidal (p), excitatory interneuron (spiny stellate) (e), external (x) or inhibitory interneuron (i) populations, respectively. By making the assumption that all excitatory synapses share the same time constants and by defining the connectivity constants, c_1, c_2, c_3 and c_4, the network of neural masses on the left side of Figure 2 can be reduced to the system depicted on the right hand side.

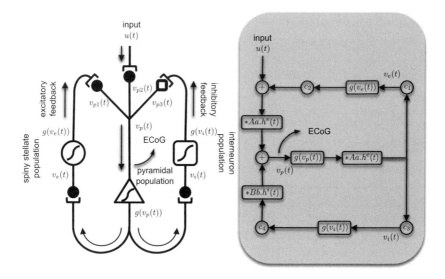

Fig. 2. **Model of a Cortical Column.** The model shows three interconnected neural masses, which are pyramidal neurons, excitatory spiny stellate cells, and inhibitory interneurons. The specific subtype of neural population is defined by the parameters that describe the post-synaptic response kernels. The input to the neural mass model is a firing rate. The symbol $*$ in the figure on the right defines the convolution operation.

2.1. Synthetic Data

The synthetic data used to test the estimation schemes employed parameters that generate alpha rhythm like activity.[10] The model was discretized using Euler's method with a time step of 1 ms. The input for the model was Gaussian noise with a standard deviation of 60 pulses per second and a mean of 90 or 220 pulses per second for the deterministic and stochastic estimators, respectively. The observation noise was also Gaussian with a mean of zero and a standard deviation of 20% of the size of the standard deviation of the simulated pyramidal membrane potential.

3. Deterministic Estimation: Adaptive Observer

This section describes the adaptive observer[21] and provides adequate details and equations for implementation. Proofs that demonstrate that the observer's parameter and state estimates converge to the true values for the Jansen and Rit model are provided in Postoyan et al.[21] In the following a vector $\begin{bmatrix} a \\ b \end{bmatrix}$ is denoted (a, b), for all $a \in \mathbb{R}^{n_a}$, $b \in \mathbb{R}^{n_b}$.

The adaptive observer considered here has been designed for systems that have the state-space form,

$$\dot{\mathbf{x}}_0 = \mathbf{M}_0 \mathbf{x}_0 + \boldsymbol{\phi}_0(y)\boldsymbol{\theta}$$
$$\dot{\mathbf{x}}_1 = \mathbf{M}_1 \mathbf{x}_1 + \boldsymbol{\phi}_1(\mathbf{x}_0, u)\boldsymbol{\theta}$$
$$y = \mathbf{C}_1 \mathbf{x}_1, \tag{20}$$

where $\mathbf{x}_0 \in \mathbb{R}^{n_0}$ and $\mathbf{x}_1 \in \mathbb{R}^{n_1}$ are the states, $\boldsymbol{\theta} \in \mathbb{R}^p$ is a vector of constant and unknown parameters, $y \in \mathbb{R}^{n_y}$ is the measurement and $u \in \mathbb{R}^{n_u}$ is the input. Note that we are assuming that the measurement noise is zero for the derivation.

The Jansen-Rit model[10] can be expressed in the state-space form of equation (20) by taking the states to be $\mathbf{x}_0 = (x_{01}, x_{02}) \in \mathbb{R}^2$ and $\mathbf{x}_1 = (x_{11}, \dots, x_{14}) \in \mathbb{R}^4$, where x_{01}, x_{11}, x_{13} are membrane potential contributions of the pyramidal neurons and the excitatory and inhibitory interneurons respectively, and x_{02}, x_{12}, x_{14} are their respective derivatives. According to the notation of Jansen and Rit,[10] $\mathbf{x}_0 = (y_0, y_3)$ and $\mathbf{x}_1 = (y_1, y_4, y_2, y_5)$. The measured output (ECoG) is $y \in \mathbb{R}$, $u \in \mathbb{R}$ is the excitatory input from neighbouring columns, which is assumed to be known and $\boldsymbol{\theta} = (A, B) \in \Theta \subseteq \mathbb{R}^2$ is a vector of *unknown* parameters, where A and B represent the synaptic gains of the excitatory and inhibitory neuronal populations, respectively. The matrices in (20) are defined as

$$\mathbf{C}_1 = \begin{pmatrix} 1 & 0 & -1 & 0 \end{pmatrix}, \ \mathbf{M}_0 = \mathbf{M}_a, \ \mathbf{M}_1 = \mathrm{diag}(\mathbf{M}_a, \mathbf{M}_b),$$

$$\text{where } \mathbf{M}_a = \begin{pmatrix} 0 & 1 \\ -a^2 & -2a \end{pmatrix}, \ \mathbf{M}_b = \begin{pmatrix} 0 & 1 \\ -b^2 & -2b \end{pmatrix}.$$

The inverse post-synaptic response time constant parameters, $a, b \in \mathbb{R}_{\geq 0}$ are assumed to be known. The nonlinear terms in (20) are given by

$$\phi_0(y) = \begin{pmatrix} 0 & 0 \\ a2e_0g(y) & 0 \end{pmatrix},$$

$$\phi_1(x_0, u) = \begin{pmatrix} 0 & 0 \\ ac_22e_0g(c_1x_{01}) + au & 0 \\ 0 & 0 \\ 0 & bc_42e_0g(c_3x_{01}) \end{pmatrix}.$$

The connectivity parameters, $c_1, c_2, c_3, c_4 \in \mathbb{R}_{\geq 0}$ are assumed to be known, g denotes the sigmoid function defined in equation (13) and $2e_0 \in \mathbb{R}_{\geq 0}$ defines the maximal firing rate. It is worthwhile to note that v_p, v_e and v_i in the right side of Figure 2 correspond to $y = x_{11} - x_{13}$, c_1x_{01}, and c_3x_{01}, respectively.

For ease of notation, we write (20) in the following form

$$\begin{aligned} \dot{\mathbf{x}} &= \mathbf{M}\mathbf{x} + \phi(y, u, \mathbf{x})\boldsymbol{\theta} \\ y &= \mathbf{C}\mathbf{x}, \end{aligned} \tag{21}$$

where $\mathbf{x} = (\mathbf{x}_0, \mathbf{x}_1)$, $\mathbf{M} = \mathrm{diag}(\mathbf{M}_0, \mathbf{M}_1)$, $\mathbf{C} = (\mathbf{0}, \mathbf{C}_1)$ and $\phi = (\phi_0, \phi_1)$. The nonlinear terms, $\phi_0 : \mathbb{R} \to \mathbb{R}^{n_0} \times \mathbb{R}^p$ and $\phi_1 : \mathbb{R}^{n_0} \times \mathbb{R}^{n_u} \to \mathbb{R}^{n_1} \times \mathbb{R}^p$, are globally Lipschitz and bounded.

We consider the following adaptive observer for system (21):

$$\begin{aligned} \dot{\hat{\mathbf{x}}} &= \mathbf{M}\hat{\mathbf{x}} + \phi(y, u, \hat{\mathbf{x}})\hat{\boldsymbol{\theta}} + \boldsymbol{\Gamma}(y - \hat{y}) \\ \hat{y} &= \mathbf{C}\hat{\mathbf{x}} \\ \dot{\hat{\boldsymbol{\theta}}} &= \bar{\boldsymbol{\Gamma}}(y - \hat{y}) \\ \dot{\boldsymbol{\Upsilon}} &= \mathbf{M}\boldsymbol{\Upsilon} + \boldsymbol{\Delta}\phi(y, u, \hat{\mathbf{x}}), \qquad \text{with } \boldsymbol{\Upsilon}(0) = 0 \\ \dot{\mathbf{Q}} &= d\mathbf{Q} - d\mathbf{Q}\boldsymbol{\Upsilon}^\top\mathbf{C}^\top\mathbf{C}\boldsymbol{\Upsilon}\mathbf{Q}, \qquad \text{with } \mathbf{Q}(0) = \mathbf{Q}^\top(0) > 0, \end{aligned} \tag{22}$$

where $\boldsymbol{\Gamma} = \boldsymbol{\Delta}^{-1}\boldsymbol{\Upsilon}\bar{\boldsymbol{\Gamma}}$, $\bar{\boldsymbol{\Gamma}} = \mathbf{Q}\boldsymbol{\Upsilon}^\top\mathbf{C}^\top$ and $\boldsymbol{\Delta} = \mathrm{diag}(\mathbf{I}_{n_0}, \frac{1}{d}\mathbf{I}_{n_1})$. The quantity $d > 0$ is a design parameter that trades off convergence speed for accuracy. The vector, $\hat{\mathbf{x}}$, denotes the estimate of $\mathbf{x}$ and $\hat{\boldsymbol{\theta}}$ the estimate of $\boldsymbol{\theta}$. The variable $\boldsymbol{\Upsilon} \in \mathbb{R}^{(n_0+n_1) \times p}$ is initialized to $\boldsymbol{\Upsilon}(0) = 0$. An essential assumption required for our adaptive observer to work is as follows. For any signals $u, y, \hat{x}$ that belong to $\mathcal{L}_\infty$, there exist $a_1, a_2 \in \mathbb{R}_{\geq 0}$, $T \in \mathbb{R}_{\geq 0}$ such that the solution to

$$\dot{\boldsymbol{\Upsilon}} = \mathbf{M}\boldsymbol{\Upsilon} + \boldsymbol{\Delta}\phi(y, u, \hat{\mathbf{x}}) \text{ with } \boldsymbol{\Upsilon}(0) = 0, \tag{23}$$

satisfies, for all $t \geq 0$,

$$a_1\mathbf{I}_2 \leq \int_t^{t+T} \boldsymbol{\Upsilon}^\top(\tau)\mathbf{C}^\top\mathbf{C}\boldsymbol{\Upsilon}(\tau)\mathrm{d}\tau \leq a_2\mathbf{I}_2. \tag{24}$$

This condition (24) is known as the persistency of excitation of the signal $\mathbf{C\Upsilon}(t)$ and is a well-known condition in the control theory literature.[22] Inequality (24) is hard to verify analytically in general, however, simulations demonstrate that this condition is satisfied for the Jansen and Rit model.

3.1. *Demonstration of Adaptive Observer using ECoG Data Simulation*

Here we demonstrate online parameter estimation for two parameters of the Jansen and Rit model, A and B, that represent the synaptic gains of the excitatory and inhibitory neuronal populations, respectively. The design parameter of the adaptive observer was set to $d = 1.5$. In Figure 3 it can be seen that the parameter estimates converge to the true estimates within 10 seconds, even though the initial estimates begin at either 60% above or 60% below the actual value in the two different simulations.

4. Stochastic Estimation

In this section, we shall switch to discrete time notation, indicated by using the superscript t to index the samples. Furthermore, we shall use the same notation f to describe the system, bearing in mind that the discrete version has different properties to the continuous version.

An alternative way of describing the model in equation (14) is to allow the parameters to be time varying, but on a much slower time scale than the states that have previously been defined. By making the assumption that the parameters are varying slowly, we can form the augmented state-space model

$$\mathbf{x}^{t+1} = f\left(\mathbf{x}^t, \boldsymbol{\theta}^t\right) + \boldsymbol{\varepsilon}^t \tag{25}$$

$$\boldsymbol{\theta}^{t+1} = \boldsymbol{\theta}^t + \boldsymbol{\varphi}^t \tag{26}$$

$$y^t = \mathbf{C}\mathbf{x}^t + e^t, \tag{27}$$

where $\boldsymbol{\varepsilon}^t$ and $\boldsymbol{\varphi}^t$ are zero mean Gaussian disturbance terms that essentially add uncertainty to the system equations when we are using the neural mass model as an estimator. In the forward model, the term $\boldsymbol{\varepsilon}^t$ would be considered an input. The term $\boldsymbol{\varphi}^t$ adds a small amount of uncertainty to the trivial dynamics of the parameters. By augmenting the state vector with parameters that are to be estimated, we can perform state and parameter estimation simultaneously. This allows the Kalman filter to provide small corrections to the model predictions with each arrival of new data.[23-25] Our goal is to estimate the states, $\mathbf{x}^t$, and the slowly varying parameters, $\boldsymbol{\theta}^t$,

74

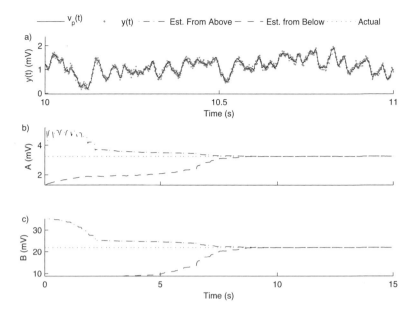

Fig. 3. **Adaptive Observer Estimation Results from Synthetic ECoG Data.**
a) An example of a 1 second segment of the synthetic ECoG data that was used, illustrating the level of noise added to the model output. Black line: the membrane potential
of the pyramidal population, $v_p(t)$. Gray dots: the ECoG signal, $y(t)$, that was used for
estimation. The estimates of the (b) excitatory gain parameter and the (c) inhibitory
gain parameter from when the initial estimate was 60% above and below the actual
value, respectively. Dotted line: the actual parameter value. Dot-dash line: the estimation results when the estimated value was initialized at 60% above. Dashed line: the
results when initialized at 60% below.

given knowledge of the biophysics of the mass action of the brain and the
noisy ECoG measurements. Therefore, we shall define the augmented state
vector as

$$\mathbf{x}_\theta^t = \begin{bmatrix} \mathbf{x}^t \ \boldsymbol{\theta}^t \end{bmatrix}^\top. \tag{28}$$

Our goal is to find

$$\hat{\mathbf{x}}_\theta^{t+} = \mathbb{E}\left[\mathbf{x}_\theta^t | y^1, y^2, \ldots, y^t\right], \tag{29}$$

which is known as the *a posteriori* augmented state estimate. This can be
found by optimally combining the *a priori* augmented state estimate, which
is defined as

$$\hat{\mathbf{x}}_\theta^{t-} = \mathbb{E}\left[\mathbf{x}_\theta^t | y^1, y^2, \ldots, y^{t-1}\right], \tag{30}$$

with the noisy measurements. The noise in the observations is modeled in
equation (27) by additive term e^t; the variance of e^t defines the confidence

we have in the measurements. The *a priori* estimate is an estimate of the same quantity as the *a posteriori* estimate, but only using the prediction from the model and not using the information from the most recent observation at time t.[23] The way the *a priori* estimate of the augmented state is corrected using the noisy observation is a trade off between the level of confidence we have in our measurement (the noise level) and the inaccuracy of our model (the disturbance level). For example, if we were certain that the *a priori* estimate was always exact, then we would set the disturbance to zero and not make use of the measurement to correct the prediction. This is the basic philosophy of the Kalman filter which formalises the trade-off between model prediction error and measure accuracy to form an optimal prediction of the trajectory of the system states.

We define the *a posteriori* and *a priori* augmented state estimate error covariances as

$$\hat{\mathbf{P}}^{t-} = \mathbb{E}\left[(\mathbf{x}_\theta^t - \hat{\mathbf{x}}_\theta^{t-})(\mathbf{x}_\theta^t - \hat{\mathbf{x}}_\theta^{t-})^\top\right] \tag{31}$$

$$\hat{\mathbf{P}}^{t+} = \mathbb{E}\left[(\mathbf{x}_\theta^t - \hat{\mathbf{x}}_\theta^{t+})(\mathbf{x}_\theta^t - \hat{\mathbf{x}}_\theta^{t+})^\top\right], \tag{32}$$

respectively.

For linear systems, the Kalman filter provides the solution to the estimation problem. However, for the nonlinear neural mass model, the integration that is required for solving the expectations has no closed-form solution. Therefore, an approximate solution is required for efficient filtering (of high dimensional systems). An appropriate method for this approximation is the unscented transform, which leads to the unscented Kalman filter.[26]

The unscented transform (UT) is a method for approximating the statistics of a random variable that undergoes a nonlinear transformation. Consider transforming an n-dimensional random variable, $\mathbf{x}_\theta$ (augmented state vector), through a nonlinear function, $\mathbf{x}_\theta^t = f\left(\mathbf{x}_\theta^{t-1}\right)$. Here we assume $\mathbf{x}_\theta^{t-1}$ is draw from a normal Gaussian distribution, such that $\mathbf{x}_\theta^{t-1} \sim \mathcal{N}(\bar{\mathbf{x}}_\theta^{t-1}, \mathbf{P}_{\mathbf{x}_\theta}^{t-1})$, where $\bar{\mathbf{x}}_\theta^{t-1}$ defines the mean. To map the statistics through the nonlinear transform, we first define the so-called $(2n_{x_\theta} + 1)$ sigma vectors, which form the sigma matrix $\mathcal{X}$, as

$$\mathcal{X}_0^{t-1} = \bar{\mathbf{x}}_\theta^{t-1} \tag{33}$$

$$\mathcal{X}_i^{t-1} = \bar{\mathbf{x}}_\theta^{t-1} + \left(\sqrt{(n_{x_\theta} + \lambda)\mathbf{P}_{\mathbf{x}_\theta}^{t-1}}\right)_i, \quad i = 1, \ldots, n_{x_\theta} \tag{34}$$

$$\mathcal{X}_i^{t-1} = \bar{\mathbf{x}}_\theta^{t-1} - \left(\sqrt{(n_{x_\theta} + \lambda)\mathbf{P}_{\mathbf{x}_\theta}^{t-1}}\right)_{i-n_{x_\theta}}, \quad i = n_{x_\theta} + 1, \ldots, 2n_{x_\theta}, \tag{35}$$

where the quantity $\lambda = \gamma^2 \left(n_{x_\theta} + \kappa\right) - n_{x_\theta}$ (usually a small positive value, e.g. $1 \geq \gamma \geq 10^{-4}$) is a scaling parameter. The constant γ determines the spread of the sigma vectors around the mean, $\bar{\mathbf{x}}^t$. The other constant, κ, is a secondary scaling parameter, which is usually set to 0 or $3 - n_{x_\theta}$. $\left(\sqrt{\left(n_{x_\theta} + \lambda\right) \mathbf{P}_{\mathbf{x}_\theta}^{t-1}}\right)_i$ is the ith column of the matrix square root (e.g. the lower triangular matrix that can be computed using the Cholesky decomposition).

The sigma vectors are propagated through the nonlinear system,

$$\mathbf{X}_i^t = f\left(\boldsymbol{\mathcal{X}}_i^{t-1}\right) \quad i = 1, \ldots, 2n_{x_\theta}, \tag{36}$$

and the mean and covariance for the transformed variable, which link back to equations (30) and (31), are approximated by

$$\bar{\mathbf{x}}_\theta^t = \hat{\mathbf{x}}_\theta^{t-} \approx \sum_{i=0}^{2n_{x_\theta}} W_i^{(m)} \boldsymbol{\mathcal{X}}_i^t \tag{37}$$

$$\mathbf{P}_{\mathbf{x}_\theta}^t = \hat{\mathbf{P}}_{\mathbf{x}_\theta}^{t-} \approx \sum_{i=0}^{2n_{x_\theta}} W_i^{(c)} \left(\boldsymbol{\mathcal{X}}_i^t - \hat{\mathbf{x}}_\theta^{t-}\right)\left(\boldsymbol{\mathcal{X}}_i^t - \hat{\mathbf{x}}_\theta^{t-}\right)^\top, \tag{38}$$

where the weights, W_i, are

$$W_0^{(m)} = \frac{\lambda}{n_{x_\theta} + \lambda} \tag{39}$$

$$W_0^{(c)} = \frac{\lambda}{n_{x_\theta} + \lambda} + \left(1 - \gamma^2 + \beta\right) \tag{40}$$

$$W_i^{(m)} = W_i^{(c)} = \frac{1}{2\left(n_{x_\theta} + \lambda\right)} \quad i = 1, \ldots, 2n_{x_\theta}, \tag{41}$$

and β is a variable that includes prior knowledge of the distribution of $\mathbf{x}_\theta$.

By using the UT to propagate the state and parameter estimates and errors through time, the standard Kalman filter update equations (since the observation equation is modeled as being linear) can be used. The Kalman gain, which is used to weight the influence of the measured data on the predicted data, is calculated by

$$\mathcal{K}^t = \hat{\mathbf{P}}_{\mathbf{x}_\theta}^{t-} \mathbf{C}_\theta^\top \left(\mathbf{C}_\theta \hat{\mathbf{P}}_{\mathbf{x}_\theta}^{t-} \mathbf{C}_\theta^\top + \sigma_e^2\right)^{-1}. \tag{42}$$

The equations that use the Kalman gain to get the *a posteriori* from *a priori* estimates of the augmented state and error are

$$\hat{\mathbf{x}}_\theta^{t+} = \hat{\mathbf{x}}_\theta^{t-} + \mathcal{K}^t \left(y - \mathbf{C}_\theta \hat{\mathbf{x}}_\theta^{t-}\right) \tag{43}$$

$$\hat{\mathbf{P}}_{\mathbf{x}_\theta}^{t+} = \left(\mathbf{I} - \mathcal{K}^t \mathbf{C}_\theta\right) \hat{\mathbf{P}}_{\mathbf{x}_\theta}^{t-}, \tag{44}$$

where $\mathbf{C}_\theta$ is the observation matrix which has been padded with zeros to account for the augmented state vector.

The UT captures the properties of the nonlinear transform of a Gaussian random variable to 3rd order Taylor series expansion for all nonlinearities (and higher order with the appropriate choice of γ and β^{27}).

4.1. Demonstration of UKF using ECoG Data Simulation

In this section, we demonstrate how the stochastic estimation framework is able to estimate the neural mass model parameters when their values are initialized 60% above and below their actual values. The results are shown in Figure 4 along with a 1 second of the data that was used.

The results show that the parameter values converge to the actual values for both initial condition cases. The discrepancy between the time it takes to converge when initialised from above compared to below is similar to the deterministic case. This effect may be due to the saturating effects of the sigmoidal nonlinearity. Alternatively, it may be due to the smaller time constants (larger reciprocals), which reduces the transition times in the system allowing the system to respond more readily to changes. It indicates that it is advantageous to initialize parameters to values in the upper region of the physiological range.

4.2. Demonstration of using Real ECoG Data

4.2.1. ECoG Data

The data that was used in this section was collected from a patient undergoing assessment for resective surgery at St. Vincent's Hospital Melbourne, and is used with patient consent and permission from the Human Research Ethics Committee (protocol HRECA-006/08). Data was recorded from a sub-dural grid electrode with electrode spacing of 0.5 cm and surface diameter of 2 mm (Ad-Tech Medical). The most focal differential channel was used, relative to the seizure onset zone. The data was sampled at a rate of 1kHz and low-pass filtered with a cut-off of 95 Hz. The data was re-scaled by a factor of 1×10^4 to have an amplitude in the same order of magnitude to the output of the neural mass model. A 5 minute epoch of the data was used, with approximately 200 seconds before electrographic seizure onset and 100 seconds post-onset.

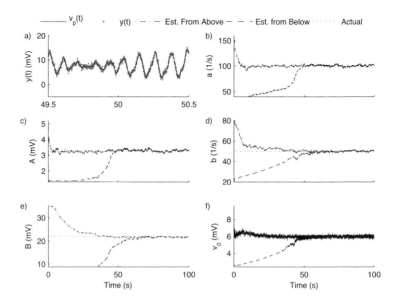

Fig. 4. **UKF Estimation Results from Synthetic Data.** a) An example of the synthetic data that was used, illustrating the level of noise added to the model output. Black line: the membrane potential of the pyramidal population. Gray dots: the ECoG signal that was used for estimation. Subplots b) to f) show the estimated parameters from when the initial guess was 60% above and below the actual value. Dotted line: the actual parameter value. Dot-dash line: the estimation results when the estimated value was initialized at 60% above. Dashed line: the results when initialized at 60% below. b) Estimate of the reciprocal of the excitatory time constant. c) Estimate of the excitatory gain parameter. d) Estimate of the reciprocal of the inhibitory synaptic time constant. e) Estimate of the inhibitory gain parameter. f) Estimate of the sigmoid threshold parameter.

4.2.2. Parameter Estimates

A major challenge in applying the method lies in initializing the estimator. The initial parameter estimates were chosen based on a trial and error approach. The Jansen and Rit parameters to simulate the alpha rhythm were initially used. If any one parameter diverged rapidly then the initial condition was adjusted in the direction of divergence in small steps until the direction changed. After some tuning, the parameters gave a steady value until approximately 40 seconds prior to seizure onset, where the inhibitory population synaptic time constant began to decrease from the base-line level.

Figure 5 shows the results from the ECoG data. As expected, the gains for both excitatory and inhibitory, A and B, populations increased during the seizure. Figure 6 demonstrates that the ratio of excitation to inhibition was fairly constant prior to the seizure, increased during the seizure, and returned to pre-seizure levels a short time after the seizure. The excitatory synaptic time constant became shorter during the seizure, which explains higher frequency activity during the event. Interestingly, the inhibitory time constant decreased approximately 40 seconds prior to the onset, reached its minimum shortly after the onset, and then increased during the seizure. This provides a new intuition into higher frequency oscillations prior to seizures and the chirping effect observed during seizures. Finally, the threshold parameter decreased at seizure onset and then increased at seizure termination. We speculate that this may be a result in a shift in the resting membrane potential due to seizure related changes in ionic concentrations; however, this remains to be tested.

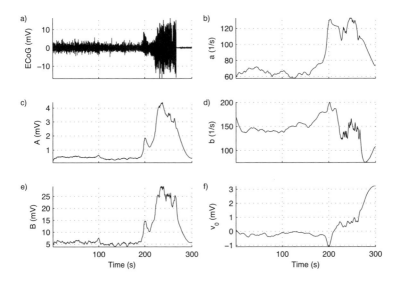

Fig. 5. **UKF Estimation Results from ECoG Data.** a) The ECoG data from a focal channel recorded from a grid array. b) Estimate of the reciprocal of the excitatory synaptic time constant. c) Estimate of the excitatory gain parameter. d) Estimate of the reciprocal of the inhibitory time constant. e) Estimate of the inhibitory gain parameter. f) Estimate of the sigmoid threshold parameter.

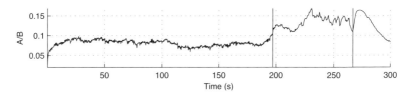

Fig. 6. **Ratio of Excitatory to Inhibitory Strength Estimated from ECoG Data.** The solid vertical lines mark the electrographic seizure onset and termination.

5. Discussion

We have presented a novel method developed by our group, the adaptive observer, and compared it to a novel application of an existing method, the augmented state UKF, for state and parameter estimation of ECoG data using a neural mass model. The purpose of the chapter was not to provide a rigorous proof of these particular algorithms, but to provide some insight and demonstrate the possibilities of a model-based data analysis approach. These methods can be used for inferring underlying brain changes based on a single ECoG recording. The stochastic estimation method relies on an extension of the UKF, while the deterministic estimation method relies on Lyapunov-based approaches for adaptive observer design. The adaptive observer estimates are guaranteed to converge to the true state and parameter values of the neural mass model provided a persistency of excitation condition holds. Although convergence is not guaranteed for the stochastic method, the UKF deals well with uncertainty and model error because it takes these into account implicitly.

Due to the Lyapunov-based design, the adaptive observer has a degree of robustness to uncertainty, and nominal robustness for small model-system mismatch. However, this needs to be analyzed further. Here we have shown in simulations that the adaptive observer is robust to a large degree of measurement noise although this is not considered in the observer design. The adaptive observer was applied to the real ECoG data, although it was not shown in the chapter, and the estimation results were unstable. This is maybe due to the mismatch between the neural mass model and the actual physical dynamics. Further work is needed to specifically design an adaptive observer that is robust to input uncertainty and model-system mismatch.

The flexibility of the UKF to uncertainties means that it performs well at estimating a larger number of parameters than the adaptive observer. This online estimation of neural mass model parameters with real seizure ECoG data is the first of its kind. Moreover, the parameter changes occurring at seizure onset, such as an increase in postsynaptic potential amplitudes (A,B) and an initial decrease in threshold v_0, appear consistent with what might be expected during seizures. The online estimation presented here contrasts with and compliments the excellent offline estimation techniques that have also been applied to epilepsy data.[28,29]

The true meaning and interpretability of parameter changes requires further study. In particular, different parameter combinations may produce similar ECoG seizure dynamics and a question needs to be answered: which parameter combination is the true combination? One way to get around this problem is to limit the complexity of the computational models to allow for reliable estimation and at the same time reduce the dimensionality of the parameter space. For more complex models, higher fidelity data acquisition and greater signal sampling is required for coping with uncertainties. To put it another way, the models can be considered as tools for interpolating missing or hidden data. To capture more complex features of the system, richer data are required or the interpolation will be overly simplified. Signal scaling, re-referencing, offsets, and DC-filtering also need to be considered in future estimator designs.

Such biologically motivated online estimator designs will likely revolutionise how we can image the underlying activity of the brain and devise improved methods for neurological monitoring, control and treatment.

Acknowledgments

This research was partly supported by the Australian Research Council (Linkage Project LP100200571). The Bionics Institute acknowledges the support it receives from the Victorian State Government through the Operational Infrastructure Support Program. Romain Rostoyan is funded by the PEPS-CNRS project APSE and by the ANR under the grant SEPICOT (ANR 12 JS03 004 01).

References

1. S. Schiff, *Neural Control Engineering: The Emerging Intersection Between Control Theory and Neuroscience* (The MIT Press, Cambridge, MA, 2011).
2. E. Marder and J. Goaillard, *Nature Reviews Neuroscience* **7**, 563 (2006).
3. F. Marten, S. Rodrigues, P. Suffczynski, M. Richardson and J. Terry, *Physical Review E* **79**, p. 21911 (2009).
4. F. Mormann, R. Andrzejak, C. Elger and K. Lehnertz, *Brain* **130**, 314 (2007).
5. L. Kuhlmann, D. Freestone, A. Lai, A. Burkitt, K. Fuller, D. Grayden, L. Seiderer, S. Vogrin, I. Mareels and M. Cook, *Epilepsy Research* **91**, 214 (2010).

6. H. Khalil, Nonlinear Systems (Prentice-Hall, Englewood Cliffs, New Jersey, U.S.A., 2002) pp. 610–625, 3rd edn.

7. G. Besançon, Nonlinear Observers and ApplicationsLecture Notes in Control and Information Sciences (Springer, 2007).

8. O. David, S. Kiebel, L. Harrison, J. Mattout, J. Kilner and K. Friston, *NeuroImage* **30**, 1255 (2006).

9. D. Freestone, P. Aram, M. Dewar, K. Scerri, D. Grayden and V. Kadirkamanathan, *NeuroImage* **56**, 1043 (2011).

10. B. Jansen and V. Rit, *Biological Cybernetics* **73**, 357 (1995).

11. G. Besançon, *Systems & Control Letters* **41**, 271 (2000).

12. S. Julier and J. Uhlmann, New extension of the kalman filter to nonlinear systems, in *AeroSense'97*, 1997.

13. R. van der Merwe, Sigma-point kalman filters for probabilistic inference in dynamic state-space models, PhD thesis, University of Stellenbosch2004.

14. O. Faugeras, J. Touboul and B. Cessac, *Frontiers in computational neuroscience* **3** (2009).

15. F. Freyer, J. Roberts, R. Becker, P. Robinson, P. Ritter and M. Breakspear, *The Journal of Neuroscience* **31**, 6353 (2011).

16. G. Deco, V. Jirsa, P. Robinson, M. Breakspear and K. Friston, *PLoS Computational Biology* **4**, p. e1000092 (2008).

17. F. L. da Silva, A. Hoek, H. Smith and L. Zetterberg, *Cybernetic* **15**, 27 (1974).

18. F. Wendling, A. Hernandez, J. Bellanger, P. Chauvel and F. Bartolomei, *Journal of Clinical Neurophysiology* **22**, 343 (2005).

19. O. David and K. Friston, *NeuroImage* **20**, 1743 (2003).

20. F. Wendling, F. Bartolomei, J. Bellanger and P. Chauvel, *European Journal of Neuroscience* **15**, 1499 (2002).

21. R. Postoyan, M. Chong, D. Nešić and L. Kuhlmann, Parameter and state estimation for a class of neural mass models, in *IEEE Conference on Decision and Control*, (Maui, Hawaii, 2012).

22. P. Ioannou and J. Sun, *Robust Adaptive Control* (Prentice-Hall, New Jersey, 1996).

23. R. Kalman, *Journal of Basic Engineering* **82**, 35 (1960).

24. E. W. Ericwan, R. V. D. Merwe and A. T. Nelson, 666 (2000).

25. V. H.U., J. Timmer and J. Kurths, *International Journal of Bifurcation and Chaos* **14**, 1905 (2004).

26. S. Haykin, *Kalman Filtering and Neural Networks* (Wiley Online Library, 2001).

27. S. Julier, The scaled unscented transformation, in *American Control Conference, 2002. Proceedings of the 2002*, 2002.

28. A. Blenkinsop, A. Valentin, M. Richardson and J. Terry, *European Journal of Neuroscience* **36**, 2188 (2012).

29. F. Wendling, F. Bartolomei, F. Mina, C. Huneau and P. Benquet, *European Journal of Neuroscience* **36**, 2164 (2012).

COMPUTATIONAL MODELLING OF MICROSEIZURES AND FOCAL SEIZURE ONSET

YUJIANG WANG[1]*, MARC GOODFELLOW[2], PETER NEAL TAYLOR[3],
DANIEL JAMES GARRY[1], AND GEROLD BAIER[4]

[1] *Manchester Interdisciplinary Biocentre.*
131 Princess Street. Manchester M1 7DN. United Kingdom
[2] *Faculty of Life Sciences*
University of Manchester. United Kingdom
[3] *School of Electrical & Electronic Engineering*
Nanyang Technological University. Singapore
[4] *Centre fo Organismal Studies, BioQuant BQ18*
University of Heidelberg, 69120 Heidelberg, Germany
* yujiang.wang-2@manchester.ac.uk

Purpose: To create a computational model on the mesoscale of a cortical sheet $(5 \times 5mm^2)$ to study the mechanisms of microseizure restriction, the recruitment of normal tissue into seizure activity and possibilities for therapeutic intervention.

Methods: We develop a model of interacting minicolumns where the dynamics of each minicolumn contains a switch between a low-activity background and high-activity seizure state. The connectivity between minicolumns is based on results from anatomical studies of the neocortex.

Results: The model reproduces the clinically observed, spatially restricted microseizures on the cortical mesoscale as transient self-terminating localised events. To model focal seizures, small regions of abnormal, hyperexcitable tissue were included, which spontaneously recruited larger regions of tissue into macroscopic seizure activity. The model predicts that severing cortico-cortical connections between scattered clusters of hyperactive microdomains could be sufficient to prevent seizure onset.

Significance: Our model provides a framework to test the organization and interactions within epileptic foci on the cortical mesoscale. In addition it allows the development and testing of suitable surgical treatment protocols *in silico*.

Keywords: Focal seizure, microseizure, spatio-temporal modelling, cortical connectivity

List of Symbols

Variables of the model:

$x(t)$: Vector of length n^2 containing the activity states of each unit of the simulated cortical surface

$x_i(t)$: The i-th element in $x(t)$

Parameters of the model:

n: The width of the simulated square sheet

d_0, d_3: Decay rates of the system below 0 and above 1, respectively

Θ_e: Excitability threshold, which upon crossing sends the system to 1 corresponding to a high-activity state

R_{bg}: Decay rate at $x_i(t) = \Theta_e$

R_{exc}: Decay rate at $x_i(t) = 1$

A_n: Afferent noise amplitude

w_L: Weight scaling of local connections

r_L: Radius of reach for local connections

δ_L: Decay rate of number of connection with distance

w_R: Weight scaling for remote connections

n_p: Number of remote patches

m_p^2: Number of minicolumns in a patch

r_p: Radius of reach for remote patches

n_S: Number of overlapping patches shared by neighbouring macrocolumns

n_O: Number of remote connections established by each minicolumn

1. Introduction

An important aspect of the generation of epileptic seizures is the recruitment of substantial regions of cortical tissue into pathological activity which underpins macroscopic electrographic recordings as well as clinical signs and symptoms. In addition to large scale spatial features of epileptic electrographic activity, as captured by terms like "focal" or "generalised", recent findings have highlighted the relevance of abnormal activity at a smaller spatial scale. Microperiodic epileptiform discharges occurring during interictal intervals were reported by Schevon et al.,[1] who used microelectrode arrays embedded into human epileptic neocortex. These electrodes were $3 - 5\mu m$ in diameter at the recording tip and $35 - 75\mu m$ at the base (i.e. the scale of a cortical minicolumn[2]). Similarly, Stead et al.[3] reported electrographic, seizure-like activity recorded in isolated microelectrodes of $40\mu m$ diameter in size. Such electrographic activity, termed "microseizures",[3] was also observed in people without epilepsy albeit less frequently, highlighting the importance of considering the role of mesoscopic abnormalities in the recruitment of large regions of tissue for clinical seizures.

Stead et al.[3] proposed the hypothesis, that "pathological microdomains" (i.e. microdomains that are able to generate and sustain isolated high activity states) might be found in healthy brains, but are more densely distributed in and around epileptogenic tissue. To test this hypothesis, one must therefore consider the anatomical cortical connectivity networks that potentially support propagating localised abnormal activity at the spatial scale of interacting minicolumns (the mesoscale[4]). At this cortical scale, local connections to neighbours are abundant, but more remote connections are also important and make up to 40% of all outgoing connections.[5] Furthermore these remote connections are structured, in that they often cluster and clusters from neighbouring regions overlap.[5]

Here, we develop a computational model to explore the restriction and spreading of abnormal activity in cortical tissue at the mesoscale using realistic cortical network topologies. Minicolumn dynamics are formulated to capture both the transient high activity (seizure) state as well as the low-activity background state. We demonstrate that localised transient high-activity events can occur in this model, without spreading to neighbouring minicolumn. Including clusters of hyperexcitable units that correspond to suggested "pathological microdomains", we show the spontaneous recruitment of farther reaching regions. We then use this model to explore a potential strategy for surgical intervention to prevent the onset of macroscopic seizures.

2. Model details

We address the spatiotemporal dynamics of pathological electrographic activity at the scale where spatially restricted microseizure activity has been reported:[3,6] the scale of minicolumns. We compartmentalise a cortical piece of tissue into interacting minicolumn nodes. We model the dynamics of a single node using a rule-based, discrete-time approach, following previous literature.[7,8] In the following we conceptualise microseizures as excitation into a high activity state and refer to model microseizures as any kind of local high activity (e.g. microperiodic epileptiform discharges, high frequency oscillations). This allows us to focus on the spatial aspect of state transitions. Modelling the details of specific temporal waveforms of subtypes of focal seizures is referred to future work.

2.1. Single unit dynamics

The single unit $x(t_k) \in \mathbb{R}, k = 0, 1, 2, 3, \ldots$ is set up to reflect the activity of a minicolumn ($50\mu m \times 50\mu m$ in size[2]) over time. The distinction between the background state and the seizure state is based on the activity level. We set the background state to 0 and the excited state to 1.

Noise input: Noise is added to the current activity of the minicolumn for the next iteration, reflecting afferent activity from other brain regions: $x(t_{k+1}) = x(t_k) + p(t_k)$, where $p(t_k)$ is normally distributed over t_k. Refer to the next section (Cortical sheet model) for details of the noise input.

Cortico-cortical input: All units are coupled via a connectivity matrix C and the input from neighbouring units is passed through a sigmoid function $S(\ldots)$ to ensure saturation in activity. Therefore, the input from other units in a simulated piece of tissue (sheet) can be written as $CS(x_i(t_k))$, where $i = 1, 2, 3, \ldots$ indicates the number of a connected node. With this addition, the general equation for a single unit becomes $x(t_{k+1}) = x(t_k) + p(t_k) + CS(x_i(t_k))$.

Decay: The activity in each unit decays according to a decay term $d(.)$ that is activity state dependent (see below). The general equation for a single unit then becomes $x(t_{k+1}) = x(t_k) + p(t_k) + CS(x_i(t_k)) - d(x(t_k))$. The state-dependent decay is designed to mimic the decay process in a dynamical system with an excitable fixed point. If such a system is perturbed within an excitability threshold (Θ_e), it returns to the fixed point in an exponential fashion. Perturbations above the threshold direct the systems trajectory away from the fixed point to some excited (seizure) state. Ultimately, however, the trajectory returns to the original fixed point. In order for our rule-based model to reflect this behaviour, three parameters are required, namely i) the excitability threshold: Θ_e; ii) a parameter controlling the amount of activation needed to switch from background to excited state: R_{bg}; and iii) a parameter controlling the amount of activation needed to remain in the activated state: R_{exc}. The decay term, d, is partitioned in a piece-wise linear fashion to implement such an excitability (see Fig. 1) and is given in detail below.

For negative activity and for positive activity values below the excitability threshold ($x(t) \leqslant \Theta_e$), the systems dynamics decay towards the stable background activity with linear dependence on current activity: $d(x) = d_0 * x$ for $x(t) \leqslant 0$ and $d(x) = d_1 x(t)$ for $0 < x(t) \leqslant \Theta_e$, respectively. For $\Theta_e < x(t) \leqslant 1$, another linear term (usually with negative slope) $d(x) = d_2 x(t) + m_2$ is used for the decay rate to allow for a transient non-background activity, which given noise will eventually return to background. For $x(t) > 1$, the decay rate is set to $d(x) = d_3 x(t) + m_3$, with positive slope for fast decay. The parameters $d_{1,2}$ can be parametrized in terms of R_{bg} and R_{exc} ($R_{bg} = d(x = \Theta_e)$ and $R_{exc} = d(x = 1)$) as shown in Fig. 1. With the assumed continuity of $d(.)$ and fixing $d_0 = d_3 = 2$, we can therefore unambiguously determine the parameters $m_{2,3}$. Therefore the only parameters for the model are set to $R_{bg} = 0.12$ and $R_{exc} = 0.08$. Finally, when a unit crosses the excitability threshold (becomes excited) at a time step, its value is set to 1, to represent the divergence of the trajectory to the excitable structure. In Fig. 2 we show exemplary behaviour of a single unit in response to subthreshold and supra-threshold perturbations.

2.2. Cortical sheet model

Arrays of interacting minicolumns are assumed to model a cortical tissue sheet. We arrange minicolumns into macrocolumns consisting of 10×10 minicolumns.[9] All extrinsic noise inputs project to a macrocolumn (i.e. subsquares of 10×10 minicolumns receive the same noise input from afferent projections). Figure 3(a) illustrates this scheme. The noise input for each macrocolumn at each time point is drawn independently from the normal distribution centred around zero and the standard deviation is A_n, which is chosen depending on R_{bg} and the desired model output.

To represent the sheet mathematically, we use the variable $x(t)$, which is a vector of length n^2 containing the states of each unit of the simulated cortical surface and n is the width of the square sheet. $x_i(t)$ denotes the i-th element in this vector. In this work we use $n = 100$, i.e. the sheet is divided up into 100 macrocolumns, and a total of 10,000 minicolumns. The whole sheet corresponds to a size of approx. $5mm \times 5mm$.

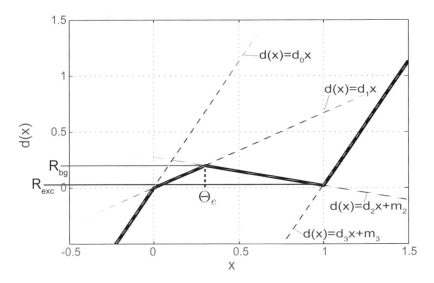

Fig. 1. The decay function $d(x)$ plotted against x. The piecewise-linear function approximates the behaviour of an excitable dynamical system (see text for details).

2.3. Connectivity between units

Following Voges et al.,[5] we include two types of connections. Anatomical (tracer injection) studies suggest that *local connectivity* is constrained within a certain radius. Voges et al.[5] suggests using $500\mu m$ (corresponding to the length of 10 minicolumns) for the radius. This is an upper limit found in anatomical studies of mammalian cortex, with reported values starting from $300\mu m$ (6 minicolumns).[5] Inspecting the tracer injection images (compare Fig. 7.3 in Levitt et al.[10]), one can additionally observe that connectivity decreases for larger radii.

Based on these considerations, we implement local connectivity using an algorithm that connects all neighbours within a certain Euclidean distance r_L. Outside this distance, the algorithm connects probabilistically to nodes based on an exponential function. The parameters of the algorithm are r_L and the exponential fall-off δ_L. Values of these parameters were chosen such that within a length of 3 minicolumns ($150\mu m$) all neighbours are connected ($r_L = 3$ minicolumns). Outside this radius, nodes in up to 6 minicolumns ($300\mu m$) distance can be connected ($\delta_L = 1$) probabilistically. Effectively, this algorithm generates connection in a $300\mu m$ radius, with less density in connectivity towards the edge of the range. Note that local connections

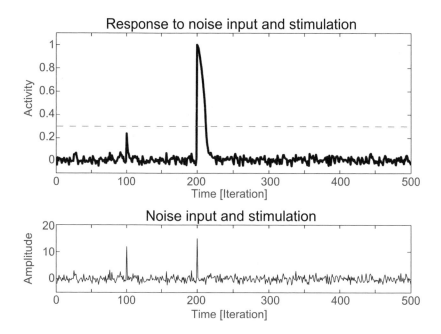

Fig. 2. Top: Sub- and supra-threshold response of a single unit $x(t)$ at t=100 and t=200, respectively, with the noise input protocol in the bottom panel. The dashed line indicates the value of the threshold Θ_e. The stimulation (t=100 and t=200) has been incorporated in the noise vector as shown in the bottom plot.

extend beyond macrocolumn boundaries. Fig. 3(b) shows an example of connections for one unit. The weight of the connections has been chosen to be proportional to distance with proportionality factor w_L. This choice reflects the underlying decrease in neuronal connections with distance as observed in the tracer injection images. Note that for different realistic values of the radius ($300 - 500\mu m$), qualitatively the same results as those reported here could be obtained, if the connection weight w_L was adjusted accordingly.

For *remote connections*, Voges et al.[5] proposes a patchy, overlapping scheme. We use an algorithm that generates n_P random patches for each macrocolumn and all minicolumns within the macrocolumn can connect to these patches with n_O outgoing connections. The patches contain m_P^2 minicolumns and are located within a distance of r_P minicolumns. Neighbouring macrocolumns share n_S patches with a randomly chosen direct neighbour. Parameters are fixed as: $n_P = 6, m_P = 10, r_P = 35(1.75mm), n_S = 3$, in line with the suggestions of Voges *et al.*,[5] see Figure 3(c). To avoid boundary effects, toroidal boundary conditions were used for both remote and local connections. The behaviour of the system is sensitive to n_O, but less to the choice of other parameters, which agrees with Ref. 11. However, our analysis also showed that adjustment of the weighting w_R of the remote connections could counter balance the effects of n_O. We set $w_R = 0.012$ and $n_O = 10$. The current parameter setting yields a system that supports spread of high-activity states via remote connections, where local connections help to sustain these states.

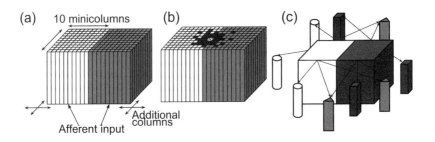

Fig. 3. (a) Scheme of two macrocolumns (white and light grey) subdivided into minicolumns and receiving subcortical projections. (b) The minicolumn at the centre labelled 'x' has connections to all neighbours within the distance of 3 minicolumns and additional random connections to neighbours up to a distance of 6 minicolumns (marked in dark grey). (c) Projections of two exemplary macrocolumns (grey and white) to 6 remote patches each. White (round) patches receive input from the white column only; dark-grey (square) patches receive input from the dark grey column only; and the light-grey (triangular) patches receive input from both columns.

In summary, the model can be generally written as

$$x(t_{k+1}) = \begin{cases} 1 & \text{if x crosses } \Theta_e \\ x(t_k) + CS(x(t_k)) + p(t_k) - d(x(t_k)) & else, \end{cases} \quad (1)$$

where x is the activity level of the units; C is the connectivity matrix; $S(.)$ is a sigmoid function; $p(.)$ is an afferent noise-process; and $d(.)$ is the piecewise linear function (Fig. 1) as discussed in the subsection for single unit dynamics.

The exact parameters we use for the result section are as follows. The sheet is 100×100 minicolumns in size, i.e. $n = 100$. The parameters controlling the single unit dynamics are $d_0 = d_3 = 2, R_{bg} = 0.12, R_{exc} = 0.08$ and Θ_e is normally distributed around 0.3, with a standard deviation of 0.03

and negative values drawn from this distribution are ignored. The afferent noise amplitude was fixed at $A_n = 0.02$. The local connectivity parameters were set to $w_L = 0.0035$, $r_L = 3$ minicolumns and $\delta_L = 1$ minicolumn. For the remote connectivity, each macrocolumn has $n_p = 6$ patches, each patch is a cluster of $m_p^2 = 10^2$ minicolumns. The patches are within $r_p = 35$ minicolumns distance and neighbouring macrocolumns have $n_S = 3$ overlapping patches. Each minicolumn establishes $n_O = 10$ remote connections, with weight $w_R = 0.012$.

3. Results

3.1. *Non-epileptic state*

The parameters indicated in the last paragraph allow the occurrence of microseizures (i.e. transient, localised, self-terminating transitions to the excited state) with a mean duration of about 98 iteration steps for the microseizures in the single units. During simulations of 10000 iteration (time) steps approximately 20% of all nodes exhibited noise-induced (spontaneous) excitation to high amplitude activity, i.e. 'microseizures'. Due to the excitability properties of the network nodes, this activity self-terminates. Fig. 4 (top) shows an exemplary time series of model output. Microseizures can be noted in different locations which would be picked up by microelectrodes only as they do not recruit neighbouring or distant nodes. They would therefore be missed by mean field potential recordings as those from standard electrocorticogram.[3] The long-term temporal average of the simulated tissue sheet is fairly homogeneous (Fig. 4 (bottom left)), although the irregular occurrence of microseizures does cluster to certain locations within the sheet (Fig. 4 (bottom right)). Also, despite the occurrence of local microseizures in various locations, no spreading or generalisation of abnormal seizure activity is observed.

3.2. *Epileptic state*

Following Stead et al.,[3] we incorporate microdomains that are intrinsically able to generate local high-activity events. These microdomains are small clusters of hyperexcitable units. To model their presence we decrease their R_{bg} value (see Fig. 5(a)). We use 25 clusters, 30 minicolumns in size, randomly scattered over the sheet with the altered value of $R_{bg} = 0.07$. This value implies that $R_{bg} < R_{exc}$ and the slope d_2 (see Fig. 1) becomes slightly positive. Hence activity of the altered units remain almost permanently in the active state.

92

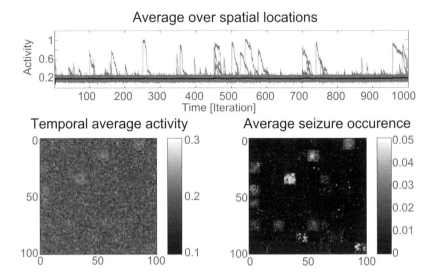

Fig. 4. Top: Thin grey lines indicate the mean of macrocolumns, thick black line indicates mean of the whole sheet. Bottom: The corresponding sheet averaged over time. The grey-coding indicates the mean activity and the mean microseizure occurrence, respectively. Note: mean microseizure occurrence refers to the percentage of time a unit spent in the excited state (i.e. $x_i(t) > \Theta_e$).

We observe that these clusters lead to the localised occurrence of hyperactivity in the simulated cortical sheet. The locations of occurrence of high activity are now distributed more densely. In contrast to the previous case, the domains of hyperactivity are now able to recruit neighbouring and distant sites to the abnormal activity and can thus lead to a generalisation throughout the whole sheet into a globally excited state (Fig.5(c)). Fig.5(d) shows snapshots of the activity in the sheet before, during and after this generalisation.

We studied how the time until recruitment of the whole sheet depends on the number of hyperexcitable clusters. Fig. 6(left) shows that the more clusters are present, the earlier the recruitment occurs. The recruitment time also depends on the cluster size and the spatial organization of the clusters. The smaller the clusters, the later the recruitment. Clusters that are denser in one area tend to recruit surrounding units and a few remote regions. If the whole sheet is covered in clusters (as is the case in Fig. 5) the whole sheet can be recruited as shown. Moreover, the value of R_{bg} for these hyperexcitable clusters play a role in the recruitment time as shown in

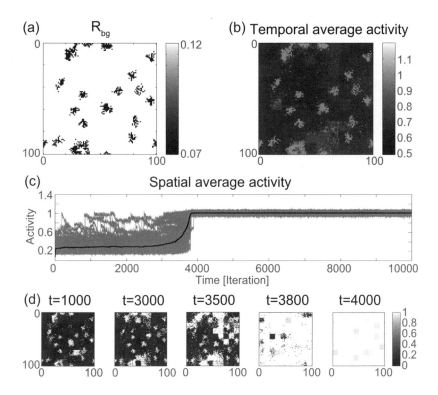

Fig. 5. (a) Position of hyperexcitable nodes (decreased value of R_{bg}). (b) The temporal average of the activity of the sheet over the whole simulated time. (c) The sheet in spatial average. Thin grey lines indicate the mean of macrocolumns, thick black line indicates mean of the whole sheet. (d) Snapshots of the activity on the sheet at different time points.

Fig. 6(right). Interestingly, this transition is not smooth but comparatively sudden.

3.3. *The effect of reducing connections*

We investigated the effect of severing cortical-cortical connections in such a sheet with hyperexcitable clusters, and observed that this could stop the recruitment process (see Fig. 7). In this case the three 'incisions' follow the schematics in Fig. 7(first column). In Fig. 7(a) the total length of the incision was $250\mu m$, i.e. 5 minicolumns. 503 local and 874 remote connections (that is 0.12% of local connections and 0.88% of remote connections) were cut in this process. This was not enough to stop recruitment and

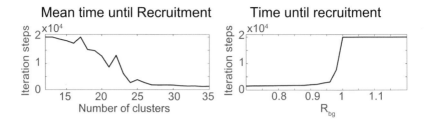

Fig. 6. Left: Recruitment time of the whole sheet averaged over 10 different randomly distributed hyperexcitable clusters at the indicated cluster numbers. Right: Recruitment time of the whole sheet of 25 (fixed) clusters for the indicated value of R_{bg}. The total simulation time was 20000 iteration steps.

global spreading of the high activity state. The second incision (Fig. 7(b)) was $500\mu m$, i.e. 10 minicolumns long. 964 (0.23%) local and 2112 (2.13%) remote connections were cut. Although this prolongs the time until the whole model is recruited into high activity, it does not stop this from happening altogether. In Fig. 7(c) the incision was $2250\mu m = 2.25mm$, i.e. 45 minicolumns long (4160 (0.99%) local and 8511 (8.59%) remote connections were cut) and this did not lead to generalised recruitment of the whole sheet (after 10^5 iteration steps). In further studies we observed that the time until recruitment of the whole sheet directly correlates with the number of connections cut (data not shown). Therefore, a significant reduction in transitions to model seizures is achieved by a localised reduction in connections which leaves the majority of the simulated tissue intact.

4. Discussion

We proposed a modelling framework to study the occurrence and spreading of activity on the mesoscopic scale of connected cortical minicolumns. We demonstrated that in a system incorporating realistic cortico-cortical connectivity micro-activities can occur which are transient and spatially restricted, i.e. microseizures. We find that the additional presence of hyperexcitable clusters of nodes can recruit the whole simulated tissue into full blown macroseizures. The recruitment depends upon the interplay between location, density and hyperexcitability of these clusters. Furthermore we demonstrated the potential of this model to study the effects of simulated surgical interventions which are less severe than conventionally practised volume resection.

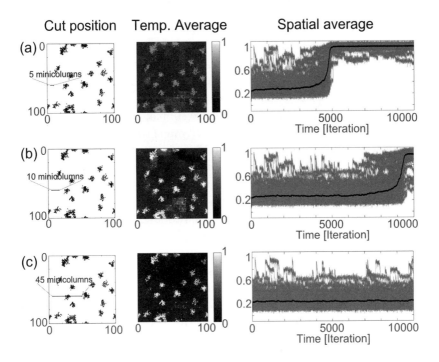

Fig. 7. Simulated incision positions (first column), temporal averages of the sheet after the incision (second column), and spatial averages (third column) are shown. (a) The incision was 5 minicolumns in length. (b) The incision was 10 minicolumns in length. (c) The incision was 45 minicolumns in length. All the cuts start from the minicolumn in position (60,5). For details regarding the number of connections cut for each incision, see text.

For the description of the onset of a focal seizure, our model shows the recruitment of otherwise healthy parts of tissue by abnormal microdomains. Abnormal localised activity has been recorded in human epileptogenic tissue during interictal states[1,3] but was also observed, albeit less frequently, in nonepileptic cortex of epileptic patients and cortex of subjects without epilepsy.[3] These studies suggest the notion that epileptogenic tissue is characterised by increased density of abnormal microdomains. The higher density of abnormal microdomains could then be the tissue correlate of the "interacting network of pathologically connected neuron clusters" as hypothesized by Bragin et al.[12] Our model allowed the investigation of this hypothesis and we observed a faster recruitment of the model into high activity levels when more clusters of hyper-excitable nodes were incorporated.

In addition, Stead et al.[3] suggested that an increased connectivity between pathological microdomains could be an underlying mechanism for recruitment. The fact that severed connections between these microdomains in our model disrupt recruitment is in line with this hypothesis. Further studies of the model along these directions can suggest optimal interactions given specified densities of abnormal nodes, and their connection, which could lead to insight into the efficacy of multiple subpial transections.[13]

To model sustained, but localised activity in networks, Kaiser and Hilgetag[8] suggested using hierarchical network topologies. However, they focused on the different hierarchies (scales) of the whole brain rather than the specific scale of local cortical tissue. Hence they did not use specific anatomical connectivities that are observed on the mesoscale (which we addressed in the current work). In comparison to the network structure of the model of Kaiser and Hilgetag,[8] our cortical network is more densely connected (number of edges per node of 0.12 vs. $\sim$ 45 in the present case) and not strictly hierarchical according to the properties in Ref 14 (the degree distribution is a skewed gaussian, and the slope of the log C(k) to log(k) plot is around -2). In addition our model is constructed such that node dynamics specifically mimic excitable dynamical systems. In this aspect our work can be seen as an alternative proposal for how networks can display local sustained activity. The exact relation between the two suggested network topologies could be resolved when incorporating multiple scales in our network.

Our model distinguishes between normal and abnormal dynamics based on two levels of activity and does not currently capture details of seizure waveforms. Using this kind of abstract model is in line with previous modelling approaches investigating network properties in the context of epilepsy.[7,8,15,16] Our approach is to describe the transitions from background to epileptiform activity in interconnected, heterogeneous tissue at a level that is applicable across the heterogeneous phenomenology of drug-resistant focal seizures.[17,18] This is consistent with the proposal that the generation of epileptic seizures due to abnormally dense microdomains might be a general principle for focal seizures of different aetiologies.[3]

In its abstraction, the model offers a range of advantages. The clear correspondence of the model parameters to dynamical properties allows for a simple model fitting. For example R_{bg} and Θ_e can be fitted to (micro)seizure occurrence rates, and R_{exc} can be fitted to (micro)seizure duration statistics. This can be performed for instance within the period of time that electrodes are implanted prior to neurosurgery. The model results can then inform about an optimal surgical protocol. Moreover, the relation of the model parameters to dynamical properties of neural mass models enables hypothesis formulation based on neural population models, using for example principles derived in Ref. 19. Finally, the ease and speed of computation using these models offers the possibility to run systems up to square-centimetres in size in real time on powerful PCs. The computational efficiency of the current framework will allow a systematic exploration of the relationship between connectivity, node dynamics, and spatial organisation of these in future work.

In summary, the proposed model can give insight into the complex organisation of epileptogenic tissue during the transition to clinical seizures by probing the relationship between the distribution and density of abnormal nodes in realistically connected brain networks. Within this framework we have demonstrated the potential of the model to test hypotheses regarding novel treatment protocols in drug resistant epilepsy.

References

1. C. A. Schevon, S. K. Ng, J. Cappell, R. R. Goodman, G. McKhann, A. Waziri, A. Branner, A. Sosunov, C. E. Schroeder and R. G. Emerson, *J Clin Neurophysiol* **25**, 321 (2008).
2. A. Peters, The morphology of minicolumns, in *The Neurochemical Basis of Autism*, ed. G. J. Blatt (Springer US, 2010) pp. 45–68.
3. M. Stead, M. Bower, B. H. Brinkmann, K. Lee, W. R. Marsh, F. B. Meyer, B. Litt, J. Van Gompel and G. A. Worrell, *Brain* **133**, 2789 (2010).
4. H. Liljenström, *Scholarpedia* **7**, p. 4601 (2012).
5. N. Voges, A. Schuz, A. Aertsen and S. Rotter, *Prog. Neurobiol.* **92**, 277 (2010).
6. C. A. Schevon, R. R. Goodman, G. McKhann and R. G. Emerson, *J Clin Neurophysiol* **27**, 406 (2010).
7. M. Goodfellow, P. N. Taylor, Y. Wang, D. J. Garry and G. Baier, *Eur. J. Neurosci.* **36(2)**, 2178 (2012).
8. M. Kaiser and C. C. Hilgetag, *Front. Neuroinf.* **4** (2010).
9. D. P. Buxhoeveden and M. F. Casanova, *Brain* **125**, 935 (2002).
10. L. J. Levitt, J., *Intrinsic connections in mammalian cerebral cortex. In: Cortical Areas: Unity and Diversity* (Taylor and Francis, 2002).
11. N. Voges and L. U. Perrinet, *Front. Comput. Neurosci.* **6** (2012).
12. A. Bragin, C. L. Wilson and J. Engel, *Epilepsia* **41 Suppl 6**, S144 (2000).
13. E. Faught, *Epilepsy Curr* **2**, p. 108 (2002).
14. E. Ravasz and A.-L. Barabási, *Phys. Rev. E* **67**, p. 026112 (2003).
15. R. D. Traub, R. Duncan, A. J. C. Russell, T. Baldeweg, Y. Tu, M. O. Cunningham and M. A. Whittington, *Epilepsia* **51**, 1587 (2010).
16. O. Benjamin, T. Fitzgerald, P. Ashwin, K. Tsaneva-Atanasova, F. Chowdhury, M. Richardson and J. Terry, *J Math Neurosci* **2** (2012).

17. W. Blume, G. Bryan Young and J. Lemieux, *Electroen. Clin. Neuro.* **57**, 295 (1984).
18. S. S. Spencer, P. Guimaraes, A. Katz, J. Kim and D. Spencer, *Epilepsia* **33**, 537 (1992).
19. Y. Wang, M. Goodfellow, P. N. Taylor and G. Baier, *Phys. Rev. E* **85**, p. 061918 (2012).

PREDICTABILITY OF SEIZURE-LIKE EVENTS IN A COMPLEX NETWORK MODEL OF INTEGRATE-AND-FIRE NEURONS

A. ROTHKEGEL* and K. LEHNERTZ

Department of Epileptology, University of Bonn, Sigmund-Freud-Str. 25, 53105 Bonn, Germany

Helmholtz-Institute for Radiation and Nuclear Physics, University of Bonn, Nussallee 14-16, 53115 Bonn, Germany

Interdisciplinary Center for Complex Systems, University of Bonn, Römerstr. 164, 53117 Bonn, Germany

* E-mail: alexander@rothkegel.de

Prediction of epileptic seizures relies on a consistent relationship between indices of brain activity on the one hand and seizure probabilities on the other hand. We study a qualitative complex network model of integrate-and-fire neurons which generates both asynchronous behavior and short seizure-like events of collective firing. The network model is interpreted as a small seizure-generating zone, which is influenced by various endogenous and exogenous factors, which possibly modulate seizure probability and which are represented by model parameters. For constant parameters the events seem unpredictable, and we find that an increase in seizure probability is accompanied by an increase of fluctuations of the asynchronous behavior, for various considered influencing factors. Using this observation, we find some predictability if the model is endowed with randomly varying model parameters, which could reflect changes in endogenous and exogenous factors that might influence ictogenesis.

Keywords: Complex networks; Neural dynamics; Extreme events; Prediction; Seizure probability

1. Introduction

Research in computational modelling of epilepsy has provided us with several approaches which allow to mimic both physiologic as well as seizure-like activity.[1-3] While some models rely on parameter changes to switch between both kinds of dynamical behaviors, recent approaches allow for self-generated and self-terminated transitions, even for constant parameters. Such self-generated transitions have been related to recurrent escapes from a quasi-stable attractor (representing the interictal brain dynamics) either by noise influences,[4-6] or via some chaotic motion.[7] Prediction of seizure-like events in such models is difficult as even sophisticated models usually have homogeneous attractors which do not allow for a large number of dynamical changes in the modelled interictal brain dynamics.

However, it can be argued that the seizure-generating brain structures in epilepsy patients usually are not subject to constant conditions. One the contrary, they are influenced by various endogenous and exogenous factors, which possibly influence seizure generation and which usually are not captured by models.[8] We assume that these factors can be modeled by varying model parameters. Attempts towards seizure prediction assume that the seizure generation process is non-stationary and mediated or influenced by gradual changes of the interictal brain activity, which are slow compared to the time scale of seizures.[9] By definition, seizure prediction approaches characterize brain activity between seizures (e.g. via time series analysis techniques). From the derived indices, these approaches attempt to estimate the probability that a seizure will occur within a given time interval. We will denote this probability as instantaneous seizure rate. As the brain is influenced by a large amount of endogenous and exogenous factors, it is a priori not clear, whether each factor changes both interictal activity and seizure probabilities in a consistent way. A consistent relationship is necessary, if we have no knowledge about influencing factors and want to estimate seizure probabilities from interictal brain activities.

We here investigate prediction in a qualitative spatial network model of integrate-and-fire neurons which exhibits self-generated events of seizure-like activity that are separated by exponentially distributed periods of asynchronous behavior, even for constant model parameters. We investigate the possibility for prediction using an approach which characterizes fluctuations in the asynchronous behavior prior to events. The modelled network is interpreted as a small seizure-generating zone, which is influenced by various factors. We make the assumption that a change of some influencing factor compares to a change of model parameters. We show that different choices of parameters influence both fluctuations in the asynchronous behavior between events and event rates in a consistent way. This consistent response allows for some predictability of seizure-like events, if we assume time-varying model parameters according to some random process.

2. The Model

The model consists of $N = 50,000$ oscillatory leaky integrate-and-fire neurons. We describe each neuron by a phase variable $\phi \in [0, 1]$ with $\dot{\phi} = 1$. If for some t_f and some neuron n the phase reaches 1 ($\phi_n(t_f) = 1$), it is reset to 0 ($\phi_n(t_f^+) = 0$) and we introduce a phase jump in all neurons n' which are connected to neuron n according to some network:

$$\phi_{n'}(t_f^+) = \phi_{n'}(t_f) + \Delta\left(\phi_{n'}(t_f)\right). \tag{1}$$

Here, $\Delta(\phi)$ denotes the phase response curve, which we define by

$$\Delta(\phi) = \begin{cases} (1-\vartheta)\Delta_c(\frac{\phi-\vartheta+\tau}{1-\vartheta}) & \vartheta - \tau < \phi < 1 - \tau, \\ 0 & \text{otherwise.} \end{cases} \tag{2}$$

where $\Delta_c(\phi)$ is given by

$$\Delta_c(\phi) = \min\left\{ -c\frac{(1-\alpha)}{\ln(\alpha)}\alpha^{-\phi}, 1 - \phi \right\}. \tag{3}$$

The parameters can be interpreted in the following way. c denotes some coupling strength, $\alpha \in [0,1]$ determines the leakage current of neurons, such that non-leaky neurons are obtained for $\alpha \to 1$. ϑ is the refractory period, in which all incoming excitations are ignored. Assuming $\tau < \vartheta$, we can interpret τ as the time delay of interactions. As network, we use a one dimensional ring in which each node is connected to its 50 nearest neighbors (25 to each side). From this configuration, we remove one half of the directed connections and replace them by connections with randomly chosen source and target nodes. In the following we choose the model parameters either as constant or as time-dependent during a single simulation of the model. To assess synchrony in the network in a time-resolved manner, we use the standard order parameter $r(t)$, which takes a value of 1 for complete synchrony and small values for asynchronous firing of neurons:

$$r(t) = 1/N \sum_{n \in N} e^{i\phi_n(t)} \tag{4}$$

A more detailed description of the model is presented elsewhere.[7] All numerical computations were done with the computational framework Conedy.[10] The model –when endowed with constant parameters– is able to produce short events of synchronous firing which may be comparable to seizures and which are separated by asynchronous firing of neurons (see Fig. 1), possibly comparable to the interictal activity of the seizure-generating zone in epileptic brains. We define the beginning t_{ev} and the end of an event as the times at which the order parameter $r(t)$ crosses the arithmetic mean of the largest and the smallest values of $r(t)$ within the observation time, and we measure the distribution of event durations and of inter-event durations

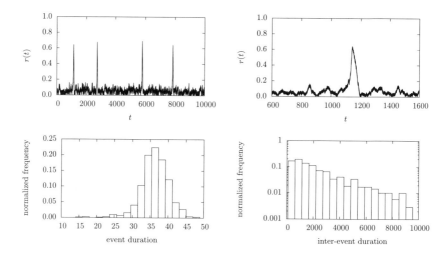

Fig. 1. Top: Rare events of partial synchrony as generated by a spatial network model[7] using constant parameters ($\tau = 0.002, \vartheta = 0.0265, \alpha = 0.85, c = 0.009$). Observation time $T = 500000$. Initial condition: uniformly distributed phases. Top left: The order parameter $r(t)$ indicates short stereotypical events of collective firing, which are separated by asynchronous behavior. Top right: closer view of the first event in the upper left plot. Bottom left: histogram of event durations. Bottom right: histogram of inter-event durations. The measured histogram is consistent with an exponential law.

(see Fig. 1). Events are stereotypical and last for about 35 collective oscillations for the chosen parameters. In contrast, the inter-event durations are highly variable. Our measurement of these durations is consistent with an exponential distribution, which can be considered as the hallmark of a process which is random and does not allow for prediction; with the notion of a Poisson process the exponential distribution can be derived from the assumption that an event occurs at every time with the same probability. In the following we discuss predictability of events for constant model parameters.

3. Constant Parameters

To test the possibility for prediction of the synchronous events, we pursue a simple time series analysis technique which characterizes fluctuations in the asynchronous interval between events by the measure $v(t)$ which is explained in Fig. 2. To investigate predictability of the events of synchronous firing, we analyze the asynchronous behavior in the interval $[t_{ev} - 1500, t_{ev}]$ before each event at time t_{ev}. In the upper part of Fig. 3 we show the time evolution of the mean fluctuation measure $\langle v(t) \rangle$, averaged over a large

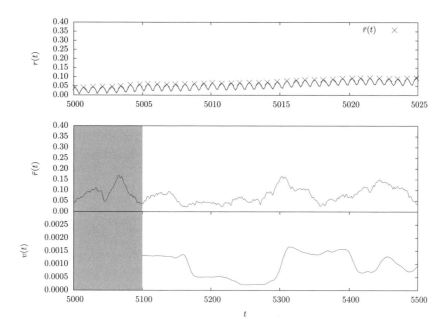

Fig. 2.   Exemplification of a fluctuation-based time series analysis approach. Upper plot: exemplary time evolution of the order parameter $r(t)$ for the asynchronous behavior of the model. $r(t)$ shows small amplitude oscillations related to the oscillator's eigenfrequency. We remove this frequency from the data by generating the series of local maxima $\bar{r}(t)$, plotted as crosses. Lower plots: time evolution of $\bar{r}(t)$ for a longer time period. We perform a moving window analysis with window size $w = 100$, calculating in each window the sample variance v of $\bar{r}(t)$, which we associate with the time point at the right boundary of the window. The window size is indicated as grey box in the plot.

number of pre-event intervals. This evolution confirms our intuition that the events, which are emerging from the chaotic asynchronous state, may indeed be non-predictable, at least for the chosen time scale and using the considered analysis technique.

For given parameters, the model produces synchronous events with a rate, which we will denote as seizure probability λ. In the asynchronous regions, we observe values of v with an expectation value denoted as $\mathbb{E}(v)$. We will now investigate, in which way λ and $\mathbb{E}(v)$ are influenced, if we use other parameters settings. Changed parameter settings are interpreted as changes in endogenous and exogenous factors which influence the seizure-generating zone that is represented by the model. We fix all but one parameter, which we vary between different realizations of the model dynamics. As initial condition, we again chose homogeneously distributed phases. We

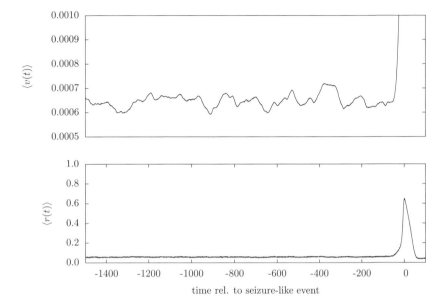

Fig. 3. Top: mean fluctuation measure $\langle v(t) \rangle$ averaged over $N = 207$ pre-event intervals $[t_{\text{ev}} - 1500, t_{\text{ev}}]$ for the spatial neuron network model with constant parameters. Data were rejected if another event occurred within the interval. Bottom: average of the order parameter $r(t)$ for the same data.

discard the initial segment $[0, 1500]$ to let transients die out. We observe $\lambda(t)$ for every parameter setting for an observation time of $T = 500000$. We remove 200 oscillations before and after each seizure-like event to ensure that the remainder is not directly influenced by the dynamics of events and calculate $\mathbb{E}(v)$. The analysis is performed for all neuron parameters $(c, \tau, \vartheta, \alpha)$ (see Fig 4). Note that in this way we only move along the axes in the 4-dimensional parameter space. We did not investigate how λ and $\mathbb{E}(v)$ are influenced if we vary two parameters at once. We observe fluctuations and seizure probabilities to covary although we have no one-to-one correspondence between them; parameter combinations which lead to increased seizure probabilities also lead to increased fluctuations in the asynchronous behavior. In principle, the observed relationship can be used to relate fluctuations to seizure rates and thus to estimate the criticality of the system with the fluctuations in the asynchronous behavior.

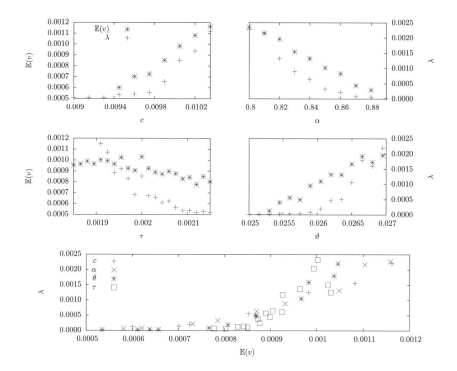

Fig. 4. Seizure rate λ and $\mathbb{E}(v)$ in dependence on model parameters. Top left: dependence on the coupling strength c, top right: dependence on the leakage constant α, middle left: dependence on the time delay τ, middle right: dependence on the refractory period ϑ. Bottom: For the same data as in the upper plots, λ is plotted against $\mathbb{E}(v)$. Parameters when not varied: $\tau = 0.002, \vartheta = 0.0265, c = 0.009, \alpha = 0.9$.

4. Time-dependent Parameters

Finally, we investigate the model with time-dependent parameters. We assume for the temporal evolution of all model parameters $x = (c, \tau, \vartheta, \alpha)$ an Ornstein-Uhlenbeck process with equilibrium x_0, drift θ_x, and diffusion σ_x. The evolution (cf. 5) is described by the following stochastic differential equation:[11]

$$dx(t) = \theta_x(x_0 - x(t))dt + \sigma_x dW. \tag{5}$$

In Fig. 6 we show histograms for event and inter-event durations. The events are stereotypical even for time-dependent parameters, and we observe a similar distribution of their durations as for constant parameters (cf. Fig. 1). However, the statistics of the non-event intervals seems changed; the distribution of these durations shows a tendency to smaller values which

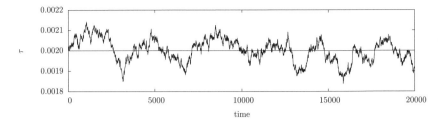

Fig. 5. Exemplary temporal evolution values of the time delay τ as generated by an Ornstein-Uhlenbeck process. The vertical line indicates the equilibrium τ_0.

is not present for constant parameters and deviates from an exponential distribution. We repeated an analysis of fluctuations during pre-event intervals (cf. Fig. 3) to investigate if the model with time-dependent parameters allows for predictability of events. We observe a increase of the fluctuation measure v before events (Fig. 6 bottom).

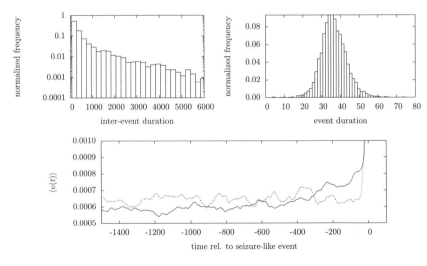

Fig. 6. Top: Statistics of events of partial synchrony in a spatial network model with time-dependent parameters from Ornstein-Uhlenbeck processes ($\theta_\tau = 0.001, \sigma_\tau = 3 \cdot 10^{-6}, \tau_0 = 0.002; \theta_\alpha = 0.001, \sigma_\alpha = 1 \cdot 10^{-6}, \alpha_0 = 0.85; \theta_\vartheta = 0.001, \sigma_\vartheta = 3 \cdot 10^{-6}, \vartheta_0 = 0.002$; cf. 4). Left: histogram of inter-event durations, right: histogram of event durations. Bottom: values of fluctuation measure $\langle v(t) \rangle$ averaged over pre-event intervals for time-dependent parameters (solid line, $N = 275$ pre-event intervals) and, for comparison, for constant model parameters (dashed line, $N = 207$ pre-event intervals).

5. Conclusions

We investigated predictability of seizure-like events in a complex network model of integrate-and-fire oscillators, which mimics both seizure-like and inter-ictal activity. When we endow the model with time-varying parameters, some prediction seems possible with an approach which characterizes fluctuations in the inter-ictal activity. The prediction relies on a consistent response of the model, such that we observe seizure rates and fluctuations to covary. In contrast, we find no indication for predictability in the model for constant parameters. Increased fluctuations near critical parameter values have been described for observables of a variety of structurally different systems in which multiple time scales are involved in the dynamics.[12,13] It is plausible, that the epileptic brain can be regarded as such a system as durations of ictal and inter-ictal states usually differ by several orders of magnitude. Therefore, it is conceivable that our findings are transferable to other computational models for ictogenesis. We claim that computational models with constant parameters may be an overly pessimistic setting to test predictability of seizure-like events, as the model dynamics is usually overly homogeneous compared to the highly non-stationary dynamics that we can observe in human brains.

References

1. F. Wendling, *J. Clin. Neurophysiol.* **22**, 285 (2005).
2. I. Soltesz and K. Staley, *Computational neuroscience in epilepsy* (Academic Press, London, UK, 2008).
3. W. W. Lytton, *Nat. Rev. Neurosci.* **9**, 626 (2008).
4. O. Benjamin, T. H. Fitzgerald, P. Ashwin, K. Tsaneva-Atanasova, F. Chowdhury, M. P. Richardson and J. R. Terry, *J. Math. Neurosci.* **2**, 1 (2012).
5. G. Baier, M. Goodfellow, P. N. Taylor, Y. Wang and D. J. Garry, *Front. Physiol.* **3**, 281 (2012).
6. W. S. Anderson, F. Azhar, P. Kudela, G. K. Bergey and P. J. Franaszczuk, *Epilepsy Res.* **99**, 202 (2012).
7. A. Rothkegel and K. Lehnertz, *Europhys. Lett.* **95**, 38001 (2011).
8. W. G. Lennox, *Science and Seizures* (Harper, New York, London, 1946).
9. F. Mormann, R. Andrzejak, C. E. Elger and K. Lehnertz, *Brain* **130**, 314 (2007).
10. A. Rothkegel and K. Lehnertz, *Chaos* **22**, 013125 (2012).
11. P. E. Kloeden and E. Platen, *Numerical Solution of Stochastic Differential Equations* (Springer, Berlin, 1999).
12. M. Scheffer, J. Bascompte, W. A. Brock, V. Brovkin, S. R. Carpenter, V. Dakos, H. Held, E. H. van Nes, M. Rietkerk and G. Sugihara, *Nature* **461**, 53 (2009).
13. C. Kuehn, *Physica D: Nonlinear Phenomena* **240**, 1020 (2011).

BURSTING AND SYNCHRONY IN NETWORKS OF MODEL NEURONS

C. GEIER[1,2,*], A. ROTHKEGEL[1,2,3], K. LEHNERTZ[1,2,3]

[1]*Department of Epileptology, University of Bonn,*
Sigmund-Freud-Straße 25, 53105 Bonn, Germany
[2]*Helmholtz-Institute for Radiation and Nuclear Physics, University of Bonn,*
Nussallee 14–16, 53115 Bonn, Germany
[3]*Interdisciplinary Center for Complex Systems, University of Bonn,*
Brühler Straße 7, 53175 Bonn, Germany
[*]*E-mail: geier@uni-bonn.de*

Bursting neurons are considered to be a potential cause of over-excitability and seizure susceptibility. The functional influence of these neurons in extended epileptic networks is still poorly understood. There is mounting evidence that the dynamics of neuronal networks is influenced not only by neuronal and synaptic properties but also by network topology. We investigate numerically the influence of different neuron dynamics on global synchrony in neuronal networks with complex connection topologies.

Keywords: Bursting, Epilepsy, Synchronization, Network, Small-World

1. Introduction

Epilepsy is a disorder of the brain characterized by an enduring predisposition to generate epileptic seizures and by the neurobiologic, cognitive, psychological, and social consequences of this condition.[1] Approximately 1% of the world's population suffers from epilepsy. An epileptic seizure is defined as a transient occurrence of signs and/or symptoms due to abnormal excessive or synchronous neuronal activity in the brain.[1,2] In about 25% of individuals with epilepsy, seizures cannot be controlled by any available therapy. During the last decades a variety of potential seizure-generating (ictogenic) mechanisms have been identified, including synaptic, cellular, and structural plasticity as well as changes in the extracellular milieu. Although there is a considerable bulk of literature on this topic (see Ref. 3 for a comprehensive overview) the exact mechanisms are not yet fully explored. On the cellular level, bursting neurons are considered to be a potential cause of over-excitability and seizure susceptibility. In regular-firing neurons, a brief depolarization causes the generation of a single action potential, whereas a prolonged depolarization induces a series of independent action potentials. In bursting neurons, threshold depolarization triggers a high-frequency, all-or-none burst of action potentials.[4,5] Although a high abundance (up to 90%) of bursting neurons can be observed in epileptic tissue[6] the functional impact of these neurons in extended epileptic networks is still poorly understood.

Over the past few years, substantial progress has been made in modeling epileptic phenomena at different scales (see Refs. 7 and 8 for an overview). Large-scale network models take into account intrinsic properties of neurons and the complex, nonrandom connectivity of cortex.[9–15] Findings obtained with these models stress the importance of both cellular and network mechanisms in the generation of seizure-like dynamics, which suggests that a single ictogenic mechanism alone may not be responsible for seizure generation.

We here investigate numerically the influence of different neuron dynamics (regular spiking, chattering, bursting) on global synchrony in neuronal networks with connection topologies of lattice, small-world, and random type.

Table 1. Model parameter settings for different neuron dynamics.

neuron dynamics	a	b	c	d
spiking	0.02	0.2	−65	8
bursting	0.02	0.2	−55	4
chattering	0.02	0.2	−50	2

2. Methods

We study networks of Izhikevich model neurons n which are described by the following two-dimensional map:[16]

$$v_n(t+1) = 0.04v_n(t)^2 + 5v_n(t) + 140 - u_n(t) + I(t)$$
$$u_n(t+1) = a_n(b_n v_n(t) - u_n(t)). \qquad (1)$$

Here v_n is considered as membrane potential and $I(t)$ specifies the total input current which is composed of three currents:

$$I(t) = I_{\text{const}} + I_{\text{noise}}(t) + I_{\text{c}}(t).$$

110

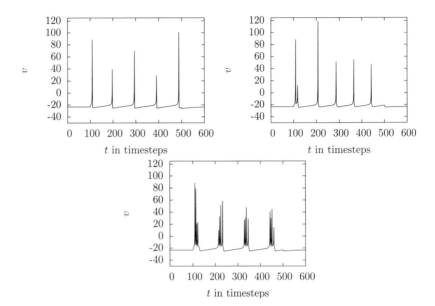

Fig. 1. Temporal evolution of the membrane potential v of different model neurons. Top-left: regular spiking neuron; top-right: bursting neuron; bottom: chattering neuron.

$I_{\text{const}} = 4$ is a constant current which is injected into all neurons. $I_{\text{c}}(t) := \epsilon \cdot (\# \text{ presynaptic neurons firing at } t - 1)$ represents the synaptic coupling, and the noisy current $I_{\text{noise}}(t)$ is used to generate asynchronous states as initial conditions.

Whenever $v_n(t)$ reaches a threshold (here 30), neuron n fires and its dynamical variables are updated in the following way:

$$\text{if } v_n(t) \geq 30 \text{ , then } \begin{cases} v_n(t) := c_n \\ u_n(t) := u_n(t) + d_n \end{cases}$$

Depending on parameters a_n, b_n, c_n, and d_n, the neuron model mimics the behavior of regular spiking, bursting, or chattering neurons (cf. Table 1 and Figure 1).

We studied networks of 10.000 model neurons (we note that we obtained similar findings for networks of 4.000, 20.000 and 50.000 neurons). We considered a one-dimensional lattice on which every neuron is connected to its k nearest neighbors (here $k = 20$) using a cyclic boundary condition. Starting from this configuration, every directed connection was removed with probability $\rho \in [0, 1]$ and a connection between two randomly chosen, previously unconnected neurons was introduced.

Besides networks consisting of only a single neuron type, we built inhomogeneous networks consisting of spiking and bursting neurons and of spiking and chattering neurons and investigated the network dynamics in dependence on the fraction of different neuron types.

As initial condition we chose asynchronous states, which were generated in the following way: To every neuron we assigned a binary noise input, which takes a value of I_{noise} with a probability of 0.1 and 0 otherwise. We began with $I_{noise} = 40$ and repeatedly decreased I_{noise} by 1 after 200 timesteps until $I_{noise} = 0$. Then we let these networks evolve for 10.000 time steps to ensure that transients died out. We then measured the fraction of firing neurons $f(t)$ for 2.000 time steps. During this time frame $f(t)$ typically exhibited regular oscillations (alternating periods of high and low values of $f(t)$). To assess synchrony in the network, we used the number of concurrently firing neurons at the periods of high values. This number can be estimated (due to the regularity) by the maximum value of $f(t)$ within the observation time $F = \max\{f(t)|0 < t < 2.000\}$.

We investigated synchrony F depending on the rewiring probability ρ and on the coupling strength ϵ for both homogeneous and inhomogeneous networks.

3. Results

3.1. *Homogeneous Networks*

In Figure 2 we show the dependence of synchrony F in homogeneous networks on the rewiring probability ρ for a fixed coupling strength ϵ. For spiking neuron networks, F slightly increased for $\rho < 0.6$ and then reached a plateau. For the other neuron networks, F attained similar values for all investigated rewiring probabilities, except for $\rho < 0.1$.

In Figure 3 we show the dependence of network synchrony F on the coupling strength ϵ for a fixed rewiring probability ρ. For networks of chattering neurons, F increased monotonously with increasing ϵ. For small coupling strength ($\epsilon \leq 0.3$), F attained similar values for networks of bursting and chattering neurons. However, for $\epsilon \geq 0.3$, F dropped for networks of bursting neurons even below the levels observed for networks of spiking neurons. For larger values of ϵ ($\epsilon \leq 1.5$) F increased again and approached the values for networks of chattering neurons.

For networks consisting of spiking neurons, we observed F to increase with increasing ϵ similarly as observed for chattering neuron networks. At

112

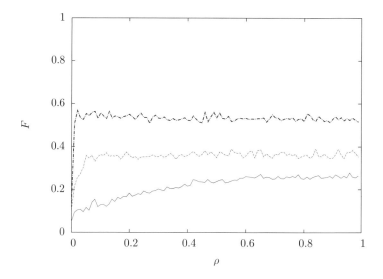

Fig. 2. Synchrony F in dependence on the rewiring probability ρ; fixed coupling strength $\epsilon = 3.0$. Solid line: spiking neuron network; darker dashed line: bursting neuron network; lighter dashed line: chattering neuron network.

$\epsilon \approx 1.7$ synchrony of spiking neuron networks decreased since these neurons sometimes showed bursting behavior due to the large input currents generated by firing neurons. For even larger values of ϵ synchrony F increased again.

3.2. Inhomogeneous Networks

In inhomogeneous networks we observed synchrony F to increase with an increasing rewiring probability ρ until $\rho \approx 0.2$ and then to approximately stay constant, irrespective of the coupling strength ϵ (see Figure 4). Similarly as observed for homogeneous networks, synchrony F attained larger values for larger coupling strength ϵ. We also observed for $\rho > 0$ higher values of F for networks containing chattering neurons than for networks containing bursting neurons, which is analogous to our finding for homogeneous networks.

For a fixed rewiring probability $\rho = 0.3$ and large coupling strength ($\epsilon = 4$) we observed an approximately linear relationship between synchrony F and the fraction of bursting or chattering neurons in a network (see Figure 5 bottom). For a small coupling strength $\epsilon = 1$, we observed synchrony F

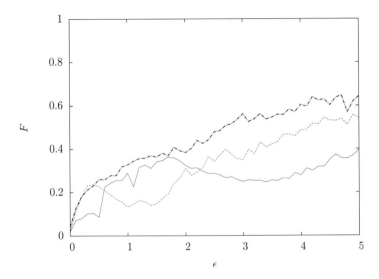

Fig. 3. Synchrony F in dependence on the coupling strength ϵ; fixed rewiring probability $\rho = 0.3$. Solid line: spiking neuron network; darker dashed line: bursting neuron network; lighter dashed line: chattering neuron network.

first to decrease with the fraction of bursting or chattering neurons and than to increase again(see Figure 5 top).

For the spiking-chattering neuron network F decreased until it reached a minimum at around 40% chattering neurons and then increased to larger values of F than for homogeneous spiking neuron networks. This was, however, not the case for spiking-bursting neuron networks. Here synchrony F decreased with the fraction of bursting neurons until it reached a minimum at about 5% bursting neurons and then increased but remained smaller than for homogeneous spiking neuron networks. This is in agreement with our findings for homogeneous networks as synchrony was larger for spiking neuron than for bursting neuron networks for coupling strength $\epsilon \in [0.75, 2.0]$.

4. Conclusion

We studied complex neuron networks with homogeneous and inhomogeneous local dynamics. We observed that chattering neuron networks exhibited higher levels of synchrony than bursting neuron networks which in turn exhibited higher levels of synchrony than spiking neuron networks. In addition, synchrony was higher for small-world and random network configurations than for lattice-like structures. In inhomogeneous networks, composed

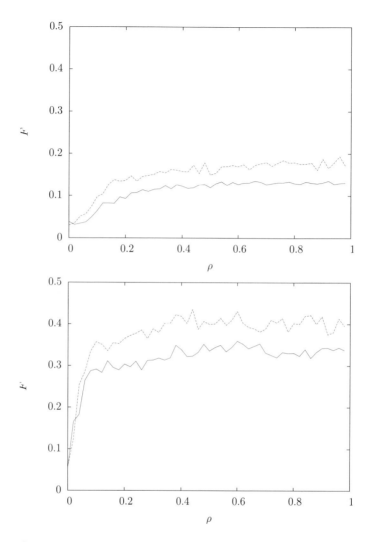

Fig. 4.   Synchrony F in dependence on the rewiring probability ρ for networks consisting of 70% spiking and 30% of bursting/chattering neurons. Solid line: spiking/bursting neuron network; dashed line: spiking/chattering neuron network. Top: $\epsilon = 1$; bottom: $\epsilon = 4$.

of both spiking and bursting neurons, we observed that synchrony may be decreased due to the influence of the bursting neurons. These observations

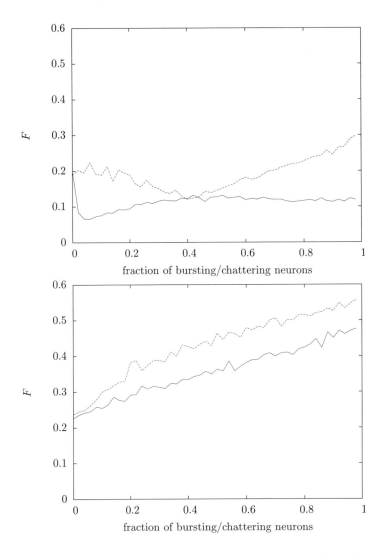

Fig. 5. Synchrony F for inhomogeneous networks with $\rho = 0.3$ in dependence on the fraction of spiking and bursting/chattering neurons. Solid line: spiking-bursting neuron network; dashed line: spiking-chattering neuron network. Top: $\epsilon = 1$; bottom: $\epsilon = 4$.

support the notion, that under certain conditions inhomogeneity, such as in the degree (connectivity) distribution,[17] in the coupling architecture,[11,18] or – as shown here – with different node dynamics, hinders synchrony.

References

1. R. S. Fisher, W. van Emde Boas, W. Blume, C. E. Elger, P. Genton, P. Lee and J. Engel Jr, *Epilepsia* **46**, 470 (2005).
2. J. Engel Jr, *Epilepsia* **47**, 1558 (2006).
3. J. J. Engel and T. A. Pedley, *Epilepsy: A Comprehensive Textbook*, 2nd edn. (Lippincott, Williams & Wilkins, Philadelphia, 2007).
4. J. E. Lisman, *Trends Neurosci.* **20**, 38 (1997).
5. H. Beck and Y. Yaari, *Nat. Rev. Neurosci.* **9**, 357 (2008).
6. Y. Yaari and H. Beck, *Brain Pathol.* **12**, 234 (2002).
7. W. W. Lytton, *Nat. Rev. Neurosci.* **9**, 626 (2008).
8. I. Soltesz and K. Staley, *Computational neuroscience in epilepsy* (Academic Press, London, UK, 2008).
9. T. I. Netoff, R. Clewley, S. Arno, T. Keck and J. A. White, *J. Neurosci.* **24**, 8075 (2004).
10. B. Percha, R. Dzakpasu, M. Zochowski and J. Parent, *Phys. Rev. E* **72**, 031909 (2005).
11. J. Dyhrfjeld-Johnsen, V. Santhakumar, R. J. Morgan, R. Huerta, L. Tsimring and I. Soltesz, *J. Neurophysiol.* **97**, 1566 (2007).
12. S. Feldt, H. Osterhage, F. Mormann, K. Lehnertz and M. Zochowski, *Phys. Rev. E* **76**, 021920 (2007).
13. R. J. Morgan and I. Soltesz, *Proc. Natl. Acad. Sci. U.S.A.* **105**, 6179 (2008).
14. A. Bogaard, J. Parent, M. Zochowski and V. Booth, *J. Neurosci.* **29**, 1677 (2009).
15. A. Rothkegel and K. Lehnertz, *Europhys. Lett.* **95**, 38001 (2011).
16. E. M. Izhikevich, *IEEE Trans. Neural Netw.* **14**, 1569 (2003).
17. A. E. Motter, C. Zhou and J. Kurths, *Phys. Rev. E* **71**, 016116 (2005).
18. M. Denker, M. Timme, M. Diesmann, F. Wolf and T. Geisel, *Phys. Rev. Lett.* **92**, 074103 (2004).

Advances in Analysis and
Measurement Techniques

SIGNAL PROCESSING OF THE EEG: APPROACHES TAILORED TO EPILEPSY

B. SCHELTER* and M. THIEL

*Institute for Complex Systems and Mathematical Biology (ICSMB),
University of Aberdeen,
Aberdeen, AB24 3UE, UK
* E-mail: b.schelter@abdn.ac.uk, m.thiel@abdn.ac.uk
http://www.fdm.uni-freiburg.de/team/schelter*

M. MADER and W. MADER

*Freiburg Center for Data Analysis and Modeling, University of Freiburg,
Eckerstrasse 1, Freiburg, 79104, Germany
E-mail: malenka.mader@fdm.uni-freiburg.de, wolfgang.mader@fdm.uni-freiburg.de*

By now seizure prediction in epilepsy has a history of more than two decades. Several alternative approaches have been suggested to predict epileptic seizures. These approaches are mainly based on signal processing of electroencephalograms. In this chapter, the basic principles of signal processing geared to seizure prediction in the framework of epilepsy will be summarised and discussed.

Keywords: Epilepsy, spectral analysis, data analysis, statistical evaluation, network reconstruction

1. Introduction

Analysing measurements, we face two different challenges. If one has formed an hypothesis about the underlying model the challenge is to characterise the data that can be produced by it. Although this challenge is already hard to address, the second situation can be considered to be even more challenging. It is to use data to generate, to characterise, and to validate a model that describes the measured data. In general, if nothing else can be assumed, the underlying model could be either deterministic or stochastic, it could be linear or non-linear. The class of non-linear stochastic models is realised by nature most frequently. Electroencephalography (EEG) measurements, in particular, are prototypical for this class.

Even in cases, in which the underlying model is known, it is typically not sufficient to generate data from this model. This is because in actual applications, one typically observes the underlying process not directly but rather transformed by a possibly unknown observation function and contaminated by observational noise. Moreover, measurements are time discrete. However, it should be emphasised here, that the time discrete nature of measurement itself is not in general a justification to model the dynamics time discretely. Using time discrete models for time continuous dynamics leads to erroneous conclusions.[1]

In epilepsy research and in particular in seizure prediction the aim is to reliably predict epileptic seizures. A good performance, i.e. a high sensitivity and specificity, could warrant a widespread application of a given seizure prediction algorithm; the discussion about the suitability of the model or the characteristics of the data would be less important.

In this Chapter, we focus on general principles and concepts that should be considered when analysing EEG data rather than elaborating on the appropriateness or inappropriateness of models for seizure prediction. We refer the interested reader to recent reviews and books,[2] and the other chapters in this book, for such discussions.

2. Referencing

EEG signals cannot be recorded without referencing the recording electrodes to a given electrode. A suitable choice for this reference electrode is subject to many discussions. Often the text book recommendation is to use a quiet reference, which is typically not trivial. This is because the reference electrode should (i) be close to the recording site, (ii) capture the same global unknown unwanted activity, (iii) not be the electrode of central interest, and (iv) an artefact free recording site. Several strategies for the selection of the reference electrode are conceivable.

When scalp and intracranial EEG recordings are measured simultaneously, the selection strategy of an appropriate reference electrode is even more challenging. A good choice for the intracranial electrodes does not necessarily require to be a good choice for the scalp electrodes. To overcome the problem of choosing a proper reference electrode, bipolar referencing presents an alternative. In bipolar referencing, the reference electrode is typically one that is close to the recording electrode. Due to the close spatial proximity the recording and the reference electrode should capture more or less the same artefacts. Thus, in this montage, artefacts are typically found less prominently in the signals as for the single electrode referencing approach. The bipolar montage suffers from the complication that also signal contents of interest could be picked up by both electrodes and therefore be removed. Moreover, neuronal activity can be modeled by electrical dipoles. Only neurons with a specific orientation can be recorded by the bipolar montage. This again hampers the interpretability of the results.

To overcome these limitations and to get closer to the single referencing electrode strategy, it has been suggested to use the average activity of all electrodes as a reference for the EEG activity. Artefacts that show up in the majority of electrodes and artefacts that are strong in some of the electrodes will be corrected for by this approach. The probability to accidentally remove some of the interesting information is considerably reduced using this procedure. But, when it comes to analysing measurements that are referenced to the common activity of all channels, one has to face a considerable predicament. Approaches that focus on the interaction between channels cannot be sensibly applied. The common average will induce a correlation of all channels to each other. Any strategy that has been suggested to infer the interaction between channels will likely reveal that all channels are highly connected. To overcome this problem, often a referencing approach, called the Laplacian, is used. The underlying idea being that the activity of interests in EEG recordings is the current source density. This is linked to the measured EEG activity by a second order spatial derivative, the Laplacian.[3-6] As it is typically very difficult to calculate the Laplacian exactly, a numerically efficient approximation is used.[7] This numerical approximation is based on the idea of local averaging. 1, The strategy to obtain the

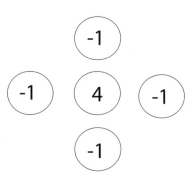

Fig. 1.   Weights of local averaging for the numerical approximation of the Laplacian.

weights for averaging to derive the Laplacian is shown in Fig. in which the weights for averaging in order to derive the Laplacian, are shown. The central electrode is weighted four-times positively, while the surrounding four electrodes are weighted with -1, each. As the Laplacian realises a very local averaging strategy, it allows further analyses, that include interaction measures. Additionally, as it characterises the current source density, it provides a physically interpretable result.

3. Spectral Analysis

Analysing the spectral properties of a given signal is one of the first steps in signal analysis. The spectral information allows for an efficient characterisation of several features of the measured signals.

Although strictly speaking a linear analysis, spectral analysis allows us to investigate (a) rhythms, (b) nonstationaries, (c) certain artefacts such as line noise, and (d), noise contents in the signals.[8,9]

Spectral analysis also provides information about filters that have been applied to the recorded signals. Some of which are indeed necessary to obtain sensible signals that can be analysed. A high pass filter typically is applied to avoid drifts in the signal. A low pass filter at half the sampling frequency, the so-called Nyquist frequency, is applied to avoid aliasing. These two filters are hardware filters that have to be applied before digitalising the signals.

Other filters are only applied because humans cannot easily remove specific spectral features when visually inspecting the data. Prototypical examples for such filters are line noise filters, which are e.g. at 50 Hz in Europe and at 60 Hz in the USA. While the 50 Hz noise causes the peak in the spectrum, see Fig. 2 (a), the filtered signal is characterised by a dip at this very same frequency, see Fig. 2 (b); so this only "inverts" the problem.

Typically, time series analysis algorithms are influenced negatively by either peaks or dips in the spectrum. There are some techniques, such as those depending on autoregressive models, that can easily cope with peaks but not with dips.[9] Prior to any analysis, one should check, which analysis technique is to be applied, and accordingly decide about possible preprocessing and filtering steps.

Similarly, naïve down sampling of data can also change the spectral characteristics of the underlying signal considerably. In Fig. 3, the effect of naïve down sampling is shown. The 50 Hz peak clearly visible in Fig. 3 (a) introduces a spurious peak in Fig. 3 (b) at a frequency of around 15 to 20 Hz. Prior to any down sampling the data needs to be filtered at half

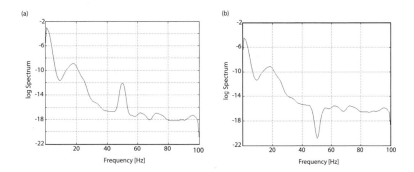

Fig. 2. Spectrum (in arbitrary units) of a signal is governed by a peak at 50 Hz coming from the line noise (a). After application of line noise filters, a dip occurs at the same frequency as the peak before (b).

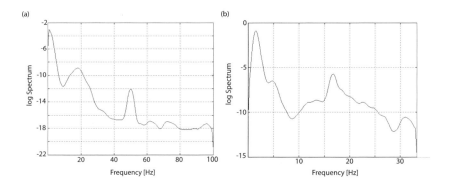

Fig. 3. Naive downsampling can change the original spectrum (in arbitrary units) (a) at various frequencies (b).

the desired sampling frequency. This filtering should be performed in the frequency domain to avoid introducing unwanted time delays.[1]

4. Data Analysis

Several approaches are conceivable to analyse the recorded, and potentially preprocessed, data sets. Related to the spectral analysis shown in the previous section there is an analysis method called coherence. Coherence is the frequency domain counterpart of the cross-correlation; it quantifies the interaction between two processes in the frequency domain. The advantage of analysing coherence rather than correlation lies in the superior statistics of coherence. As seen in Fig. 4, coherence reveals interactions at a particu-

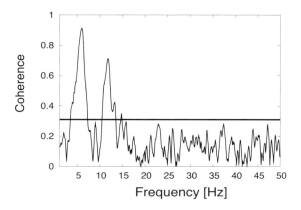

Fig. 4. Coherence as a measure of linear interaction in the frequency domain between two processes. The horizontal line is the significance level which can be derived analytically.

lar frequency. It is normalised to $[0, 1]$ showing higher values for stronger linear interactions. The horizontal line in Fig. 4 shows the critical value for the absence of a linear interaction for the level of significance of 5%. In particular for EEG signals which are typically interpreted in the frequency domain at particular frequency ranges or bands, coherence is an optimal choice to estimate the linear interaction between two signals.

Coherence analysis is a purely linear approach. Non-linear extensions and approaches such as synchronisation[10] are also conceivable. Most non-linear approaches are hampered by the fact that they require exquisite measurements to be estimated reliably. The amount to which non-linear approaches typically outperform linear approaches does often not warrant their application in several circumstances. Arguing that the EEG can be modelled using a non-linear stochastic dynamics does not imply that linear approaches cannot be applied to investigate certain characteristics of the signal.

Synchronisation-based approaches first estimate the phase content of a given signal. Various approaches are suggested to estimate the phase of a given signal. The Hilbert transform of a real valued signal $x(t)$

$$\mathcal{H}\{x\}(t) = \frac{1}{\pi} P.V. \int \frac{x(\tau)}{t - \tau} \, \mathrm{d}\tau \qquad (1)$$

with P.V. Cauchy's principal value is one of the most frequently applied transformations to this end. Defining the analytic signal

$$x(t) + i\mathcal{H}\{x\}(t) = A(t)e^{i\Phi(t)} \qquad (2)$$

it provides both the phase Φ as well as the envelope $A(t)$ of the signal. In the presence of phase synchronisation two phases are linked by some functional relationship to one another. This allows characterising the bivariate interaction. Thus, phase synchronisation analysis is similar to coherence analysis in this respect. We mention here that there are also discussions related to the definition of phase synchronisation and the analytic signal.[11–13]

The drawback of bivariate approaches, such as coherence and synchronisation, lies in the fact that it is basically impossible to infer the network structure based on these approaches. This is true as both approaches cannot distinguish direct from indirect interactions. Multivariate counterparts of both do exist in the literature.[14,15]

Even if it was possible to distinguish direct and indirect interactions, one still needs to be able to infer the direction of information flow. Granger in 1969[16] suggested a mathematical framework based on the idea of predictability to introduce his concept of causality. Granger causality is based on the common sense conception that causes need to precede their effects in time. He mathematically formulated this based on the predictability in the framework of autoregressive models.[14–17]

5. Network Analysis

Networks are often used to characterise complex systems such as the brain. In particular in the framework of epilepsy analysis, growing interest has been on the investigation of the brain as a network. Therefore network analysis is necessary, see the chapter in this book "From time series to complex networks: an overview" by Bialonski and Lehnertz.

Renormalized partial directed coherence is a method that has proven to be powerful in the reconstruction of networks and has a huge potential for EEG analysis. Therefore we will review this method briefly.[14,15]

Network reconstruction based on the renormalised partial directed coherence (rPDC) of an n-dimensional system consists of autoregressive modelling. That is, coefficients of an n-dimensional vector autoregressive process of order p (VAR[p])

$$\vec{x}(t) = \sum_{r=1}^{p} \mathbf{a}_r \vec{x}(t-r) + \vec{\varepsilon}_x(t), \quad \vec{\varepsilon}_x(t) \sim \mathcal{N}(\vec{0}|\mathbf{\Sigma}), \qquad (3)$$

where $\vec{\varepsilon}_x$ denotes independent Gaussian noise with zero-mean and covariance matrix Σ, need to be fitted. Parameter matrices $\mathbf{a}_r$ contain the parameters of the VAR[p]. Each component of such a vector autoregressive process can be interpreted physically as a combination of stochastically driven relaxators and damped oscillators.[18]

The renormalised partial directed coherence is the squared absolute value of the estimator of the Fourier transform of the parameter matrices $\mathbf{a}_r$ normalised by a multiple of its covariance. This is mathematically described by

$$\lambda_{i\leftarrow j}(\omega) = \mathbf{X}_{ij}(\omega)' \left(\mathbf{V}_{ij}(\omega)\right)^{-1} \mathbf{X}_{ij}(\omega) \in [0, \infty) \qquad (4)$$

with

$$\mathbf{X}_{ij}(\omega) = \begin{pmatrix} \mathrm{Re}(\bar{\mathbf{A}}_{ij}(\omega)) \\ \mathrm{Im}(\bar{\mathbf{A}}_{ij}(\omega)) \end{pmatrix}, \ \mathbf{X}_{ij}(\omega)'\mathbf{X}_{ij}(\omega) = |\bar{\mathbf{A}}_{ij}(\omega)|^2 = \mathbf{I}_n - \mathbf{A}^*(\omega), (5)$$

where $(\cdot)'$ denotes matrix transposition and $\mathbf{A}^*$ the Fourier transform of the parameter matrices, and

$$\frac{\mathbf{V}_{ij}(\omega)}{N} = \frac{\Sigma_{ii}}{N} \sum_{l,m=1}^{p} \mathbf{R}_{jj}^{-1}(l,m) \begin{pmatrix} \cos(l\omega)\cos(m\omega) & \cos(l\omega)\sin(m\omega) \\ \sin(l\omega)\cos(m\omega) & \sin(l\omega)\sin(m\omega) \end{pmatrix} \quad (6)$$

with $\mathbf{R}$ the covariance matrix of the VAR process.[19]

If $\lambda_{i\leftarrow j}(\omega) = 0$, a Granger-causal, linear influence from x_j to x_i can be excluded at the frequency ω, when considering all processes. We have shown that the α-significance level for zero-Granger-causal linear influence, $\lambda_{i\leftarrow j}(\omega) = 0$, is given by $\chi^2_{2,1-\alpha}/N$.[14] High values of rPDC correspond to strong connections.

If interaction between processes varies with time, the time-resolved estimation of parameters is essential.

Blockwise Estimation

As a first approach, the data can be cut into blocks and the parameters can be estimated blockwise. One drawback of this approach is that the result highly depends on the relation of chosen blocksize and time scale on which the parameters vary. The appropriate blocksize is therefore difficult to determine based on data analysis.

State Space Model and Kalman Filter Based Estimation

To overcome the problem of choosing a fixed blocksize in order to get time-resolved interaction measures, a non-stationary model can be used in the first place. To this end, the non-stationary state space model is a good choice. Parameter estimation in this model can be based on the Kalman filter.[20]

We first introduce the stationary state space model (SSM)

$$\vec{y}(t) = \mathbf{B}\vec{y}(t-1) + \vec{\epsilon}_y(t) \tag{7}$$

$$\vec{z}(t) = \mathbf{C}\vec{y}(t) + \vec{\epsilon}_z(t), \tag{8}$$

which consists of a linear dynamics equation, Eq. (7), and a linear observation equation, Eq. (8). The hidden process $\vec{y}(t)$ is an vector autoregressive process. It is observed according to Eq. (8) by the observation matrix $\mathbf{C}$ and independent Gaussian observational noise $\vec{\epsilon}_z(t)$ with mean $\vec{0}$ and covariance $\mathbf{\Gamma}$.

A vector autoregressive process of order p (VAR[p]) and dimension n, Eq. (3), can be rewritten as a process of first order by augmenting its dimensions to n^2p such that it meets the conditions of dynamics equation of the state space model.[15] To include nonstationary dynamics the parameter matrix $A(t)$ rewritten into a vector, is modelled in the dynamics equation

$$\mathbf{A}(t) = \mathbf{A}(t-1) + \epsilon_A(t) \tag{9}$$

with the process matrix $\mathbf{B}$ as the identity matrix. The parameters are influenced by Gaussian white noise $\epsilon_A(t)$ with zero-mean and covariance $\mathbf{Q}_A$. For the implementation, the matrix $\mathbf{A}(t)$ is rewritten as a vector of size $(n^2p \cdot n^2p)$.

The nonstationary process $\vec{u}(t) = \mathbf{A}(t)\vec{u}(t-1) + \vec{\epsilon}_u(t)$ is modelled in the observation equation, Eq. (8), as a function of the previous observation $\vec{u}(t-1)$ and the process parameters

$$\vec{u}(t) = \mathbf{C}\mathbf{A}(t) + \epsilon_u(t). \tag{10}$$

The observation matrix has to be replaced by $\mathbf{C} = \mathbf{A}(t)\vec{u}(t-1)$ such that the vector of parameters $\mathbf{A}(t)$, which corresponds to the parameter matrix map $\vec{u}(t-1)$ onto $\vec{u}(t)$ except for the noise term $\vec{\epsilon}_u(t)$.

In order to estimate the parameters of the nonstationary SSM Eqs. (9) and (10), the Kalman filter has been proposed.[21] The Kalman filter then uses two steps in the estimation procedure. In a first step, the process at time t is predicted from the past $t' = \{1, \ldots, t-1\}$ steps, and a second step, in which the prediction is corrected according to the observation $\vec{u}(t)$. The Kalman filter estimates the most likely trajectory given the observations.[15]

In order to obtain the optimal parameters of the State Space Model the Expectation-Maximization algorithm can be used.[22]

128

Example

In order to demonstrate that the State Space Model (SSM) and Kalman-Filter based estimation is more superior to the blockwise approach, we simulated 5 000 data points of a 2-dimensional VAR[2]-process

$$\vec{x}(t) = (x_1(t), x_2(t))' = \sum_{r=1}^{2} \mathbf{a}_r \vec{x}(t - r) + \varepsilon_x(t)$$

with parameters $\mathbf{a}_1 = \begin{pmatrix} 1.3 & c \\ 0 & 1.7 \end{pmatrix}$, $\mathbf{a}_2 = \begin{pmatrix} -0.8 & 0 \\ 0 & -0.8 \end{pmatrix}$ and sinosoidally varying causal strength

$$c(t) = \sin(25 \cdot t/N), \tag{11}$$

of an influence from x_2 onto x_1. Process x_1 oscillates at $\omega_1 = 0.12$ Hz, x_2 at $\omega_2 = 0.05$ Hz.

In Fig. 5 the renormalised partial directed coherence at the main fre-

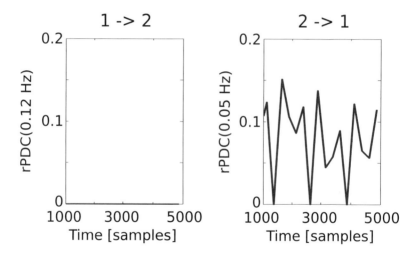

Fig. 5. Blockwise estimated rPDC for two AR[2] processes with oscillating coupling from x_2 onto x_1. Values reflect the absent (left) and present (right) interaction at the respective main frequency of the influencing process.

quency of the driving process is shown based on a blockwise estimation for an order of $p = 10$ on 20 non-overlapping segments . The rPDC is capable of quantifying the strength of interaction within each block, but it fails to reveal the sinusoidal structure of the coupling strength.

However, the temporal evolution of the sinusoidal coupling is detected when employing the state space model (SSM) combined with the Kalman filter for estimating the process parameters (Fig. 6, right) at the respective main frequencies, 0.05 Hz and 0.12 Hz, of the influencing processes x_1 (left) and x_2 (right), respectively.

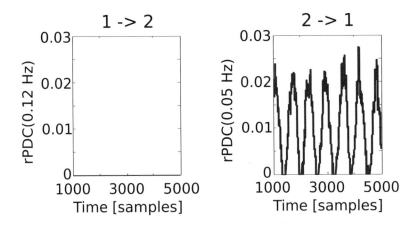

Fig. 6. rPDC estimated employing SSM and Kalman filtering, evaluated at the main frequency of the influencing process. Even the dynamics of the absent (left) and present (right) interaction is revealed.

At the same time, the absent interaction from x_1 onto x_2 is found to be nonsignificant (left).

6. Summary

In this Chapter, we haven given a short overview over existing methods and preprocessing steps to process EEG data in the framework of seizure prediction in epilepsy. It should be noted again, that in epilepsy, in particular when it comes to seizure prediction, the underlying model and data analysis approach might eventually be less important. If seizures can by any means be predicted reliably, i.e. with high sensitivity and specificity, it is not necessary to justify the model or analysis technique by medical, biological, or physical processes.

The idea of a seizure prediction device would be to take the raw EEG signal, perform some feature extraction potentially based on some of the ideas and concepts mentioned above, raise alarms using the features, and

130

trigger a warning or automatic intervention. In this process, the violation of any of the assumptions made by the analysis techniques or mathematical models is of course acceptable, if seizures can be predicted reliably. Important guidelines for seizure prediction irrespective of the model or analysis technique were suggested. It was proposed, firstly, to use long-term, non-preselected EEG signals, secondly, to evaluate seizure prediction performance based on training and testing data, thirdly, to report the results separately for the training and testing data, and fourthly, to statistically validate the results.[23,24] Many approaches for the statistical validation of the results have been discussed in the literature.[23,25]

In summary, in this chapter some analysis techniques and preprocessing steps have been introduced and summarised that are potentially applicable in seizure prediction studies. A detailed discussion and ranking of methods for seizure prediction, however, is beyond the scope of this chapter. When reporting seizure prediction studies, it is vital that the statistical validation is provided and comprehensible. Without such a statistical validation no seizure prediction algorithm should be suggested or introduced.

References

1. J. Honerkamp, *Statistical Physics*, 3 edn. (Springer, Berlin, 2012).
2. B. Schelter, J. Timmer and A. Schulze-Bonhage *Seizure Prediction in Epilepsy. From Basic Mechanisms to Clinical Applications*, 1 edn. (Wiley-VCH, Weinheim, 2008).
3. B. Hjorth, *Electroenceph Clin Neurophys* **39**, 526 (1975).
4. P. Nunez, *Brain Topog* **2**, 141 (1989).
5. S. Law, P. Nunez and R. Wijesinghe, *IEEE J BME* **40**, 145 (1993).
6. H. Ramoser, J. Müller-Gerking and G. Pfurtscheller, *IEEE J RE* **8**, 441 (2000).
7. R. Bortel and P. Sovjka, *Clin Neurophysiol* **online** (2012).
8. J. Timmer, M. Lauk and G. Deuschl, *Electroenceph Clin Neurophys* **101**, 461 (1996).
9. M. Priestley, *Spectral Analysis and Time Series* (Academic Press, London, 1989).
10. A. Pikovsky, *Synchronization: A universal concept in nonlinear sciences* (Cambridge University Press, Cambridge, 2001).
11. M. Le van Quyen,J. Foucher, J. Lachaux, E. Rodriguez, A. Lutz, J. Martinerie, and F. Varela, *J Neurosci Meth* **111**, 83 (2001).
12. G. Osipov, B. Hu, C. Zhou, M. Ivanchenko and J. Kurths *Phys rev let* **91**, 24101, (2003)
13. A. Politi, F. Ginelli, S. Yanchuk, and Y. Maistrenko *Physica D* **244**, 90, 2006
14. B. Schelter, J. Timmer and M. Eichler, *J Neurosci Meth* **179**, 121 (2009).

15. M. Killmann, L. Sommerlade, W. Mader, J. Timmer and B. Schelter, *Biomed Tech (Berl)* (2012).
16. C. W. J. Granger, *Econometrica* **37** 424 (2012).
17. W. Mader, D. Feess, R. Lange, D. Saur, V. Glauche, C. Weiller, J. Timmer and B. Schelter, *IEEE J Sel Top Sig Proc* **2**, 965 (2008).
18. J. Honerkamp, *Stochastic Dynamical Systems* (VCH, New York, 1993).
19. H. Lütkepohl, *Introduction to Multiple Time Series Analysis* (Springer, Berlin, 1993).
20. L. Sommerlade, M. Thiel, B. Platt, A. Plano, G. Riedel, C. Grebogi, J. Timmer and B. Schelter, *J Neurosci Meth* **203**, 173 (2012).
21. E. Wan and A. Nelson, Neural dual extended Kalman filtering: applications in speech enhancement and monaural blind signal separation, in *IEEE Proceedings in Neural Networks for Signal Processing: VII. Proceedings of the 1997 IEEE Workshop*, 1997.
22. R. Shumway and D. Stoffer, *Time Series Analysis and Its Application* (Springer, New York, 2000).
23. B. Schelter, R. Andrzejak and F. Mormann, *Seizure Prediction in Epilepsy. From Basic Mechanisms to Clinical Applications* (Wiley-VCH, Weinheim, 2008), ch. Can Your Prediction Algorithm Beat a Random Predictor?, pp. 237–248.
24. F. Mormann, R. Andrzejak, C. Elger and K. Lehnertz, *Brain* **130**, 314 (2007).
25. B. Schelter, M. Winterhalder, T. Maiwald, A. Brandt, A. Schad, A. Schulze-Bonhage and J. Timmer, *Chaos* **16**, p. 13108 (2006).

FROM TIME SERIES TO COMPLEX NETWORKS: AN OVERVIEW

S. BIALONSKI* and K. LEHNERTZ

Department of Epileptology, University of Bonn,
Sigmund-Freud-Straße 25, 53105 Bonn, Germany
Helmholtz Institute for Radiation and Nuclear Physics, University of Bonn,
Nussallee 14–16, 53115 Bonn, Germany
Interdisciplinary Center for Complex Systems, University of Bonn,
Brühler Straße 7, 53175 Bonn, Germany
* E-mail: bialonski@gmx.net

The network approach towards the analysis of the dynamics of complex systems has been successfully applied in a multitude of studies in the neurosciences and has yielded fascinating insights. With this approach, a complex system is considered to be composed of different constituents which interact with each other. Interaction structures can be compactly represented in *interaction networks*. In this contribution, we present a brief overview about how interaction networks are derived from multivariate time series, about basic network characteristics, and about challenges associated with this analysis approach.

Keywords: interaction networks, network characterization, time series analysis, spatial sampling, temporal sampling

1. Introduction

Understanding, predicting, and controlling the dynamics of complex systems lies at the heart of many scientific challenges. A case in point is the human brain which is composed of an overwhelming number of interacting parts. While during the last decades, remarkable progress has been made in the neurosciences in advancing our knowledge about these individual parts (subsystems), the challenge to characterize and understand the dynamics of the brain as a whole has sparked the development of sophisticated data analysis techniques. Recent multivariate analysis approaches adopted concepts from *network theory*[1–4] and take into account the complex interrelation structures between many subsystems. Such interrelation structures can be derived from analyses of multivariate time series and are reflected in the topology of *interaction networks*. To this respect, interaction networks can be considered as a means to characterize the dynamics of a complex system. Properties of interaction networks can be investigated via a plethora of methods which is by now available.[5–10]

In the neurosciences, the network approach has already led to a number of intriguing results. Specific aspects of interaction networks were reported to differentially reflect physiologic processes (e.g. sleep,[11–13] aging,[14,15] daily rhythms[16]) as well as pathological states associated e.g. with schizophrenia,[17–19] Alzheimer's disease,[20–23] or epilepsy.[16,24–32] Interaction networks differ between epilepsy patients and healthy controls[30,33–37] and were reported to possess more lattice-like topologies during epileptic seizures[16,24–28] than prior to or after seizures. It remains to be shown whether the network approach can help to improve the characterization of the interictal-to-preictal-to-ictal transition.[16]

In this contribution, we provide basic definitions and notions used in applied network science and present a brief overview of methods—frequently used in the neurosciences—to derive interaction networks from multivariate time series. Finally, we discuss challenges of the network analysis approach and point to possible ways of how to meet them.

2. Inferring interaction networks from multivariate time series

Various methods have been proposed to derive interaction networks from empirical data, and each of these methods comes along with various advantages and disadvantages. Being aware of the chosen method is an important prerequisite for evaluating, comparing, and interpreting analysis results. Broadly speaking, with approaches most frequently used in the neurosciences, sensors (e.g., EEG electrodes or voxels in fMRI data) are associated with network nodes, and network edges are inferred using bivariate time series analysis techniques that aim at quantifying the strength and/or the direction of an interaction. We note that methods for deriving networks from single time series are covered in a different review.[38] In the following, we recall basic concepts from network theory as well as from bivariate time series analysis, and present approaches used to derive interaction networks.

2.1. Network basics

Networks are studied in graph theory in which they are represented as *graphs*. A graph is a non-empty set of nodes and a set of pairs of elements of the set of nodes, i.e., the set of edges.[3,4] A node i is said to be a neighbor of node j if there exists an edge between i and j. A graph is said to be directed (undirected) if edges (do not) carry a direction, i.e., the set of edges is a set of ordered (unordered) pairs of elements of the set of nodes. A *weighted graph* can be defined by introducing a set of values (most frequently real numbers) which represent weights attached to the edges.

A graph is usually represented by an $N \times N$ square matrix $\boldsymbol{A}$ (*adjacency matrix*), where N denotes the number of nodes of the graph (also known as the *size* of the graph[3]). Let $i, j \in \{1, \ldots, N\}$. If i and j are neighbors, $A_{ij} = 1$. Otherwise, if i and j are not neighbors, $A_{ij} = 0$. Whether nodes are defined as self-connected ($A_{ii} = 1 \forall i$) or not ($A_{ii} = 0 \forall i$) varies across the literature, and here we follow the second and commonly used definition. The adjacency matrix is symmetric for undirected graphs, $A_{ij} = A_{ji}$. For directed graphs, the adjacency matrix is usually not symmetric, and $A_{ij} = 1$ implies that an edge has a direction and points from node i to node j. Weighted graphs are usually described by an adjacency matrix $\boldsymbol{A}$ and a *weight matrix* $\boldsymbol{W}$ which is an $N \times N$ square matrix containing the weights of the edges. In the following, we will focus on undirected unweighted graphs.

A basic property of a graph is the degree of nodes. The *degree* k_i of a node i is defined as the number of neighbors of i, and the *mean degree* $\bar{k}$ is defined as the mean of the degrees of all nodes of a graph,

$$k_i = \sum_{j=1}^{N} A_{ij}, \qquad \bar{k} = N^{-1} \sum_{i=1}^{N} k_i. \tag{1}$$

Another important property of a graph is its *edge density* ϵ. The edge density is defined as the fraction of edges which exist among all possible edges of the graph. Let E denote the number of edges of a graph. Since $E = (\sum_{i,j} A_{ij})/2$ and since the number of all possible edges of a graph of size N is $N(N-1)/2$, we obtain

$$\epsilon = \frac{2E}{N(N-1)} = \frac{\bar{k}}{N-1}. \tag{2}$$

Different aspects of a graph can be characterized by investigating its *paths*. A path between two distinct nodes i and j is a sequence of neighboring nodes starting with i and ending with j which contains no node more then once.[3] The number of edges traversed in a given path is known as the *path length*. If the latter is finite, the path is said to be finite. A path between nodes i and j is called the *shortest path* if there does not exist any other path between i and j with a smaller path length. The length of the shortest path between i and j is frequently denoted as l_{ij}.

The concept of paths allows one to further characterize a graph. For instance, if a finite path exists for every pair of distinct nodes, the graph is called to be *connected*. If the opposite is true, the graph is said to be *disconnected*. A connected subgraph is called a *component* of the graph.[4] Two distinct components of a graph are disconnected if there is no path connecting any of the nodes of the first with any of the nodes of the second component.

In addition to the characteristics described above, a plethora of methods is available which allows one to assess a variety of graph properties.[3,4,10,39] We restrict the following brief discussion to those frequently employed in the neurosciences and to the case of unweighted graphs. Generalizations of the discussed characteristics to weighted graphs are presented in a number of different reviews.[3,4,39] In accordance with the majority of field studies, we will use the notions *graph* and *network* interchangeably in the following.

Many natural networks show a tendency that neighbors of a node are also connected to each other. This *transitivity* can be assessed using various methods among which the *clustering coefficient* C is frequently employed in field studies.[2,3,40] It is defined as the average of the local clustering coefficients C_i,

$$C = \frac{1}{N} \sum_{i=1}^{N} C_i, \qquad C_i = \begin{cases} \frac{1}{k_i(k_i-1)} \sum_{j,m} A_{ij} A_{jm} A_{mi}, & \text{if } k_i > 1 \\ 0, & \text{if } k_i \in \{0, 1\}, \end{cases} \tag{3}$$

where C_i is defined as the fraction of existing edges among all possible edges between the neighbors of i. Networks showing large values of C are often considered to be robust against a random removal of nodes.

The efficiency of a network to transport information can be characterized by the average shortest path length L,[2]

$$L = \frac{2}{N(N+1)} \sum_{i \leq j} l_{ij}, \tag{4}$$

where we included the shortest paths from each node to itself ($l_{ii} = 0 \forall i$) in the average.[2] Low values of L indicate a network to be very efficient because only a small number of edges have to be traversed on average in order to reach any node. If the network is not connected, L will become infinitely large since $l_{ij} = \infty$ for some i and j. Thus, it has been proposed to either replace the l_{ij} values in the above definition with their inverse values l_{ij}^{-1} leading to a network characteristic called *efficiency*,[41,42] or to simply exclude infinite values from the summation.[43]

Within the small-world framework,[40] networks can be classified into different network classes. So called *small-world networks*[40,44] combine desirable features, namely robustness and efficiency. In a network theoretic sense, a small-world network is characterized by a large clustering coefficient together with an average shortest path length scaling at most logarithmically with N (the latter is often denoted as the small-world *property* in the mathematics literature).[3] Reliably determining the scaling behavior of L cannot typically be achieved in field studies since such an investigation comes along with altering the number of nodes over several orders of magnitudes. Instead, it is common practice to compare values of C and L with mean values C_r and L_r obtained from ensembles of corresponding random networks. Whereas large values of C ($C \gg C_r$) and low values of L ($L \approx L_r$) are considered to be indicative of small-world networks, $C \gg C_r$ and $L \gg L_r$ are assumed to indicate a lattice topology and $C \approx C_r$ and $L \approx L_r$ are considered to be indicative of a random network topology.

To close this section, we mention methods to assess the relative importance of a node within a network, the node-*centrality*. Different concepts of centrality have been proposed during the last decades[3,45] which differ in the way how "relative importance" can be defined. Most important nodes are usually called *hubs*. For instance, the *degree centrality*,[3] which is defined as the degree of a node, assumes that nodes with many neighbors are more important than those with a lower number of neighbors. *Closeness centrality* scores those nodes to be very important which possess the shortest paths to every other node in the network.[46] Finally, according to the concept of *betweenness centrality*, nodes are considered to be more important the more shortest paths connecting other nodes are running through them.[46]

2.2. *Estimating signal interdependencies*

Edges in interaction networks are assumed to represent interactions between different (sub-)systems (nodes). Interactions can be determined in *active experiments*,[47] in which all constraints are known and fixed, parameters of the studied systems are altered in a controlled way, and changes in the dynamics of systems are recorded via repeated measurements. This approach, however, is often not feasible in the human brain. Instead, inference of interactions relies on estimates of interdependencies between signals recorded by sensors.

A plethora of bivariate time series analysis techniques is available[47-56] which allow one to estimate signal interdependencies and to assess the strength or direction of interactions. Well-known methods from linear time series analysis[48] (among which we mention the Pearson correlation coefficient and cross spectral density estimates) characterize linear aspects of the dynamics and have found widespread use. Time series analysis techniques developed during the last decades and recent years have largely increased the number of accessible characteristics of the dynamics and allow one to assess different aspects, including non-linear or stochastic ones. Such time series analysis methods are based on synchronization theory,[47,49] on non-linear dynamics,[50,53] on information theory,[52] or on the theory of stochastic processes.[55] Many of these methods have already been successfully applied in the neurosciences.[51,54,56]

When estimating signal interdependencies using any of the methods above, several constraints and considerations should be taken into account. For instance, methods may largely differ with respect to their statistical efficiency (the amount of required data) and robustness (against noise contaminations). Constraints imposed by the acquisition technology and by the temporal scales on which the dynamics unfold usually limit the amount of available data. Furthermore, the aforementioned methods normally require time series reflecting at least approximate *stationary* periods of the systems' dynamics. This leads to a trade-off between the stationarity of a period (mostly calling for short data segments) and the required statistical accuracy of the method at hand (calling for long data segments). Recent developments may even allow for the inference of strength or direction of interactions from transient dynamics.[57–59] Finally we mention that many studies pursue a time-resolved analysis using a sliding window approach in order to account for the non-stationarity of the dynamics of the human brain.

2.3. *Identifying nodes and edges*

In most studies in the neurosciences, the definition of nodes is straightforward: each single sensor capturing the dynamics of the system is associated with a node of the interaction network. The identification of edges, however, varies largely across the literature. Let ρ_{ij} denote a value of an estimator of signal interdependence. We assume that $\rho_{ij} \geq 0$ and that large values indicate strong signal interdependencies while values approaching 0 indicate no interdependencies. In the following we present methods used for identifying edges in unweighted networks, followed by methods to infer weighted networks.

2.3.1. *Unweighted interaction networks*

θ-**thresholding.** A straightforward way to infer an edge is to require the estimate of signal interdependence to be larger than a specified threshold θ. The adjacency matrix A of the unweighted interaction network is then defined as

$$A_{ii} = 0; \qquad A_{ij} = H(\rho_{ij} - \theta) \quad \forall i \neq j; i, j \in \{1, \ldots, N\}, \qquad (5)$$

where $H(x) = 1$ for $x > 0$ and $H(x) = 0$ else. This approach is not only frequently used in the neurosciences[6,27,60–62] but also in climate science,[63] quantitative finance,[64] and seismology.[65] How to choose the threshold in a meaningful way is still subject of ongoing debates (see, e.g., references 5 and 66). One approach is to determine θ by requiring the resulting network to possess specific properties (coined *"adaptive thresholding"* in reference 26) which is described below.

Range of thresholds. Another strategy which allows one to avoid the choice of a single threshold is based on investigating networks obtained for a whole range of thresholds.[20,21,27,30,67,68] Network characteristics which do not largely vary over a range of thresholds are considered to be robust (with respect to the threshold) and can then further be interpreted.

Adaptive thresholding.

- In $\bar{k}$-*thresholding*, instead of defining a fixed value of θ directly, the threshold θ is chosen such that the resulting network possesses a predefined mean degree $\bar{k}$.[30,69] For instance, this approach might be valuable if network characteristics that sensitively depend on the degrees are to be assessed from the derived networks. Moreover, if properties of different networks are to be compared with each other, a varying mean degree might introduce a bias into such a comparison.

- ϵ-*thresholding.* It has been demonstrated that network characteristics can decisively depend on the edge density ϵ.[68,70] These observations lead to another strategy to determine the threshold by requiring the resulting network to possess a predefined edge density ϵ.

- *Requirement of connectedness.* Some network characteristics may not be well defined for disconnected networks or may crucially depend on the connectedness of a network (e.g. synchronizability[71]). For such cases, it has been proposed to choose the threshold θ in such a way that the network possesses a minimum number of edges but is still connected.[26,30]

In time-resolved analyses, the aforementioned strategies are likely to yield different values of θ for different interaction networks. Put another way, θ is "adapted" to the matrix of signal interdependencies, which leads to the notion "adaptive thresholding" for such methods.

Significance testing. The definition of a threshold (dsirectly or parametrized by $\bar{k}$, ϵ, or the requirement of connectedness) as described above, which is applied to estimates of signal interdependencies between all pairs of time series, comes along with the risk of spuriously inferring edges (false positives) or spuriously missing edges (false negatives). To overcome this problem, it has been suggested to employ significance testing and to convert only those estimates of signal interdependence into edges which are found to be significant.[72–74] This strategy involves the definition of appropriate null models on the level of time series (see, e.g., references 75 and 72) as well as techniques counteracting the problem of multiple testing. Controlling the family-wise error rate (the probability of detecting spurious edges among all possible pairs of nodes) is a well established multiple testing technique (with its well-known incarnation, the *Bonferroni correction*) but is known to go hand in hand with a high risk of false negatives.[76] More recent methods may lower this risk by controlling the false discovery rate (the probability of false positives among all derived edges).[72,77,78]

Other approaches have been developed to infer edges, but are not frequently used in the neuroscience literature. Among these methods, we mention approaches involving the construction of minimum spanning trees[79]— a method popular in the studies inferring financial networks—, methods based on rank-ordered network growth,[80] or strategies which combine some of the aforementioned thresholding techniques.[81]

2.3.2. *Weighted interaction networks*

For weighted interaction networks, in addition to the adjacency matrix, a weight matrix has to be obtained from the data. In its simplest form, the network is considered to be fully connected, i.e., the adjacency matrix A reads

$$A_{ij} = \begin{cases} 1 & , i \neq j \\ 0 & , i = j \end{cases} \qquad i, j \in \{1, \dots, N\}, \tag{6}$$

while the weight matrix W equals the matrix of estimates of signal interdependencies,

$$W_{ij} = \begin{cases} \rho_{ij} & , i \neq j \\ 0 & , i = j \end{cases} \qquad i, j \in \{1, \dots, N\}. \tag{7}$$

One variations of this approach is to set $W_{ij} = 0, i \neq j$ in cases for which the corresponding estimate of signal interdependence ρ_{ij} was determined to be not significant.[33]

Since the distribution of edge weights alone might already strongly influence characteristics of such networks,[30,37,82] some strategies have been proposed to approach this issue. For instance, when deriving weighted networks, the first moment and/or the second central moment of the weight distribution can be set to desired fixed values, which can be achieved by simple transforms of the estimates of signal interdependence,

$$W_{ij} = \rho_{ij} - \bar{\rho} + 1, \qquad \text{or} \qquad W_{ij} = \frac{\rho_{ij} - \bar{\rho}}{\sigma_\rho} + 1, \qquad (8)$$

where $\bar{\rho}$ and σ_ρ denote the mean and the standard deviation of the values ρ_{ij}, respectively.[30] In the above equations, the weight distribution is centered around the mean value 1.

Instead of only defining moments of the distribution, one may also define the whole weight distribution. This can be achieved by sorting $\{\rho_{ij} | i < j\}$ in ascending order and determining their ranks ν_{ij} ($\nu_{ij} = \nu_{ji}$). Values obtained from the specified weight distribution are rank-ordered and then assigned to edges according to the rank-order of the ρ_{ij} values. A special case of this approach is proposed in reference 83, where the weight matrix directly reflects scaled ranks and is defined as

$$W_{ij} = \begin{cases} 2\nu_{ij}/(N(N-1)) & , i \neq j \\ 0 & , i = j \end{cases} \qquad i,j \in \{1, \dots, N\}. \qquad (9)$$

3. Challenges

Various challenges of the network analysis approach have been discovered during the last years and are associated with the issues of how the dynamics of the investigated system is spatially and temporally sampled, how nodes and edges are inferred from the measurements, how results can be interpreted, and how their significance can be reliably assessed.[43,84-89] All of the latter issues are closely interrelated with the first one, the spatial and temporal sampling of the dynamics.[90]

The *spatial sampling* of the dynamics plays a central role for the identification of nodes and edges. Since each sensor is usually associated with a node, the identification of nodes directly translates into the challenge of defining a suitable spatial sampling scheme which allows one to capture the dynamics in a meaningful way. The assumption often made implicitly is that each node represents the dynamics of a different subsystem. This can be challenging for systems characterized by physical fields for which a decomposition into subsystems represents a coarse graining of the dynamics. Depending on how meaningful the system can be decomposed into subsystems and how well their dynamics can be captured by the recording devices, there is a risk that the dynamics of the same subsystem may be recorded with two or more sensors, reflected by *common sources* in the recorded signals and leading to *redundant nodes*. It could also be that the dynamics of some subsystems may not be recorded at all (*missing nodes*). Common sources can lead to *spurious edges* since most time series analysis techniques will indicate two signals to be strongly interdependent if common sources are present. These spurious edges then do not represent mutual interactions between different subsystems but are nonetheless likely to artificially increase the clustering coefficient of derived interaction networks. Another mechanism leading to artificially increased clustering coefficients is that most time series analysis techniques cannot distinguish between direct and indirect interactions. If system *1* interacts with system *2*, and system *2* with *3*, then most time series analysis techniques will also indicate strong signal interdependencies between systems *1* and *3*, an *indirect interaction*. Together with unavoidable noise contributions which can introduce spurious shortcuts in the network and thus decrease the average shortest path length, interaction networks are likely classified as small-world networks even if the underlying interaction structure is not small-world.[43] If sensors capture dipolar patterns produced by generators in the brain, nodes associated with spatially close sensors will be strongly interconnected (large clustering coefficient) and edges (shortcuts) will exist which connect remote nodes at the respective extrema of the dipolar pattern (low average shortest path length).[84] Thus, such a network would also be classified as a small-world network.

Some strategies have been developed during the last years to approach the aforementioned issues. A straightforward way to investigate the influence of the spatial sampling on network characteristics would be to gather data with altered sensor placements. Instead of modifying sensor placements, which may not always be feasible due to technical or other constraints, some studies assessed the influence of the *spatial scale* on network characteristics by employing different coarse graining schemes.[86,91,92] Other approaches aim at developing and employing time series analysis techniques which may help to reduce spurious edges in derived interaction networks and may help to diminish or even to eliminate an artificial increase of the clustering coefficient. For instance, time series analysis techniques were proposed[93-96] which might be able to distinguish between interdependencies due to interacting different subsystems and those due to common source contributions. Other methods might be capable of distinguishing between direct and indirect interactions.[48,97-103] Another approach is to refrain from absolute interpretations of network characteristics but instead to assess *relative changes* of network characteristics in a time-resolved analysis (e.g., by pursuing a sliding window analysis).[16,26,30,88,104-107] The key idea is that relative changes over time should not be influenced by the spatial arrangement of sensors since the latter does not change during the measurements. For instance, this ansatz may be particularly useful when looking for potential seizure precursors.

The *temporal sampling* of the dynamics is important for the identification of edges. The choice of the observation duration and the temporal sampling frequency already determines the time scale at which the dynamics is studied as well as the amount of data available for subsequent steps of analysis. It has been demonstrated that the finite length of time series as well as a large amount of low frequency contributions in time series can lead to spurious properties in interaction networks if common methods for edge inference are employed.[88] As an important consequence, characteristics of interaction networks likely deviate significantly from those obtained from classical random network models (e.g. Erdős-Rényi graphs[108] or degree-preserving randomized networks[109,110]), leading to a classification as small-world networks even in cases in which the underlying finite time series just consisted of (low-pass filtered) noise. In such cases, interaction networks would represent an overly complicated description of what can be directly assessed by univariate time series analysis techniques (e.g. power spectral density estimates). To distinguish aspects from the network dynamics from those spuriously induced by the way of network inference, it has been suggested to compare characteristics of interaction networks with those of random networks generated according to a specific null model.[88,111] This null model takes into account the way how interaction networks are derived from empirical data and is based on random time series that preserve length, spectral content and amplitude distribution of the empirical time series.[75] Another null model addressing this issue is based on generating random matrices of signal interdependencies where some distributional properties of matrix entries match the ones in the observed matrix of signal interdependencies.[112] Finally, in a recent study, it was reported that interaction networks derived using the Pearson correlation coefficient can show non-trivial properties even for infinite time series.[113] This may point towards intrinsic properties of such estimators which can—regardless of the analyzed empirical data—already leave an imprint in the topology of derived interaction networks. These results call for a careful interpretation of network characteristics which take into account the whole chain of analysis.

4. Conclusion

In this contribution, we presented a brief overview about how interaction networks can be derived from multivariate time series, about basic network characteristics, and about challenges arising from the network approach. We restricted our presentation to methods which have been frequently used in the neurosciences and which are based on bivariate time series analysis techniques (methods based on analyzing single time series are covered in reference 38).

The network approach allows one to analyze dynamical systems which can be considered as networks of interacting constituents. It facilitates the assessment of complex interaction structures and their characterization in a compact way (down to a single number!). The usefulness of this approach has been repeatedly demonstrated in a multitude of studies published in various sciences, ranging from the neurosciences to earth and climate science. Challenges associated with the network analysis approach are the reliable assessment of the significance of findings and their interpretation as well as the network construction (identification of nodes and edges) which is non-trivially connected with the spatial and temporal sampling of the studied dynamics. To this respect, recent contributions indicate that future efforts will address and likely meet these challenges. Such work will enable us to gain a better characterization and deeper understanding of the dynamics of complex systems.

Acknowledgments

This work was supported by the Deutsche Forschungsgemeinschaft (Grants Nos. LE660/4-2 and LE660/5-2).

References

1. S. H. Strogatz, *Nature* **410**, 268 (2001).
2. M. E. J. Newman, *SIAM Rev.* **45**, 167 (2003).
3. S. Boccaletti, V. Latora, Y. Moreno, M. Chavez and D.-U. Hwang, *Phys. Rep.* **424**, 175 (2006).
4. A. Barrat, M. Barthélemy and A. Vespignani, *Dynamical Processes on Complex Networks* (Cambridge University Press, New York, USA, 2008).

5. J. C. Reijneveld, S. C. Ponten, H. W. Berendse and C. J. Stam, *Clin. Neurophysiol.* **118**, 2317 (2007).
6. E. Bullmore and O. Sporns, *Nat. Rev. Neurosci.* **10**, 186 (2009).
7. D. S. Bassett and E. T. Bullmore, *Curr. Opin. Neurol.* **22**, 340 (2009).
8. M. Rubinov and O. Sporns, *NeuroImage* **52**, 1059 (2010).
9. C. J. Stam, *Int. J. Psychophysiol.* **77**, 186 (2010).
10. O. Sporns, *Networks of the Brain* (MIT Press, Cambridge, Massachusetts, 2011).
11. R. Ferri, F. Rundo, O. Bruni, M. G. Terzano and C. J. Stam, *Clin. Neurophysiol.* **118**, 449 (2007).
12. R. Ferri, F. Rundo, O. Bruni, M. G. Terzano and C. J. Stam, *Clin. Neurophysiol.* **119**, 2026 (2008).
13. A. Bashan, R. P. Bartsch, J. W. Kantelhardt, S. Havlin and P. C. Ivanov, *Nat. Commun.* **3**, 702 (2012).
14. D. Meunier, S. Achard, A. Morcom and E. Bullmore, *NeuroImage* **44**, 715 (2009).
15. D. J. A. Smit, M. Boersma, C. E. M. van Beijsterveldt, D. Posthuma, D. I. Boomsma, C. J. Stam and E. J. C. de Geus, *Behav. Genet.* **40**, 167 (2010).
16. M.-T. Kuhnert, C. E. Elger and K. Lehnertz, *Chaos* **20**, 043126 (2010).
17. S. Micheloyannis, E. Pachou, C. J. Stam, M. Breakspear, P. Bitsios, M. Vourkas, S. Erimaki and M. Zervakis, *Schizophr. Res.* **87**, 60 (2006).
18. Y. Liu, M. Liang, Y. Zhou, Y. He, Y. Hao, M. Song, C. Yu, H. Liu, Z. Liu and T. Jiang, *Brain* **131**, 945 (2008).
19. D. S. Bassett, E. Bullmore, B. A. Verchinski, V. S. Mattay, D. R. Weinberger and A. Meyer-Lindenberg, *J. Neurosci.* **28**, 9239 (2008).
20. C. J. Stam, B. F. Jones, G. Nolte, M. Breakspear and P. Scheltens, *Cereb. Cortex* **17**, 92 (2007).
21. K. Supekar, V. Menon, D. Rubin, M. Musen and M. D. Greicius, *PLoS Comput. Biol.* **4**, e1000100 (2008).
22. W. de Haan, Y. A. L. Pijnenburg, R. L. M. Strijers, Y. van der Made, W. M. van der Flier, P. Scheltens and C. J. Stam, *BMC Neuroscience* **10**, 101 (2009).
23. C. J. Stam, W. de Haan, A. Daffertshofer, B. F. Jones, I. Manshanden, A. M. van Cappellen van Walsum, T. Montez, J. P. A. Verbunt, J. C. de Munck, B. W. van Dijk, H. W. Berendse and P. Scheltens, *Brain* **132**, 213 (2009).
24. H. Wu, X. Li and X. Guan, Networking property during epileptic seizure with multi-channel EEG recordings, in *Lecture Notes in Computer Science*, ed. J. Wang (Springer, Berlin, 2006) 573–578.
25. S. C. Ponten, F. Bartolomei and C. J. Stam, *Clin. Neurophysiol.* **118**, 918 (2007).
26. K. Schindler, S. Bialonski, M.-T. Horstmann, C. E. Elger and K. Lehnertz, *Chaos* **18**, 033119 (2008).
27. M. A. Kramer, E. D. Kolaczyk and H. E. Kirsch, *Epilepsy Res.* **79**, 173 (2008).
28. S. C. Ponten, L. Douw, F. Bartolomei, J. C. Reijneveld and C. J. Stam, *Exp. Neurol.* **217**, 197 (2009).

29. E. van Dellen, L. Douw, J. C. Baayen, J. J. Heimans, S. C. Ponten, W. P. Vandertop, D. N. Velis, C. J. Stam and J. C. Reijneveld, *PLoS ONE* 4, e8081 (2009).
30. M.-T. Horstmann, S. Bialonski, N. Noennig, H. Mai, J. Prusseit, J. Wellmer, H. Hinrichs and K. Lehnertz, *Clin. Neurophysiol.* 121, 172 (2010).
31. M. Richardson, *Clin. Neurophysiol.* 121, 1153 (2010).
32. D. Gupta, P. Ossenblok and G. van Luijtelaar, *Med. Biol. Eng. Comput.* 49, 555 (2011).
33. M. Chavez, M. Valencia, V. Navarro, V. Latora and J. Martinerie, *Phys. Rev. Lett.* 104, 118701 (2010).
34. W. Liao, Z. Zhang, Z. Pan, D. Mantini, J. Ding, X. Duan, C. Luo, G. Lu and H. Chen, *PLoS ONE* 5, e8528 (2010).
35. M. C. G. Vlooswijk, M. J. Vaessen, J. F. A. Jansen, M. C. F. T. M. de Krom, H. J. M. Majoie, P. A. M. Hofman, A. P. Aldenkamp and W. H. Backes, *Neurology* 77, 938 (2011).
36. Z. Zhang, W. Liao, H. Chen, D. Mantini, J.-R. Ding, Q. Xu, Z. Wang, C. Yuan, G. Chen, Q. Jiao and G. Lu, *Brain* 134, 2912 (2011).
37. G. Ansmann and K. Lehnertz, *J. Neurosci. Methods* 208, 165 (2012).
38. R. V. Donner, Y. Zou, J. F. Donges, N. Marwan and J. Kurths, *New J. Physics* 12, 033025 (2010).
39. L. da F. Costa, F. A. Rodrigues, G. Travieso and P. R. V. Boas, *Adv. Phys.* 56, 167 (2007).
40. D. J. Watts and S. H. Strogatz, *Nature* 393, 440 (1998).
41. V. Latora and M. Marchiori, *Phys. Rev. Lett.* 87, 198701 (2001).
42. V. Latora and M. Marchiori, *Eur. Phys. J. B* 32, 249 (2003).
43. S. Bialonski, M.-T. Horstmann and K. Lehnertz, *Chaos* 20, 013134 (2010).
44. A. Barrat and M. Weigt, *Eur. Phys. J. B* 13, 547 (2000).
45. S. P. Borgatti and M. G. Everett, *Soc. Networks* 28, 466 (2006).
46. L. C. Freeman, *Soc. Networks* 1, 215 (1979).
47. A. S. Pikovsky, M. G. Rosenblum and J. Kurths, *Synchronization: A universal concept in nonlinear sciences* (Cambridge University Press, Cambridge, UK, 2001).
48. D. Brillinger, *Time Series: Data Analysis and Theory* (Holden-Day, San Francisco, USA, 1981).
49. S. Boccaletti, J. Kurths, G. Osipov, D. L. Valladares and C. S. Zhou, *Phys. Rep.* 366, 1 (2002).
50. H. Kantz and T. Schreiber, *Nonlinear Time Series Analysis*, 2nd edn. (Cambridge University Press, Cambridge, UK, 2003).
51. E. Pereda, R. Quian Quiroga and J. Bhattacharya, *Prog. Neurobiol.* 77, 1 (2005).
52. K. Hlaváčková-Schindler, M. Paluš, M. Vejmelka and J. Bhattacharya, *Phys. Rep.* 441, 1 (2007).
53. N. Marwan, M. C. Romano, M. Thiel and J. Kurths, *Phys. Rep.* 438, 237 (2007).
54. K. Lehnertz, S. Bialonski, M.-T. Horstmann, D. Krug, A. Rothkegel, M. Staniek and T. Wagner, *J. Neurosci. Methods* 183, 42 (2009).

146

55. R. Friedrich, J. Peinke, M. Sahimi and M. R. R. Tabar, *Phys. Rep.* **506**, 87 (2011).
56. K. Lehnertz, *Physiol. Meas.* **32**, 1715 (2011).
57. T. Wagner, J. Fell and K. Lehnertz, *New J. Physics* **12**, 053031 (2010).
58. S. Hempel, A. Koseska, J. Kurths and Z. Nikoloski, *Phys. Rev. Lett.* **107**, 054101 (2011).
59. M. Martini, T. A. Kranz, T. Wagner and K. Lehnertz, *Phys. Rev. E* **83**, 011919 (2011).
60. V. M. Eguiluz, D. R. Chialvo, G. A. Cecchi, M. Baliki and A. V. Apkarian, *Phys. Rev. Lett.* **94**, 018102 (2005).
61. F. Bartolomei, I. Bosma, M. Klein, J. C. Baayen, J. C. Reijneveld, T. J. Postma, J. J. Heimans, B. W. van Dijk, J. C. de Munck, A. de Jongh, K. S. Cover and C. J. Stam, *Ann. Neurol.* **59**, 128 (2006).
62. M. P. van den Heuvel, C. J. Stam, R. S. Kahn and H. E. Hulshoff Pol, *J. Neurosci.* **29**, 7619 (2009).
63. A. A. Tsonis and P. J. Roebber, *Physica A* **333**, 497 (2004).
64. V. Boginski, S. Butenko and P. M. Pardalos, *Comput. Stat. Data An.* **48**, 431 (2005).
65. A. Jiménez, K. F. Tiampo and A. M. Posadas, *Nonlinear Proc. Geoph.* **15**, 389 (2008).
66. E. T. Bullmore and D. S. Bassett, *Annu. Rev. Clin. Psychol.* **7**, 113 (2011).
67. S. Micheloyannis, E. Pachou, C. J. Stam, M. Vourkas, S. Erimalo and V. Tsirka, *Neurosci. Lett.* **402**, 273 (2006).
68. B. C. M. van Wijk, C. J. Stam and A. Daffertshofer, *PLoS ONE* **5**, e13701 (2010).
69. C. J. Stam, *Neurosci. Lett.* **355**, 25 (2004).
70. B. S. Anderson, C. Butts and K. Carley, *Soc. Networks* **21**, 239 (1999).
71. M. Barahona and L. M. Pecora, *Phys. Rev. Lett.* **89**, 054101 (2002).
72. M. A. Kramer, U. T. Eden, S. S. Cash and E. D. Kolaczyk, *Phys. Rev. E* **79**, 061916 (2009).
73. J. F. Donges, Y. Zou, N. Marwan and J. Kurths, *Europhys. Lett.* **87**, 48007 (2009).
74. F. Emmert-Streib and M. Dehmer, *Complexity* **16**, 24 (2010).
75. T. Schreiber and A. Schmitz, *Physica D* **142**, 346 (2000).
76. A. C. Tamhane, *Handbook of Statistics 13: Design and Analysis of Experiments* (Elsevier Science Ltd, 1996), ch. Multiple comparisons, 587–629.
77. Y. Benjamini and Y. Hochberg, *J. Roy. Stat. Soc. B* **57**, 289 (1995).
78. Y. Benjamini and D. Yekutieli, *Ann. Stat.* **29**, 1165 (2001).
79. R. N. Mantegna, *Eur. Phys. J. B* **11**, 193 (1999).
80. J. P. Onnela, K. Kaski and J. Kertesz, *Eur. Phys. J. B* **38**, 353 (2004).
81. D. S. Bassett, A. Meyer-Lindenberg, S. Achard, T. Duke and E. Bullmore, *Proc. Natl. Acad. Sci. U.S.A.* **103**, 19518 (2006).
82. G. Ansmann and K. Lehnertz, *Phys. Rev. E* **84**, 026103 (2011).
83. M. Kuhnert, C. Geier, C. E. Elger and K. Lehnertz, *Chaos* **22**, 023142 (2012).
84. A. A. Ioannides, *Curr. Opin. Neurobiol.* **17**, 161 (2007).

85. C. T. Butts, *Science* **325**, 414 (2009).
86. A. Zalesky, A. Fornito, I. H. Harding, L. Cocchi, M. Yücel, C. Pantelis and E. T. Bullmore, *NeuroImage* **50**, 970 (2010).
87. L. Antiqueira, F. A. Rodrigues, B. C. M. van Wijk, L. da F. Costa and A. Daffertshofer, *NeuroImage* **53**, 439 (2010).
88. S. Bialonski, M. Wendler and K. Lehnertz, *PLoS ONE* **6**, e22826 (2011).
89. J. D. Power, A. L. Cohen, S. M. Nelson, G. S. Wig, K. A. Barnes, J. A. Church, A. C. Vogel, T. O. Laumann, F. M. Miezin, B. L. Schlaggar and S. E. Petersen, *Neuron* **72**, 665 (2011).
90. S. Bialonski, *arXiv* **1208.0800** (2012).
91. F. Giorgi, *Geophys. Res. Lett.* **29**, 2101 (2002).
92. S. Hayasaka and P. J. Laurienti, *NeuroImage* **50**, 499 (2010).
93. P. L. Nunez, R. Srinivasan, A. F. Westdorp, R. S. Wijesinghe, D. M. Tucker, R. B. Silberstein and P. J. Cadusch, *Electroencephalogr. Clin. Neurophysiol.* **103**, 499 (1997).
94. G. Nolte, O. Bai, L. Wheaton, Z. Mari, S. Vorbach and M. Hallett, *Clin. Neurophysiol.* **115**, 2292 (2004).
95. C. J. Stam, G. Nolte and A. Daffertshofer, *Hum. Brain Mapp.* **28**, 1178 (2007).
96. M. Vinck, R. Oostenveld, M. van Wingerden, F. Battaglia and C. M. A. Pennartz, *NeuroImage* **55**, 1548 (2011).
97. W. Gersch, *Math. Biosci.* **14**, 177 (1972).
98. R. Dahlhaus, *Metrika* **51**, 157 (2000).
99. M. Eichler, *Phil. Trans. Roy. Soc. Lond. B Biol Sci* **360**, 953 (2005).
100. B. Schelter, M. Winterhalder, R. Dahlhaus, J. Kurths and J. Timmer, *Phys. Rev. Lett.* **96**, 208103 (2006).
101. S. Frenzel and B. Pompe, *Phys. Rev. Lett.* **99**, 204101 (2007).
102. V. A. Vakorin, O. A. Krakovska and A. R. McIntosh, *J. Neurosci. Methods* **184**, 152 (2009).
103. J. Nawrath, M. C. Romano, M. Thiel, I. Z. Kiss, M. Wickramasinghe, J. Timmer, J. Kurths and B. Schelter, *Phys. Rev. Lett.* **104**, 038701 (2010).
104. S. I. Dimitriadis, N. A. Laskaris, V. Tsirka, M. Vourkas, S. Micheloyannis and S. Fotopoulos, *J. Neurosci. Methods* **193**, 145 (2010).
105. M. A. Kramer, U. T. Eden, K. Q. Lepage, E. D. Kolaczyk, M. T. Bianchi and S. S. Cash, *J. Neurosci.* **31**, 15757 (2011).
106. S. Schinkel, G. Zamora-López, O. Dimigen, W. Sommer and J. Kurths, *J. Neurosci. Methods* **197**, 333 (2011).
107. C. J. Chu, M. A. Kramer, J. Pathmanathan, M. T. Bianchi, M. B. Westover, L. Wizon and S. S. Cash, *J. Neurosci.* **32**, 2703 (2012).
108. P. Erdős and A. Rényi, *Publ. Math. Debrecen* **6**, 290 (1959).
109. J. M. Roberts, *Soc. Networks* **22**, 273 (2000).
110. S. Maslov and K. Sneppen, *Science* **296**, 910 (2002).
111. M. Paluš, D. Hartman, J. Hlinka and M. Vejmelka, *Nonlinear Proc. Geoph.* **18**, 751 (2011).
112. A. Zalesky, A. Fornito and E. Bullmore, *NeuroImage* **60**, 2096 (2012).
113. J. Hlinka, D. Hartman and M. Paluš, *Chaos* **22**, 033107 (2012).

VISUALIZING AND QUANTIFYING EEG COMPLEXITY ON THE BASE OF ORDINAL PATTERN DISTRIBUTIONS

K. KELLER*

*Institute of Mathematics, University of Lübeck,
23562 Lübeck, Germany
* E-mail: keller@math.uni-luebeck.de
www.math.uni-luebeck.de/keller*

Ordinal time series analysis which is based on analyzing distributions of ordinal patterns is a new promising approach to the exploration of long and complex time series. This paper reviews applications of this approach to EEG analysis and discusses and illustrates some ideas for visualizing and quantifying EEG complexity. Moreover, the central concept of permutation entropy is considered from the modeling viewpoint.

Keywords: EEG analysis; ordinal time series analysis; permutation entropy.

1. Introduction

Since Bandt and Pompe[5] have introduced the concept of permutation entropy in 2002, it has been applied for analyzing real world data from different fields and there is some increasing effort to understand the nature of this quantity. The approach behind permutation entropy, however, is more general. It is based on determining the distribution of ordinal patterns, which describe the up and down in a time series at the different time points, and on analyzing the obtained distribution. For a general reference, see Amigo.[2]

Although the metrical information is lost by this procedure, there are many advantages like robustness with respect to noise, invariance with respect to monotone scale changes, existence of fast and flexible algorithms and good interpretability of the results. In order to be able to extract enough information from the system behind a time series, it is necessary to have a large number of values in the series. The approach called ordinal time series analysis seems to be well adapted for detecting and analyzing structural and complexity changes. So it is not surprising that it has found some interest in EEG analysis.

For example, in anesthesiology ordinal time series analysis has been applied for detecting and distinguishing different brain states related to anesthesia (Anier et al.,[4] Bretschneider et al.,[8] Jordan et al.,[14] Kortelainen et al.,[22] Li et al.,[23] Li et al.,[25] Nicolaou et al.,[29] Olofsen et al.,[30] Silva et al.[33-35]), and there are similar applications in sleep analysis (Nicolaou and Georgiou[28]) and Alzheimers disease (Morabito[27]). In all these applications permutation entropy has been central. Marvan et al.[26] utilized an ordinal version of recurrence plots for analyzing event related potentials.

An important field of application is data from epileptic patients. The first who discussed permutation entropy in this context was Cao et al.[10] Keller and Lauffer[16] illustrated changes in brain dynamics related to vagus stimulation by permutation entropy, and Faul et al.,[12] Gudmundsson[13] and Jouny and Bergey[15] studied permutation entropy in comparison to other quantities in different contexts. The detection of preictal states and predictability of absence seizures are in the focus of papers by Bruzzo et al.[9] and Li,[24] repectively. Ouyang et al.[31] proposed distinguishing between interictal, preictal and ictal states on the base of a novel ordinal dissimilarity measure.

In this following, we want to discuss ordinal time series analysis from the conceptional viewpoint and want to give some theoretical background and EEG examples illustrating ordinal time series analysis. Special emphasize is put on the theoretical foundation of permutation entropy and its relation to the Kolmogorov-Sinai entropy.

2. Ordinal patterns

In the following $(x_t)_{t \in \mathbb{Z}}$ is a time series of values x_t in the set $\mathbb{R}$ of real numbers. Here the time points t are taken from the set of integers in order to guarantee that each time point has a predecessor, which simplifies the following discussion.

For given $d \in \mathbb{N}$ and $\tau \in \mathbb{N}$ consider the *delay vector* $(x_t, x_{t-\tau}, x_{t-2\tau}, \ldots, x_{t-d\tau})$. By the *ordinal pattern* of *order* d and *delay* τ *at time* t one understands the order type of this delay vector. Originally, it was described by a permutation.

$$(r_0, r_1, r_2, \ldots, r_d)$$

of $\{0, 1, 2, \ldots d\}$ with

$$x_{t-r_0\tau} \geq x_{t-r_1\tau} \geq \ldots \geq x_{t-r_{d-1}\tau} \geq x_{t-r_d\tau} \tag{1}$$

150

and

$$r_{l-1} > r_l \text{ if } x_{t-r_{l-1}\tau} = x_{t-r_l\tau}. \tag{2}$$

Considering t as the 'present' or '0-th past', $t - \tau$ as the '1-st past', ..., and $t - d\tau$ as the 'd-th past', this permutation codes that the value at the 'r_0-th past' is not less than the value at the 'r_1-th past', the value at the 'r_1-th past' is not less than the value at the 'r_2-th past', ..., and the value at the 'r_{d-1}-th past' is not less than the value at the 'r_d-th past', according to (1). In case that there are equal values, (2) ensures uniqueness of the permutation.

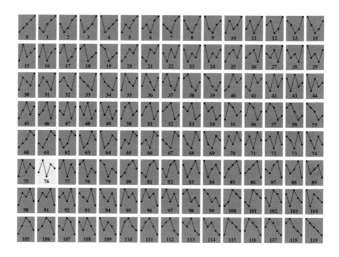

Fig. 1. All $(d+1)! = 120$ ordinal patterns of order $d = 4$

Since there are $(d+1)!$ such permutations (compare Fig. 1), the possible ordinal patterns can be enumerated by $0, 1, 2, \ldots (d+1)! - 1$. Mainly for visualization purposes, we want to use a natural way of enumeration, which is described now. For more details, see Keller et al.[17]

For $l = 1, 2, \ldots, d$, consider the *inversion number*

$$i_l^\tau(t) = \#\{r \in \{0, 1, \ldots, l-1\} \mid x_{t-l\tau} \geq x_{t-r\tau}\} \tag{3}$$

saying how often the value at the l-th past is not less then a value in the delay vector being more in the future.

Then a number $x^*_{d,\tau}(t) \in \{0,1,2,\dots (d+1)! - 1\}$ coding the ordinal pattern of order d and delay τ at time t is given by

$$x^*_{d,\tau}(t) = \sum_{l=1}^{d} i_l \frac{(d+1)!}{(l+1)!}.$$

One easily shows that the obtained numbers are different when corresponding ordinal patterns are different. $x^*_{d,\tau}(t)$ is called *number representation* of the corresponding ordinal pattern.

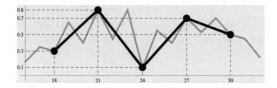

Fig. 2. Ordinal pattern of order 4 and delay 3

Example 2.1. Figure 2 illustrates an ordinal pattern of order $d = 4$ for delay $\tau = 3$ and time $t = 30$. Here the original time series is given in grey and the ordinal pattern in black.

Since $x_{t-\tau} \geq x_t$, one has $i_1 = 1$, since $x_{t-2\tau} < x_{t-\tau}, x_t$, one has $i_2 = 0$, and, since $x_{t-3\tau} \geq x_{t-2\tau}, x_{t-\tau}, x_t$, one has $i_3 = 3$. Moreover, one easily sees that $i_4 = 1$. Therefore,

$$x^*_{d,\tau}(t) = x^*_{4,3}(30) = \sum_{l=1}^{d} i_l \frac{(d+1)!}{(l+1)!} = 1 \cdot \frac{5!}{2!} + 0 \cdot \frac{5!}{3!} + 3 \cdot \frac{5!}{4!} + 1 \cdot \frac{5!}{5!}$$
$$= 76.$$

Note that for fixed $\tau \in \mathbb{N}$, the number $\frac{x^*_{d,\tau}(t)}{(d+1)!}$ is stabilizing for d approaching to infinity, in other words that

$$\lim_{d \to \infty} \frac{x^*_{d,\tau}(t)}{(d+1)!} \text{ exists.}$$

This is interesting for visualizing ordinal pattern distributions. The limit belonging to the interval $[0,1]$ can be considered as (the number representation of) an ordinal pattern of order ∞.

3. Visualization of ordinal pattern distributions

In the following, we want to present some plots for visualizing the ordinal pattern distribution underlying a finite time series $(x_t)_{t=m}^n$ (which one can consider as a part of a time series $(x_t)_{t \in \mathbb{Z}}$). In this context, we also refer to Keller et al.[17]

Two interesting model classes. A simple idea is to utilize the number representation of ordinal patterns for visualizing their distribution. Considering ordinal patterns of some order d, it is useful to divide the obtained numbers by $(d+1)!$ as described at the end of Section 2. Then, for sufficiently large d, the dependence of the obtained plots on d is marginal. (Here $d = 6$ is enough.) First we want to visualize ordinal pattern distributions for two parameter-dependent systems and $\tau = 1$.

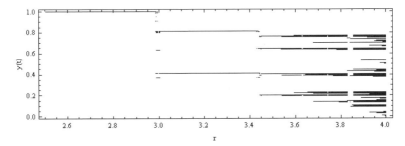

Fig. 3. Ordinal pattern distribution for logistic maps in dependence on the growth factor r

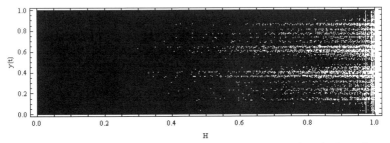

Fig. 4. Ordinal pattern distribution for fractional Brownian motions in dependence on the Hurst parameter H

The first one is the well known family of logistic maps $f_r : [0,1] \to [0,1]$ with $f_r(x) = rx(1-x)$ for $x \in [0,1]$ in dependence on the parameter $r \in$

[2.5, 4] (see Fig. 3). For fixed r, the numbers $y(2001) = \frac{x^*_{6,1}(2001)}{7!}$, $y(2002) = \frac{x^*_{6,1}(2002)}{7!}, \ldots, y(3000) = \frac{x^*_{6,1}(3000)}{7!}$ obtained from the time series $(x_t)^{3000}_{t=0} = (f_r^{\circ t}(x))^{3000}_{t=0}$ are plotted in vertical direction, illustrating the ordinal pattern distribution of a 'typical orbit' of f_r. Here $f_r^{\circ t}(x)$ denotes the t-th iterate of a random value $x \in [0, 1]$. The resulting plot can be considered as an 'ordinal Feigenbaum diagram'.

Fig. 4 shows a similar plot for the family of fractional Brownian motions in dependence on the Hurst parameter H. For $0 < H < 1$, a fractional Brownian motion is a centered real-valued Gaussian stochastic process on $[0, \infty[$ which has covariance function $\frac{1}{2}(s^{2H} + t^{2H} - |t - s|^{2H})$ for $s, t \in [0, \infty[$ and continuous realizations with probability 1 (see e.g. Embrechts and Maejima[11]). For each H, the ordinal pattern distribution of a simulated random realization of length 1000 is plotted in vertical direction. Note that for increasing H the realizations get smoother, which is reflected by a thinner pattern distribution in the picture. Note that for each H the probability for each ordinal pattern is different from 0, but, roughly speaking, in finite parts of realizations of the same length the number of ordinal patterns is decreasing for increasing H.

The two figures illustrate the difference of a deterministic and a stochastic system. Whereas usually in a deterministic systems only a few of ordinal patterns is possible, in the (Gaussian) stochastic system the distribution is extremely rich. This is also interesting in relation to the EEG data which we consider now.

EEG data sets. Figs. 5 and 6 illustrate scalp EEG data of a 36-years-old patient with a brain malformation, which are obtained from The European Epilepsy Database.[39] Data set 1 (Fig. 5) is related to an unclassified seizure during awake state with seizure patterns being rhythmic theta waves, and data set 2 (Fig. 6) is related to a complex partial seizure during awake state with seizure patterns being rhythmic delta waves. The original data recorded from electrode F3 and sampled with 256 Hz are shown at the top of the given figures. In both graphics the duration of the given epileptic seizure is indicated.

Given a long time series, the course of ordinal patterns in their number representation and in dependence of time provides insights into changes of the dynamics of a time series, in particular, when the plot is extremely truncated in the time direction. Corresponding plots for $d = 6$ and $\tau = 4$ are given as ORDINAL PATTERN DISTRIBUTION 1 in Figs. 5 and 6. Here only the occurrence of an ordinal pattern is presented, but not its frequency.

ORDINAL PATTERN DISTRIBUTION 2 presents the relative frequencies. For each time t the ordinal pattern distribution for $d = 3$ and $\tau = 4$ of the time series $x_{t-523} = x_{t-511-d\tau}, x_{t-522}, x_{t-521}, \ldots, x_t$ is considered. Principally, the values taken belong to a window of 2 seconds $= 512$ points, we however have extended the window in left direction by some values, in order to be able to compute the ordinal pattern at the left side. The plot presented shows $23 = 4! - 1$ curves. For fixed time t they divide the vertical interval $[0, 1]$ into subintervals of lengths $p_0, p_1, \ldots, p_{23}$ from above to below standing for the obtained relative frequencies of ordinal patterns $0, 1, \ldots, 23$ in their number representation. In this way local changes of the pattern distribution can be seen. Note that often it is assumed stationarity of an EEG in a period of 2 seconds.

Both ORDINAL PATTERN DISTRIBUTION 1 and ORDINAL PATTERN DISTRIBUTION 2 show that during the considered epileptic seizure and moreover for data set 2 some time interval before the seizure and in some parts after the seizure the concentration of ordinal patterns is higher than at other times. Further, one can see that in particular the patterns 0 and 23 related to monotonically decreasing and increasing delay vectors, respectively, are dominating at the considered times. Also note that ORDINAL PATTERN DISTRIBUTION 1 shows dynamical changes at times not related to the seizures.

Permutation entropy. As already mentioned, the permutation entropy introduced by Bandt and Pompe[5] is the central quantity for measuring complexity on the base of ordinal patterns. In its empirical version for a finite time series $(x_t)_{t=m}^{n}$ (which can be considered as a part of a time series $(x_t)_{t \in \mathbb{Z}}$) it is defined as follows:

The *permutation entropy* of *order d* and delay τ of $(x_t)_{t=m}^{n}$ is

$$h_{d,\tau} = -\sum_{i=0}^{(d+1)!-1} p_i \ln p_i,$$

where p_i is the relative frequency of ordinal patterns i in its number representation among $x_{d,\tau}^*(m + d\tau), x_{d,\tau}^*(m + 1 + d\tau), \ldots, x_{d,\tau}^*(n)$. In Figs. 5 and 6 the empirical permutation entropies related to a time windows of 2 seconds as described above are shown in dependence on time. Clearly, permutation entropy reflects the degree of concentration of ordinal patterns. The higher the concentration is, the lower is the entropy.

Note that a right choice of the parameters d and τ in ordinal time series analysis is a nontrivial problem. It is related to statistical aspect and to the

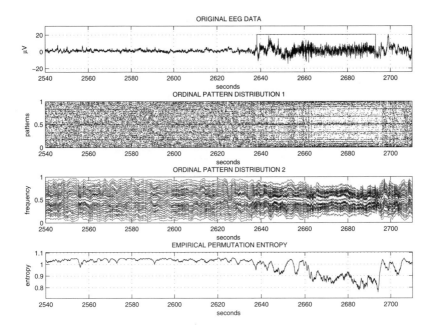

Fig. 5. Visualization of EEG data set 1

question how strong parts of a time series are adapted to ordinal patterns of some special delay, in particular, what periodicities are underlying the data. For a first attempt to tackle the problem, see Staniek and Lehnertz.[36]

4. Modeling

Stochastic Processes. In order to explain ordinal time series analysis from the viewpoint of modeling, let $(\Omega, \mathcal{A}, \mu)$ be a fixed probability space. Here Ω is interpreted as the set of the possible states of a system which are considered to be abstract in a certain sense and not necessarily 'visible' from outside. As usual, $\mathcal{A}$ is a σ-algebra which consist of the events being of interest and μ a probability measure on $\mathcal{A}$. The latter describes the distribution of the states, roughly speaking, it quantifies the chances that one finds the system in a given state.

For modeling measurement processes we consider *observables* X assigning to each state ω a *value* in $\mathbb{R}$, which can be considered as a detail of the state ω getting visible by a measurement. From the mathematical viewpoint, such observables X are random variables on Ω with values in $\mathbb{R}$ (equipped with the Borel sets).

156

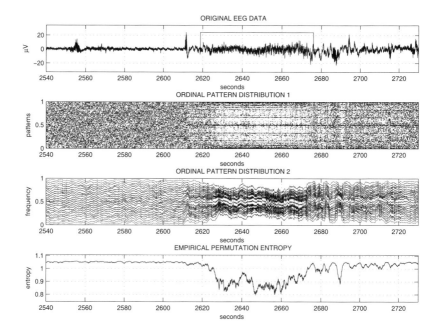

Fig. 6. Visualization of EEG data set 2

Providing an observable X_t for each time $t \in \mathbb{N}$, one gets a *stochastic* process

$$(X_t)_{t \in \mathbb{N}_0},$$

which is *stationary* if the distribution of $(X_{s_1+t}, X_{s_2+t}, \ldots, X_{s_m+t})$ does not depend on $t \in \mathbb{N}_0$ for all $s_1, s_2, \ldots, s_m \in \mathbb{N}_0$.

Determinism and dynamical systems. We are especially interested in the case that the observables X_t are linked in a deterministic way, meaning that there exists an observable X on $(\Omega, \mathcal{A}, \mu)$ and an $\mathcal{A} - \mathcal{A}$-measurable map $T : \Omega \to \Omega$ such that

$$X_t = X \circ T^{\circ t} \text{ for all } t \in \mathbb{N}_0,$$

where $X \circ T^{\circ t}(\omega) = X(\overbrace{T(T(\ldots(T(\omega))\ldots)))}^{t \text{ times}}$.

If conversely $T : \Omega \to \Omega$ is a $\mathcal{A} - \mathcal{A}$-measurable map, then an observable X on Ω defines the stochastic 'measuring' process

$$(X_t)_{t \in \mathbb{N}_0} = (X \circ T^{\circ t})_{t \in \mathbb{N}_0},$$

which is stationary if T is *invariant* with respect to μ, i.e. $\mu(T^{-1}(A)) = \mu(A)$ for all $A \in \mathcal{A}$. This case, in which $(\Omega, \mathcal{A}, \mu, T)$ is called a *measure-preserving dynamical system*, is of some special interest in the following.

5. Symbolic dynamics and measuring complexity

Entropy rate. Many complexity measures for dynamical systems are based on the concept of Shannon entropy, which for a probability space can be defined equivalently on the base of partitions (see e.g. Walters[38]) and finite-valued observables. Here we want to follow the latter approach.

Let $S_1, S_2, \ldots, S_k$ be observables on Ω, such that $S_l(\Omega)$ is contained in a finite set $\mathcal{S}$. Then the diversity of sequences of the k values accessed by the k measurements is quantified on the base of the *Shannon entropy*

$$H_\mu(S_1, S_2, \ldots, S_k) = - \sum_{s_1, s_2, \ldots, s_k \in \mathcal{S}} \mu(S_1 = s_1, S_2 = s_2, \ldots, S_k = s_k)$$
$$\ln \mu(S_1 = s_1, S_2 = s_2, \ldots, S_k = s_k).$$

Such sequences can be considered as words of length k over the *symbol set* $\mathcal{S}$ and so the Shannon entropy can be considered as the corresponding word distribution complexity.

Given a finite-valued observable X on a measure-preserving dynamical system $(\Omega, \mathcal{A}, \mu, T)$, the dynamics induced by T produces a language with 'words' $(X(\omega), X(T(\omega)), X(T^{\circ 2}(\omega)), \ldots, X(T^{\circ t-1}(\omega)))$ of length t over $\mathcal{S} = X(\Omega)$. The distribution of such words gives some insight into the system and its complexity. By the *entropy rate* of T with respect to X one understands the quantity

$$h_\mu(T, X) = \lim_{t \to \infty} \frac{H_\mu(X, X \circ T, X \circ T^{\circ 2}, \ldots, X \circ T^{\circ t-1})}{t}. \tag{4}$$

In the language of information theory, it provides the mean information on the dynamical system per symbol $s \in \mathcal{S}$.

For observables $X_1, X_2, \ldots, X_n$ on $(\Omega, \mathcal{A}, \mu, T)$, let more generally

$$h_\mu(T; X_1, X_2, \ldots, X_N) = \lim_{t \to \infty} \frac{1}{t} H_\mu(X_1, X_1 \circ T, \ldots, X_1 \circ T^{\circ t-1}, \tag{5}$$
$$X_2, X_2 \circ T, \ldots, X_2 \circ T^{\circ t-1}, \ldots$$
$$X_N, X_N \circ T, \ldots, X_N \circ T^{\circ t-1}).$$

$X_1, X_2, \ldots, X_n$ induce a finite partition of the state space Ω, where two states ω, ω' belong to the same part of the partition iff $S_1(\omega) = S_1(\omega'), S_2(\omega) = S_2(\omega'), \ldots, S_k(\omega) = S_k(\omega')$. Note that given T, the quantity h_μ only depends on the partition associated to the observables. Since each finite partition can be reached by a finite-valued observable, (5) produces the same value set as (4) when varying over all possible finite-valued observables.

The Kolmogorov-Sinai entropy. Different finite-valued observables are differently adapted to the dynamics of a system. Therefore, a complete quantification of complexity is given by considering all such variables, leading to the quantity $h_\mu(T)$ of *Kolmogorov-Sinai entropy* (*KS entropy*):

$$h_\mu(T) = \sup_{X \text{ finite-valued observable on } \Omega} h_\mu(T, X) \qquad (6)$$

$$= \sup_{X_1, X_2, \ldots, X_N \text{ finite-valued observables on } \Omega} h_\mu(T; X_1, X_2, \ldots, X_N).$$

A standardized determination of KS entropy. Looking at (6), the question is whether all possible finite-valued observables have to be considered for obtaining the KS entropy, or whether there is a natural choice on which base this can be done. Despite in a few cases there exist so called generating partitions allowing determination of the KS entropy on the base of a single finite-valued observable (see e.g. Walters[38]), finding generating partitions is however highly non-trivial. Keller and Sinn[18-20] have given a characterization of the KS entropy on the base of the ordinal structure of a system, which we describe now.

If X is an observable on $(\Omega, \mathcal{A}, \mu, T)$ and $\omega \in \Omega$, then $(x_t)_{t \in \mathbb{N}_0} = (X(T^{\circ t}(\omega)))_{t \in \mathbb{N}_0}$ is a time series (which for consistence with the presumptions at the beginning of Section 2 can be be considered as a part of a time series $(x_t)_{t \in \mathbb{Z}}$). For $d \in \mathbb{N}$, let

$$X_d^*(\omega) = x_{d,1}^*(t + d)$$

be the corresponding ordinal pattern of order d and delay 1 at time $t + d$. (Here the considered ordinal pattern is assumed to start at time t and to end at time $t + d$ in contrast to Section 2, where the ending time is t. Otherwise, the pattern would not be defined for $t = 0, 1, \ldots, d - 1$. Also note that we restrict to delay 1 here.) The observable $X_d^* : \Omega \to \mathbb{R}$ defined in this way has its values in the ordinal patterns of order d given in their number representation.

The interesting fact is that under relatively weak assumptions on observables $X_1, X_2, \ldots, X_N$ on $(\Omega, \mathcal{A}, \mu, T)$ the following holds:

$$h_\mu(T) = \lim_{d \to \infty} h_\mu(T; (X_1)_d^*, (X_2)_d^*, \ldots, (X_N)_d^*)$$

$$= \sup_{d \in \mathbb{N}} h_\mu(T; (X_1)_d^*, (X_2)_d^*, \ldots, (X_N)_d^*). \qquad (7)$$

Roughly speaking, the KS entropy can be approached by quantifying ordinal pattern distributions.

Some details. Here is some further information for those readers who want to see some mathematical details (compare Ref. 20).

Theorem 5.1. *Let* $(\Omega, \mathbb{B}(\Omega), \mu, T)$ *be a measure-preserving dynamical system, where* Ω *is a Borel subset of* $\mathbb{R}^n$ *for* $n \in \mathbb{N}$. *Further, for* $i = 1, 2, \ldots, N$, *let* X_i *be the ('coordinate') observable defined by* $X_i(x_1, x_2, \ldots, x_N) = x_i$ *for* $(x_1, x_2, \ldots, x_N) \in \Omega$. *Then* (7) *is valid.*

Theorem 5.2. *Let* $(\Omega, \mathbb{B}(\Omega), \mu, T)$ *be a measure-preserving dynamical system, where* Ω *is a compact Hausdorff space. Further, let* $X_1, X_2, \ldots, X_N$ *be continuous observables on* Ω *such that for all* ω, ω' *there exist some* i *with* $X_i(\omega) \neq X_i(\omega')$. *Then* (7) *is valid.*

In many cases one observable is sufficient for determining entropy on the base of (7), which can be shown on the base of embedding theory (see Takens[37] and Sauer et al.[32]). For more details, we refer to Keller.[20]

Permutation entropy. Although the characterization of KS entropy by (7) provides a structural simplification of the KS entropy determination, yet the corresponding approach comes along with a double limit (see (5) and (7)).

An alternative approach for measuring complexity is based on the theoretical (multivariate) analogues of (empirical) permutation entropies and was introduced and discussed by Bandt et al. (see Ref. 5,6) in the case of a one-dimensional dynamical system. Here we give a definition in the language used above.

For observables $X_1, X_2, \ldots, X_N$ on a measure-preserving dynamical system $(\Omega, \mathbb{B}(\Omega), \mu, T)$, let

$$h_\mu^*(T; X_1, X_2, \ldots, X_N) = \limsup_{d \to \infty} \frac{1}{d} H_\mu((X_1)_d^*, (X_2)_d^*, \ldots, (X_N)_d^*).$$

The $H_\mu((X_1)_d^*, (X_2)_d^*, \ldots, (X_N)_d^*)$ are the multivariate theoretical analogues of the empirical permutation entropies of order d and delay τ. The quantity $h_\mu^*(T)$ can be interpreted as the information of ordinal patterns obtained by the observables on the system relative to their order and is called *permutation entropy (rate)*.

Taking equation (7) into account, Kolmogorov-Sinai entropy and the permutation entropy are looking very similar. Actually, Bandt et al.[6] have shown equality of both entropies in a special case. We don't want to go in the detail, but we note that this is the case with T being a piecewise monotone interval map and with only one observable being the identity. (Here Ω is an interval and ordinal patters are directly observed form the points of the interval.) Generally, for observables $X_1, X_2, \ldots, X_N$, the following may be shown:

If (7) is valid, then $h_\mu(T) \leq h_\mu^*(T; X_1, X_2, \ldots, X_N)$.

It is an open problem answering to the question regarding under which general conditions both entropies coincide. In Keller et al.,[21] this problem is discussed from the structural viewpoint. Note that Amigo et al.[1,3] have considered a theoretical version of permutation entropy, which is coinciding with the Kolmogorov-Sinai entropy, but is similarly defined as the latter one since it needs refining partitions or equivalently 'refining' finite-valued observables. From the practical viewpoint, this approach is justified because of the finite precision of computers.

Acknowledgment

The author would like to thank Valentina Unakafova and Anton Unakafov for their contributions to the graphics given in this paper.

References

1. J. M. Amigo, M. B. Kennel and L. Kocarev, *Physica D* **210**, 77 (2005).
2. J.M. Amigo, *Permutation Complexity in Dynamical Systems* (Springer-Verlag, Berlin-Heidelberg, 2010).
3. J.M. Amigo, *Physica D* **241**, 789 (2012).
4. A. Anier, T. Lipping, V. Jantti, P. Puumala, A.M. Huotari., *Entropy of the EEG in transition to burst suppression in deep anesthesia: Surrogate analysis*, in *Conf. Proc. IEEE Eng. Med. Biol. Soc. 2010*, pp. 2790-2793.
5. C. Bandt and B. Pompe, *Phys. Rev. Lett.* **88**, 174102 (2002).
6. C. Bandt, G. Keller and B. Pompe, *Nonlinearity* **15**, 1595 (2002).
7. C. Bandt and F. Shiha, *Journal of Time Series Analysis* **28**, 646 (2007).
8. M. Bretschneider, M. Kreuzer, B. Drexler, H. Hentschke, B. Antkowiak, C. Schwarz, E. Kochs and G. Schneider, *Journal of Neurosurgical Anesthesiology* **18** 309 (2006).
9. A.A. Bruzzo, B. Gesierich, M. Santi, C.A. Tassinari, N. Birbaumer and C.C. Rubboli. *Neurol. Sci.* **29**, 3 (2008).
10. Y. H. Cao, W. W. Tung, J. B. Gao, V. A. Protopopescu and L. M. Hively, *Phys. Rev. E* **70**, 046217 (2004).
11. P. Embrechts and M. Maejima, *Selfsimilar Processes* (Princeton University Press, Princeton and Oxford, 2002).

12. S. Faul, G. Boylan, S. Connolly, W. Marnane and G. Lightbody, *Chaos Theory Analysis of the Newborn EEG: Is it Worth the Wait?*, in *Proc. IEEE Int. Workshop on Intelligent Signal Processing (WISP'05)*, (Faro, Portugal, 2005).
13. S. Gudmundsson, T.P. Runarsson, S.Sigurdsson, G. Eiriksdottir, K. Johnsen, *Clin. Neurophysiol.* **118**, 2162 (2007).
14. D. Jordan D, G. Stockmanns, E.F. Kochs, S. Pilge and G. Schneider, *Anesthesiology* **109**, 1014 (2008).
15. C.C. Jouny and G.K. Bergey, *Clin. Neurophysiol.* **123**, 658 (2012).
16. K. Keller and H. Lauffer, *Int. J. Bifurcation Chaos* **13**, 2657 (2003).
17. K. Keller, M. Sinn and J. Emonds, *Stoch. Dyn.* **7**, 247 (2007).
18. K. Keller and M. Sinn, *Nonlinearity* **22**, 2417 (2009).
19. K. Keller and M. Sinn, *Physica D* **239**, 997 (2010).
20. K. Keller, *Discrete and Continuous Dynamical Systems A* **32**, 891 (2011).
21. K. Keller, A.M. Unakafov, V.A. Unakafova, *Physica D* **241**, 1477 (2012).
22. J. Kortelainen, M. Koskinen, S. Mustola, T. Seppanen, *Effect of remifentanil on the nonlinear electroencephalographic entropy parameters in propofol anesthesia*, in *Conf. Proc. IEEE Eng. Med. Biol. Soc. 2009*, pp. 4994-4997.
23. D. Li, X. Li, Z. Liang, L.J. Voss, J.W. Sleigh, *J. Neural. Eng.* **7**, 046010 (2010).
24. X. Li, G. Ouyang and D. A. Richards, *Epilepsy Research* **77**, 70 (2007).
25. X. Li, S. Cui, L.J. Voss, *Anesthesiology* **109**, 448 (2008).
26. N. Marwan, A. Groth and J. Kurths, *Chaos and Complexity Letters* **2**, 301 (2007).
27. F.C. Morabito, D. Labate, F. La Foresta, A. Bramanti, G. Morabito and I. Palamara, *Entropy* **14**, 1186 (2012).
28. N. Nicolaou and J. Georgiou, *Clin. EEG Neurosci.* **42**, 24 (2011).
29. N. Nicolaou, S. Houris, P. Alexandrou and J. Georgiou, *Entropy measures for discrimination of 'awake' vs 'anaesthetized' state in recovery from general anesthesia*, in *Conf. Proc. IEEE Eng. Med. Biol. Soc. 2011*, pp. 2598-2601.
30. E. Olofsen, J.W. Sleigh, A. Dahan, *Br. J. Anaesth.* **101**, 810 (2008).
31. G. Ouyang, C. Dang, D.A. Richards, X. Li, *Clin. Neurophysiol.* **121**, 694 (2010).
32. T. Sauer, J. Yorke and M. Casdagli, *J. Stat. Phys.* **65**, 579 (1991).
33. A. Silva, H. Cardoso-Cruz, F. Silva, V. Galhardo, L. Antunes, *Anesthesiology* **112**, 255 (2012).
34. A. Silva, S. Campos, J. Monteiro, C. Venâncio, B. Costa, P. Guedes de Pinho, L. Antunes, *Anesthesiology* **115**, 303 (2011).
35. A. Silva, D.A. Ferreira, C. Venâncio, A.P. Souza, L.M. Antunes, *Br. J. Anaesth.* **106**, 540 (2011).
36. M. Staniek and K. Lehnertz, *Int. J. Bifurcation Chaos* **17**, 3729 (2007).
37. F. Takens, *Detecting strange attractors in turbulence*, in *Dynamical Systems and Turbulence*, eds. D.A. Rand and L.S. Young, *Lecture Notes in Mathematics* 898 (Springer-Verlag, Berlin-New York, 1981), pp. 366-381.
38. P. Walters, *An Introduction to Ergodic Theory* (Springer-Verlag, New York, 2000).
39. *http://epilepsy-database.eu*

DYNAMICS OF LINEAR AND NONLINEAR INTERRELATION NETWORKS IN PERI-ICTAL INTRACRANIAL EEG: SEIZURE ONSET AND TERMINATION

C. RUMMEL[1*], M. MÜLLER[2], M. HAUF[1,3], R. WIEST[1] and K. SCHINDLER[4]

[1] *Support Center for Advanced Neuroimaging, University Institute for Diagnostic and Interventional Neuroradiology, Inselspital, Bern University Hospital and University of Bern, Switzerland*
[2] *Facultad de Ciencias, Universidad Autónoma del Estado de Morelos, 62209 Cuernavaca, Morelos, Mexico*
[3] *Klinik Bethesda Tschugg, Switzerland*
[4] *Department of Neurology, Inselspital, Bern University Hospital and University of Bern, Switzerland*
E-mail: crummel@web.de

During epileptic seizures a large number of neurons are recruited into a collective dynamics. Rather than being simply monolithic "hyper-synchronous states" seizures show a complex and often patient specific evolution in multichannel EEG. Here, we summarize recent approaches to a multivariate description of the whole interacting network by diagonalization of interrelation matrices. Equal-time cross-correlation and mutual information are used to estimate linear and nonlinear interrelations and appropriate surrogates are employed for hypothesis testing.

It has been found that focal onset seizures stop after an increase of cross-correlation on the largest spatial scale accessible by intracranial EEG. On smaller scales a pronounced rearrangement of correlation patterns is observed during seizures. Ictogenic brain tissue may differ from the non-ictogenic one with respect to its degree of significantly nonlinear interrelations that cannot be explained by linear correlation alone. Nonlinear interrelation tends to be higher during seizures than inter-ictally.

We conclude that multivariate methods and a separation of nonlinear from linear effects may give new insights into spatio-temporal seizure dynamics. These approaches might contribute to a better understanding of seizure generation and termination as well as to a better delineation of ictogenic brain tissue. Thus, they may ultimately be relevant for novel diagnostic and therapeutic approaches.

Keywords: peri-ictal intracranial EEG; linear and nonlinear interrelation; networks; seizure onset; seizure termination.

1. Introduction

Despite considerable effort over the past years, in epileptology the fundamental questions how seizures start, propagate and stop are yet unresolved. Whereas the first question might have implications on early seizure detection and potentially even seizure prediction, the last two are important for intervention and seizure abortion. In diagnosis of epilepsy the electroencephalogram (EEG) remains the key examination. Focal onset seizures typically exhibit strong temporal asymmetry in EEG recordings. Epileptiform activity starts in only a few contacts (seizure onset zone, SOZ) before it spreads and eventually generalizes. This gradual spreading is contrasted by an often abrupt seizure termination, when epileptiform activity stops in all EEG channels at the same time. It is still unclear how complex systems as the human brain communicate to spontaneously achieve a synchronous signal change in all channels. As an example we show an intracranial EEG (iEEG) recorded from an 18 year old male patient suffering from temporal lobe epilepsy in Fig. 1. The EEG data was recorded during a seizure of four minutes duration. A single channel shows epileptiform activity already several seconds before generalization (channel 19 from top).

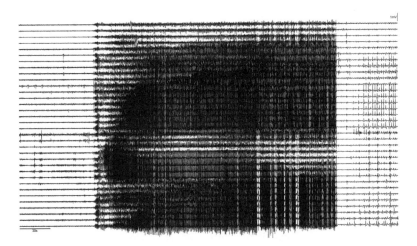

Fig. 1. Complex partial seizure recorded by iEEG: Pronounced temporal asymmetry between focal onset of seizure activity (channel 19 from top) and "generalized" seizure termination.

Epileptic seizures are commonly understood as monolithic "hypersynchronized" events.[1] The role of synchrony in seizure evolution has not yet been unambiguously described, which is at least partly due to using the same notion of synchrony to describe effects taking place at dramatically different spatial scales.[2] On the smallest scale probed by intracranial EEG (single contact) epileptiform activity is characterized by rapid low-amplitude or slower high-amplitude electrical signals. To generate these EEG signals, synchronous firing of tens of thousands of nearby neurons is required. Also on larger spatial scales, as probed by a set of intracranial or scalp EEG contacts, synchronization phenomena can be observed. However, their temporal and spatial evolution may be different. To better understand these phenomena it is essential to investigate network properties as well as the relation between the whole network and its parts.

2. Seizures and information processing as network phenomena

Another characteristic of epileptic seizures is that normal information processing is affected. Consciousness may be impaired (e.g. in generalized seizures or by defintion in so-called complex partial seizures) or may be preserved (e.g. in simple partial seizures). Importantly, impairment of consciousness can occur even during partial seizures where electrographic seizure activity remains confined to the temporal lobes. To explain these differences Englot and Blumenfeld have formulated the so-called "network inhibition hypothesis".[3] In the non-seizure state, the upper brainstem diencephalic systems activate the cerebral cortex, which maintains consciousness and enables normal information processing. Seizures starting in the mesial temporal lobe may occur without impairment of consciousness (simple partial seizures) if they remain mesial and unilateral. If, however, the seizure propagates to the ipsilateral lateral temporal lobe and finally to the contralateral temporal lobe, the activating functions of subcortical structures may be disrupted. As a result activity in bilateral frontoparietal association cortex is suppressed, leading to loss of consciousness in complex partial seizures.

A general observation in various states of impaired information processing and consciousness like seizures but also deep sleep, coma and deep anaesthesia is the presence of slow waves, especially in frontoparietal cortex. In all these conditions the brain continues being active; it is sensitive and even responsive to inputs. Rather than a simple cessation of activity, it is conjectured that information processing and consciousness themselves – as well as their impairment – are network phenomena.[4] Tononi and Massimini for example conclude that "what is critical for consciousness is not firing rates, sensory input or synchronization per se, but rather the ability of a system to integrate information".[5] It has been reported recently, that the degree of loss of consciousness in parietal seizures is associated with increased nonlinear correlation between brain regions.[6]

The brain is a complex system operating at a delicate balance between segregation and integration of information. Different input and information is processed in anatomically distinct areas (= segregation, specialization) but information must also be effectively shared among the segregated areas (= information integration). Many approaches of network analysis have been developed recently accounting for the fact that the whole system may exhibit more complex behavior than the sum of its isolated parts. We here review aspects of two approaches to quantify network effects. The first is through Graph Theory[7–9] and the second is multivariate analysis of inter-relation matrices via decomposition into eigenvalues and eigenvectors as motivated by Principal Component Analysis (PCA[10]) or Random Matrix Theory (RMT[11,12]).

3. Graph theoretical approaches

A time resolved, graph theoretical approach to epileptic seizures as recorded with iEEG has been made by Schindler et al.[13] Based on thresholding of finite-lag cross-correlation matrices that ensured connected graphs, they found a peri-ictal evolution from more random towards more regular and then back to more random network configurations. In addition, an ictal increase of synchronizability – defined as the stability of the globally synchronized state – was observed. It was conjectured that the higher synchronizability of random networks could promote seizure termination by simultanously overloading the network hubs and thereby stop the propagation of seizure activity.

Kramer et al.[14] conducted a similar study using a bootstrap approach to assess significance of links of iEEG networks.[15] They found ictal fragmentation of the network as manifested by an increased number of components. Towards seizure termination the fragments coalesced and the major component of the functional network acquired a considerable part of the nodes (> 60%). At the same time number and size of smaller components as well as the number of independent nodes decreased. The authors summarized that "... at the macroscopic spatial scale, epilepsy is not so much a manifestation of hypersynchrony but instead of network reorganization".[14] Fragmentation and decorrelation of iEEG signals during seizure are also in good agreement with previous studies[16–18] and so is formation of strong correlation before seizure termination.[18,19]

Applying similar surrogate based methods[20] to scalp EEG revealed different network evolution. Group results for twelve focal onset seizures of five patients suffering from temporal lobe epilepsy (see 21 for details) showed a decreasing fraction P_0 of significant links (left panel of Fig. 2) in the ictal and early post-ictal period. Several minutes after seizure termination P_0 moved back towards the pre-ictal situation. An opposite dynamics was observed for the average absolute strength $\langle |\mathrm{CCS}_{ij}| \rangle$ of the retained links, which increased in the early post-ictal phase (right panel of Fig. 2). In contrast to iEEG findings the dynamical rearrangement of scalp EEG networks is consistent with a network fragmentation immediately after seizure termination.

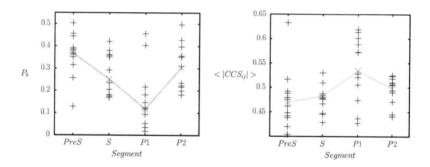

Fig. 2. Peri-ictal evolution of the fraction of significant links (left) and the average absolute strength of the retained links (right) in scalp EEG networks. The segments are pre-ictal (PreS), ictal (S), early post-ictal (P1) and late post-ictal (P2). Black pluses (+) denote the average over these phases for individual seizures, while grey crosses (x) connected by lines denote the median over all seizures.

4. Approaches based on matrix decomposition

Another multivariate approach to network phenomena is based on the decomposition of interrelation matrices by diagonalization. Symmetric matrices of dimension M yield M real eigenvalues λ_l (which can be given an order $\lambda_{l+1} \geq \lambda_l$) and corresponding eigenvectors $\mathbf{v}_l$, $(l = 1, \ldots, M)$. In the idealized case of independent systems and an infinite amount of data all eigenvalues are equal: $\lambda_l \equiv 1$. For systems where correlation is dominated by the finite length of available data the eigenvalues are randomly distributed around 1. In contrast, for genuinely interacting systems the largest eigenvalues increase. As the sum is conserved $\sum_l \lambda_l = M$ this must be compensated by a decrease of small eigenvalues ("repulsion"). Using cross-correlation as underlying interrelation measure the eigenvalues are a measure for the explained variance and involvement of data channels can be read off in principle from the eigenvectors. In PCA this is exploited by concentrating on a few largest eigenvalues, whereas in RMT different selection criteria are used, see work by Müller and colleagues[22,23] for a discussion at the example of EEG.

Using the repulsion of eigenvalues of equal-time cross-correlation matrices it has been shown by Schindler et al.[18] that seizures are not monolithic "hyper-synchronous states" but rather exhibit a complex dynamical evolution. Total correlation not sizably increased in the first half of complex partial seizures or even decreased slightly in seizures with secondary generalization. Decorrelation at seizure onset has previously also been found by Wendling et al.[16] as well as by Schiff et al.[17]

Schindler and colleagues in addition analyzed several recordings of status epilepticus (SE) using eigenvalue repulsion.[19] If SE was a hypersynchronous state, the authors expected pronounced eigenvalue repulsion throughout the status. However, they found marked eigenvalue repulsion (i.e. high global correlation) only before and after termination of SE. During SE global correlation was smaller. Correlation increased after application of seizure suppressing drugs. In one case anti-convulsant drugs were unsuccessfully applied several times during several hours (lorazepam and phenytoin), each time leading to a transient correlation increase. Only after application of diazepam correlation started to increase continuously and SE could finally be stopped.

Similar to what we discussed already in the context of graph analysis the finding is different for scalp EEG. Using the eigenvalue based approach Müller and colleagues[21,24] found that the strength of genuine, non-random cross-correlations decreases significantly during seizures and in the immediate post-seizure period for broad band data. The authors concluded that in terms of genuine zero-lag cross-correlations the ictal electrical brain activity as assessed by scalp electrodes shows spatial fragmentation. Apparently this finding is not limited to epileptic seizures. Using an adaption of the method[24] to phase synchronization Lee et al.[25] observed a decrease of genuine, non-random phase synchronization during general anaesthesia.

After discussing examples of global correlation dynamics as assessed by the eigenvalues of cross-correlation matrices we turn to more localized effects, which are reflected by the eigenvector structure. Here we report on findings obtained from the eigenvector $\mathbf{v}_M$ corresponding to the largest eigenvalue λ_M of the equal-time cross-correlation matrix calculated from the first derivatives of ieEG signals ("slope cross-correlation", SCC).[26] As the EEG slope increases both for large amplitudes and high frequencies it has previously been used to objectively define epileptiform activity.[18,27]

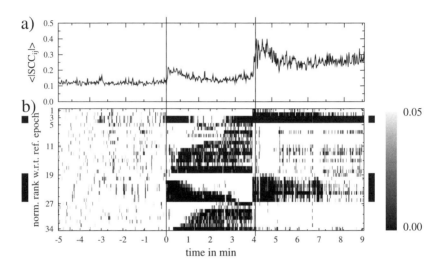

Fig. 3.   Peri-ictal evolution of SCC based quantifiers for the complex partial seizure of Fig. 1. a) Average slope cross-correlation. b) Regional decrease in the contribution of ieEG channels to the eigenvector of the largest eigenvalue is coded in dark. The channel arrangement is identical to Fig. 1. Visually defined seizure onset and termination are marked by vertical lines. The visually defined SOZ is indicated by black bars at the left and right margin of panel b.

In panel a of Fig. 3 the peri-ictal evolution of the average SCC matrix element is shown for the seizure of Fig. 1. At seizure onset the average correlation rises immediately. A second and even more pronounced increase appears at seizure termination, thereby confirming the finding that seizures terminate when the total correlation of the whole system is largest.[18,19] After seizure termination the average correlation starts to decrease slowly. Panel b displays the relative ranking of the contribution v_{iM}^2 of individual ieEG signals "i" to the eigenvector $\mathbf{v}_M$ with respect to a pre-ictal reference epoch of two minutes duration starting five minutes before seizure (zero if the present v_{iM}^2 is smaller than all values in the reference epoch and one if it is larger). Here, dark values indicate that for the corresponding channels large changes occur in the sense that their contribution to the correlation pattern described by $\mathbf{v}_M$ becomes much weaker than in the reference epoch. At seizure onset a pronounced "depletion" of contribution to $\mathbf{v}_M$ occurs for eight out of ten channels that were visually identified as the SOZ (black bars at the figure margins). Post-ictally local SCC eigenvector "depletion" persists and correlates with the SOZ. Based on the abrupt change at seizure onset it was argued by Rummel et al.[26] that the seizure generating brain tissue "decouples" from the collective dynamics and starts to follow independent evolution in time. A similar finding has been made recently by Schindler et al.[28] using symbolic estimators for signal entropy and mutual information.

Finally, we discuss a recent application of the matrix decomposition approach to a family of matrices that is capable of distinguishing between non-random ("genuine") linear correlation between pairs of EEG signals on the one hand and significantly nonlinear[a] interrelation on the other (i.e. pairwise signal associations that cannot be explained by linear correlation alone).[29] As interrelation measures linear equal-time cross-correlation and nonlinear (normalized) mutual information are used. Univariate and multivariate IAAFT surrogates[32] are employed to probe the null hypotheses of entirely random correlation given the power spectra and amplitude distributions of the signals and of entirely linearly correlated data, respectively.

The results for the matrix, which is exclusively sensitive to nonlinear interrelations are shown in Fig. 4 at the example of the EEG of Fig. 1. Before seizure the average significantly nonlinear interrelation coefficient is very small (panel a) and mainly confined to channels of the SOZ (panel b). After seizure onset significantly nonlinear interrelations increase and in the first minute nonlinearities are clearly dominated by the SOZ. After seizure termination significantly nonlinear interrelation is still present, although with reduced strength and without clear spatial pattern. An exception is channel 19 from the top of panel b, which was the first to show epileptiform activity at seizure onset, cf. Fig. 1.

To estimate the agreement between iEEG channels showing nonlinear interrelation and ictogenic brain tissue we applied the method to peri-ictal

---

[a]One has to be aware that strictly speaking these interrelations reject a well defined multivariate null hypothesis, see Rummel et al.[29] for details. Rejection is in general *not* restricted to nonlinear interrelations but can also occur for nonlinear or non-stationary univariate dynamics among others.[30] As Andrzejak et al.[31] have shown recently that these options do not necessarily imply rejection of the multivariate null hypothesis we use the simplified term "significant nonlinearities" here.

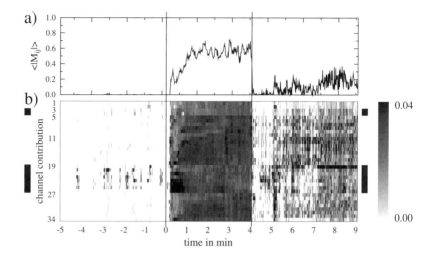

Fig. 4. Peri-ictal evolution of significant nonlinearities for the complex partial seizure of Fig. 1. a) Average significantly nonlinear interrelation. b) Contribution of iEEG channels to a weighted sum of eigenvectors.[29] The channel arrangement is identical to Fig. 1. Visually defined seizure onset and termination are marked by vertical lines. The visually defined SOZ is indicated by black bars at the left and right margin of panel b.

pieces of iEEG containing the first three seizures occurring during intracranial long-term monitoring in a group of five patients suffering from temporal lobe epilepsy (3 males, 2 females, age 18–36 years, epilepsy duration 14–23 years, 4–19 seizures recorded per patient, follow up 1–3 years). All patients became completely seizure free after epilepsy surgery for at least one year. The significance of Pearson correlation between the squared weighted eigenvectors[29] and channels corresponding to resected brain tissue was calculated. Fig. 5 shows that in general, agreement is higher for significantly nonlinear interrelation than for non-random linear correlation. With the exception of patient 4 all patients show significant correlation between contribution to nonlinear interrelation patterns and resected brain tissue in at least one of the four epochs. For non-random correlation significant agreement is found only in patient 1 in the pre-ictal and ictal phase.

5. Discussion

From the network perspective epileptic seizures exhibit a complex temporal evolution. Evaluation of graph and eigenvalue based measures for peri-ictal EEG revealed an apparent contradiction between intracranial (network in-

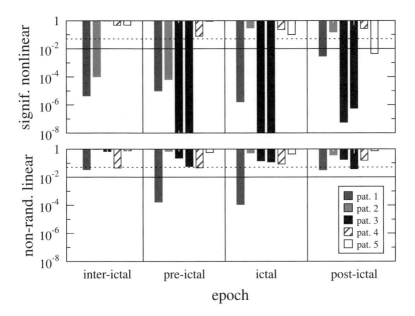

Fig. 5. Patient-wise significances of Pearson correlation between strength of channel contribution to significantly nonlinear interrelation (top) and non-random linear correlation (bottom) and surgical resection area in different epochs of peri-ictal iEEG. For patient 3 seizures starting in the left and the right hemisphere were evaluated separately. The horizontal lines represent the significance levels of $\alpha = 0.01$ (fully drawn) and $\alpha = 0.05$ (dotted), respectively.

tegration at seizure termination,[14,18,19,26] see also Fig. 3a) and scalp data (network fragmentation during seizure and in the early post-ictal phase,[21] see also Fig. 2). The question arises, how this can be explained. There are several possible answers:

(1) The spatial scale of observation is different. While scalp EEG covers a considerable fraction of the brain's surface, iEEG contacts can be implanted only to a limited region of interest, which has been previously defined on clinical grounds. Effects that appear "global" from the perspective of iEEG are indeed only valid locally and what happens in the other parts of the brain escapes from measurement.

(2) The signal quality is different. Intracranial EEG has the important advantage of a much better signal to noise ratio and high spatial resolution (tens of square millimeters as compared to several square centimeters). This may facilitate detection of "genuine", non-random correlations as

defined by Müller and colleagues.[21,24]

(3) The influence of volume conduction is different. It may more strongly confound the interpretation of cross-correlation estimates from scalp EEG than from iEEG.

Whatever the reasons for this difference will turn out to be, it is highly conceivable that there is a late ictal information exchange that allows to coordinate activity on larger spatial scales and which is possibly missed by scalp EEG due to technical issues. Otherwise, it would be hard to explain why electrographical seizure activity often stops synchronously, a finding that is common also for scalp EEG.

Ultimately, graph and matrix diagonalization based approaches to network dynamics might be relevant for novel diagnostic and therapeutic approaches. First, the observed decoupling of the dynamics of the SOZ from the global behavior at seizure onset[26,28] (see Fig. 3b) might turn out to characterize the ictogenic brain regions more objectively than visual iEEG analysis, which is still the gold standard. Second, we found indications that multivariate analysis of matrices containing significantly nonlinear interrelations only[29] might help to characterize epileptogenic brain tissue in terms of eigenvectors, see Fig. 4b. This observation is consistent with previous findings by Andrzejak and colleagues. For univariate analysis of interictal EEG they found that surrogate corrected nonlinear measures outperformed linear and nonlinear measures alone by better lateralizing the ictogenic zone.[33] The same was found for bivariate re-evaluation of the same data.[30] Third, our eigenvector based analyses presented in Figs. 3b, 4b and 5 indicate that the post-ictal phase could potentially be useful for localization of ictogenic tissue. It might turn out that this phase has wrongfully been neglected so far.

Based on recent findings that seizures stop when the total iEEG correlation is large[14,18,19,26] (see Fig. 3a) and that the SOZ ceases to contribute to the global correlation pattern at seizure onset[26,28] (see Fig. 3b) novel concepts for brain stimulation of epilepsy patients become conceivable. For patients with well defined SOZ for whom resective therapy is impossible, speculation about the following approach appears sensible. The global correlation pattern is monitored by the largest eigenvector of the SCC matrix. If the contacts corresponding to the SOZ show eigenvector depletion[26] these brain areas receive electrical feedback from the iEEG signals measured in the rest of the brain. This strategy is supposed to prevent the SOZ from developing its own decoupled dynamics and to increase global correlation.

Whereas this system analysis based paradigm would fail to prevent seizures, it could help to abort them early on.

Interestingly, there is little data about the effects that seizure suppressive drugs have on the scale of larger neuronal networks. Traditionally, these drugs are still categorized according to their main mechanism on the cellular or even molecular level. One refers for example to groups of drugs as "sodium channel blockers" or "GABA agonists" etc. However, it might turn out that the effects these drugs have on network synchronization are at least as important for guiding rational therapy as their characteristics on the more reductionist level. Thus, maybe in the future novel classification systems for drug effects will be established, consisting of classes like "temporal lobe synchronizers".

In conclusion, our findings imply that multivariate methods of signal analysis and a separation of nonlinear from linear EEG chararacteristics may ultimately lead to a better understanding of the pathophysiology of epileptic seizures.

Acknowledgment

This work was supported by Schweizerischer Nationalfonds, Switzerland (projects 320030-122010, 3200B0-1108018 and 33CM30-124089) and Consejo Nacional de Ciencia y Tecnología, Mexico (project 156667).

References

1. W. Penfield and H. Jasper, *Hypersynchrony. Epilepsy and the functional anatomy of the human brain* (Little, Brown and Company, Boston, 1954).
2. M. G. Frei, H. P. Zaveri, S. Arthurs, G. K. Bergey, C. C. Jouny, K. Lehnertz, J. Gotman, I. Osorio, T. I. Netoff, W. J. Freeman, J. Jefferys, G. Worrell, M. Le Van Quyen, S. J. Schiff and F. Mormann, *Epilepsy Behav.* **19**, 4 (2010).
3. D. J. Englot and H. Blumenfeld, *Prog. Brain Res.* **177**, 147 (2009).
4. G. Tononi, *Prog. Brain Res.* **150**, 109 (2005).
5. G. Tononi and M. Massimini, *Ann. N. Y. Acad. Sci.* **1129**, 330 (2008).
6. I. Lambert, M. Arthuis, A. McGonigal, F. Wendling and F. Bartolomei, *Epilepsia* **53**, 2104 (2012).
7. S. Boccaletti, V. Latora, Y. Moreno, M. Chavez and D.-U. Hwang, *Phys. Rep.* **424**, p. 175 (2006).
8. C. J. Stam and J. C. Reijneveld, *Nonlin. Biomed. Phys.* **1**, p. 3 (2007).
9. M. A. Kramer and S. S. Cash, *Neuroscientist* **18**, 360 (2012).
10. I. T. Jolliffe, *Principal Component Analysis* (Springer, Berlin, 1986).
11. T. Brody, J. Flores, J. French, P. Mello, A. Pandey and S. Wong, *Rev. Mod. Phys.* **53**, 385 (1981).

12. T. Guhr, A. Müller-Groeling and H. A. Weidenmüller, *Phys. Rep.* **299**, 189 (1998).
13. K. Schindler, S. Bialonski, M.-T. Hostmann, C. E. Elger and K. Lehnertz, *Chaos* **18**, p. 033119 (2008).
14. M. A. Kramer, U. T. Eden, E. D. Kolaczyk, R. Zepeda, E. N. Eskandar and S. S. Cash, *J. Neurosci.* **30**, 10076 (2010).
15. M. A. Kramer, U. T. Eden, S. S. Cash and E. D. Kolaczyk, *Phys. Rev. E* **79**, p. 061916 (2009).
16. F. Wendling, F. Bartolomei, J. Bellanger, J. Bourien and P. Chauvel, *Brain* **126**, 1449 (2003).
17. S. J. Schiff, T. Sauer, R. Kumar and S. L. Weinstein, *NeuroImage* **28**, 1043 (2005).
18. K. Schindler, H. Leung, C. E. Elger and K. Lehnertz, *Brain* **130**, 65 (2007).
19. K. Schindler, C. E. Elger and K. Lehnertz, *Clin. Neurophysiol.* **118**, 1955 (2007).
20. C. Rummel, M. Müller, G. Baier, F. Amor and K. Schindler, *J. Neurosci. Meth.* **191**, 94 (2010).
21. M. F. Müller, G. Baier, Y. López Jiménez, A. O. Marín García, C. Rummel and K. Schindler, *J. Clin. Neurophysiol.* **28**, 450 (2011).
22. M. Müller, G. Baier, A. Galka, U. Stephani and H. Muhle, *Phys. Rev. E* **71**, p. 046116 (2005).
23. M. Müller, G. Baier, C. Rummel, K. Schindler and U. Stephani, A multivariate approach to correlation analysis based on random matrix theory, in *Seizure Prediction in Epilepsy: From Basic Mechanisms to Clinical Applications*, eds. A. Schulze-Bonhage, J. Timmer and B. Schelter (Wiley, 2008).
24. M. Müller, G. Baier, C. Rummel and K. Schindler, *Eur. Phys. Lett.* **84**, p. 10009 (2008).
25. U. Lee, H. Lee, M. Müller, G.-J. Noh and G. A. Mashour, *PLoS ONE* **7**, p. e46313 (2012).
26. C. Rummel, M. Goodfellow, H. Gast, M. Hauf, F. Amor, A. Stibal, L. Mariani, R. Wiest and K. Schindler, *Neuroinform.* (2012).
27. K. Schindler, R. Wiest, M. Kollar and F. Donati, *Clin. Neurophysiol.* **112**, 1006 (2001).
28. K. Schindler, H. Gast, M. Goodfellow and C. Rummel, *Epilepsia* **53**, 1658 (2012).
29. C. Rummel, E. Abela, M. Müller, M. Hauf, O. Scheidegger, R. Wiest and K. Schindler, *Phys. Rev. E* **83**, p. 066215 (2011).
30. R. G. Andrzejak, D. Chicharro, K. Lehnertz and F. Mormann, *Phys. Rev. E* **83**, p. 046203 (2011).
31. R. G. Andrzejak, K. Schindler and C. Rummel, *Phys. Rev. E* **86**, p. 046206 (2012).
32. T. Schreiber and A. Schmitz, *Physica D* **142**, 346 (2000).
33. R. G. Andrzejak, F. Mormann, G. Widman, T. Kreuz, C. Elger and K. Lehnertz, *Epilepsy Res.* **69**, p. 30 (2006).

ON THE CENTRALITY OF THE FOCUS IN HUMAN EPILEPTIC BRAIN NETWORKS

G. GEIER[1,2,*], M.-T. KUHNERT[1,2,3], C. E. ELGER[1], K. LEHNERTZ[1,2,3]

[1]*Department of Epileptology, University of Bonn,*
Sigmund-Freud-Straße 25, 53105 Bonn, Germany
[2]*Helmholtz-Institute for Radiation and Nuclear Physics, University of Bonn,*
Nussallee 14–16, 53115 Bonn, Germany
[3]*Interdisciplinary Center for Complex Systems, University of Bonn,*
Brühler Straße 7, 53175 Bonn, Germany
E-mail: geier@uni-bonn.de

There is increasing evidence for specific cortical and subcortical large-scale human epileptic networks to be involved in the generation, spread, and termination of not only primary generalized but also focal onset seizures. The complex dynamics of such networks has been studied with methods of analysis from graph theory. In addition to investigating network-specific characteristics, recent studies aim to determine the functional role of single nodes—such as the epileptic focus—in epileptic brain networks and their relationship to ictogenesis. Utilizing the concept of betweenness centrality to assess the importance of network nodes, previous studies reported the epileptic focus to be of highest importance prior to seizures, which would support the notion of a network hub that facilitates seizure activity. We performed a time-resolved analysis of various aspects of node importance in epileptic brain networks derived from long-term, multi-channel, intracranial electroencephalographic recordings from an epilepsy patient. Our preliminary findings indicate that the epileptic focus is not consistently the most important network node, but node importance may drastically vary over time.

Keywords: Centrality; Epileptic Focus; Epileptic Brain Network; Complex Networks.

1. Introduction

Over the last decade network analysis has proven to be an invaluable tool to advance our understanding of complex dynamical systems in diverse scientific fields[1-7] including the neurosciences.[8-11] Specific aspects of functional brain networks—with nodes that are usually associated with sensors capturing the dynamics of different brain regions and with links representing interactions[12-19] between pairs of brain regions—were reported to differ between epilepsy patients and healthy controls[20–22] which supports the concept of an epileptic network.[23–27] Moreover, epileptic networks during generalized and focal seizures (including status epilepticus) were shown to possess topologies that differ from those during the seizure-free interval.[28–36] Most of the aforementioned studies investigated network-specific characteristics such as the average shortest path length or the clustering coefficient. Network theory, however, also provides concepts and tools to assess various aspects of importance (e.g. centralities) of a node in a network,[37–41] but by now, there are only a few studies that investigated node-specific characteristics of epileptic networks,[42–44] and these studies investigated the dynamics of functional brain networks during seizures only. Refs. 43 and 44 reported on highest centrality values for the (clinically defined) epileptic focus which would support the notion of a crucial network node that facilitates seizure activity.

We here report preliminary findings obtained from a time-resolved analysis of node importance in functional brain networks derived from long-term, multi-channel, intracranial electroencephalographic (iEEG) recordings from an epilepsy patient. Investigating various centrality aspects, we provide first evidence that the epileptic focus is not consistently the most important node (i.e., with highest centrality), but node importance may drastically vary over time.

2. Methods

2.1. *Inferring Weighted Functional Networks*

We analyzed iEEG data from a patient who underwent presurgical evaluation of drug-resistant epilepsy of left mesial-temporal origin and who is completely seizure free after selective amygdalohippocampectomy. The patient had signed informed consent that the clinical data might be used and published for research purposes. The study protocol had previously been approved by the local ethics committee. iEEG was recorded from $N = 60$ channels (chronically implanted intrahippocampal depth and subdural grid and strip electrodes) and the total recording time amounted to about 1.7 days, during which three seizures were observed. iEEG data were sampled at $200\,\mathrm{Hz}$ using a 16 bit analog-to-digital converter, filtered within a frequency band of 0.1–$70\,\mathrm{Hz}$, and referenced against the average of two recording contacts outside the focal region.

Following previous studies[21,22,33,41] we associated each recording site with a network node and defined functional network links between any pair of nodes j and k—regardless of their anatomical connectivity—using the mean phase coherence $R_{j,k}$ as a measure for signal interdependencies.[45] We used a sliding window approach with non-overlapping windows of $M = 4096$ data points (duration: 20.48 s) each to estimate $R_{j,k}$ in a time-resolved fashion, employing the Hilbert transform to extract the phases Φ from the windowed iEEG. The elements of the interdependence matrix $\mathbf{I}$ then read:

$$R_{jk} = \left| \left(\frac{1}{M} \sum_{m=0}^{M-1} \exp i \left(\Phi_j(m) - \Phi_k(m) \right) \right) \right|. \tag{1}$$

In order to derive an adjacency matrix $\mathbf{A}$ from $\mathbf{I}$ (i.e, an undirected, weighted functional network) and to account for the case that the centrality metrics could reflect trivial properties of the weight collection[46] we sort $\{R_{jk} \mid j < k\}$ in ascending order and denote with v_{jk} the position of R_{jk} in this order (rank). We then consider $A_{jk} = 2v_{jk}/(N(N-1))$, $j \neq k$, and $A_{jj} = 0$. This approach leads to a weight collection with entries being uniformly distributed in the interval $[0, 1]$.

2.2. *Estimating Centrality*

The importance of a network node may be assessed via centrality metrics.[37–40] Degree, closeness, and betweenness centrality are frequently used for network analyses, and for these metrics generalizations to weighted networks have been proposed (see Ref. 41 for an overview).

If a node is adjacent to many other nodes, it possesses a high degree centrality. When investigating weighted networks, however, the number of neighboring nodes is not a sensible measure and one may consider *strength centrality* of node j instead[47]

$$\mathcal{C}^S(j) = \frac{\sum_k a_{jk}}{N-1}. \tag{2}$$

Assessing node importance in weighted networks via closeness and betweenness centrality requires the definition of shortest paths. This can be achieved by assuming the "length" of a link to vary inversely with its weight.[48] The *closeness centrality* of node j is defined as

$$\mathcal{C}^C(j) = \frac{N-1}{\sum_k d_{jk}}, \tag{3}$$

where d_{jk} denotes the length of the shortest path from node j to node k.

The *betweenness centrality* of node j is the fraction of shortest paths running through that node.

$$C^B(j) = \frac{2}{(N-1)(N-2)} \sum_{h=0}^{N} \sum_{\substack{k=0 \\ k \neq j}}^{N} \frac{\eta_{hk}(j)}{\eta_{hk}}. \quad (4)$$

Here, $\eta_{hk}(j)$ denotes the number of shortest paths between nodes h and k running through node j, and η_{hk} is the total number of shortest paths between nodes h and k. We used the algorithm proposed by Brandes[49] to estimate the aforementioned centralities. Fig. 1 illustrates the centrality metrics C^S, C^C, and C^B for the nodes of an exemplary network.

3. Results

In Figs. 2, 3, and 4 we show the temporal evolutions of C^S, C^C and C^B over 41 h for three selected nodes from the exemplary epileptic brain networks investigated here. We chose one node from within the epileptic focus (upper plots of figures), another node from the immediate surrounding of the epileptic focus (middle plots of figures), and a third one which was associated with a recording site far off the epileptic focus (lower plots in figures). All centrality metrics exhibited large fluctuations over time, both on shorter and longer time scales. The temporal evolutions of C^S and C^C were quite similar, while C^B behaved differently from the two other metrics. The similarity between C^S and C^C was to be expected, at least to some degree (see the discussion in Ref. 41), since they characterize the role of a node as a starting or end point of a path. On the other hand, C^B characterizes a node's share of all paths between pairs of nodes that utilize that node.

For this patient, we could not observe any clear cut changes of the centrality metrics prior to seizures that would indicate a preictal state. Moreover, none of the metrics exhibited features in their temporal evolutions that would constantly indicate the network nodes associated with the epileptic focus (or its immediate neighborhood) as important nodes. Rather, their importance may drastically vary over time.

To demonstrate that our exemplary results hold for all nodes of the epileptic brain networks investigated here, we show, in Fig. 5, findings obtained from an exploratory data analysis. The main statistical characteristics of centralities of each node (maximum and minimum value, the median, and the quartiles estimated from the respective temporal evolutions) indicated that neither the epileptic focus nor its immediate surrounding can be

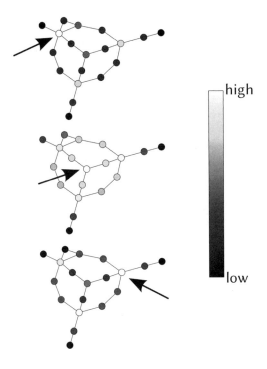

Fig. 1.   Values of degree centrality (top), closeness centrality (middle) and betweenness centrality (bottom) for nodes of an exemplary binary network. The most important node (highest centrality) is indicated by an arrow.

considered as important, and that the different centrality metrics ranked different nodes as most important.

4. Conclusion

We have investigated various aspects of centrality of individual nodes in epileptic brain networks derived from long-term, multi-channel iEEG recordings from an epilepsy patient. Utilizing different centrality metrics, we observed nodes far from the clinically defined epileptic focus and its immediate surrounding to be the most important ones. Although our findings must, at present, be regarded as preliminary, they are nevertheless in stark contrast to previous studies[43,44] that reported highest node centralities for the epileptic focus only. It remains to be investigated whether the different findings can be attributed to the dynamics of different epileptic brains or

180

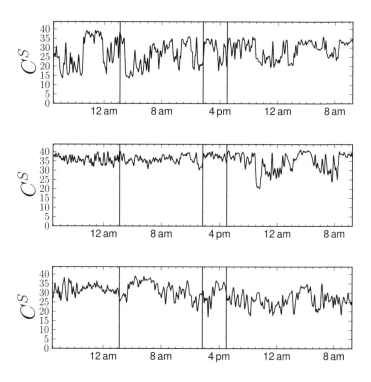

Fig. 2. Temporal evolution of strength centrality for a node located within the clinically defined epileptic focus (top), for a node located in its immediate surrounding (middle), and for a distant node (bottom). Recording time was 41 h, during which three seizures occurred. Moving average over 4096 windows corresponding to 20.48 s. Black vertical lines mark the times of electrical seizure onsets. For legibility, all curves were smoothed using a Gaussian kernel ($\sigma = 5$ min).

to, e.g., differences in network inference. One also needs to take into account that there are a number of potentially confounding variables whose impact on estimates of different centrality metrics is still poorly understood.

Acknowledgments

This work was supported by the Deutsche Forschungsgemeinschaft (Grant No. LE660/4-2).

References

1. S. H. Strogatz, *Nature* **410**, 268 (2001).

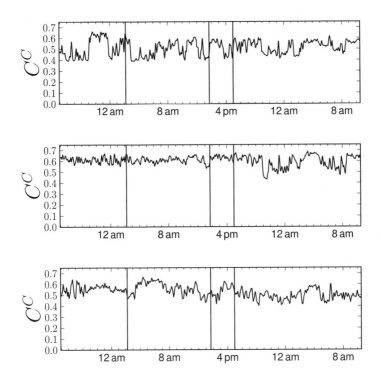

Fig. 3.　Same as Fig. 2 but for closeness centrality.

2. R. Albert and A.-L. Barabási, *Rev. Mod. Phys.* **74**, 47 (2002).
3. M. E. J. Newman, *SIAM Rev.* **45**, 167 (2003).
4. S. Boccaletti, V. Latora, Y. Moreno, M. Chavez and D.-U. Hwang, *Phys. Rep.* **424**, 175 (2006).
5. A. Arenas, A. Díaz-Guilera, J. Kurths, Y. Moreno and C. Zhou, *Phys. Rep.* **469**, 93 (2008).
6. S. Fortunato, *Phys. Rep.* **486**, 75 (2010).
7. M. E. J. Newman, *Nat. Phys.* **8**, 25 (2012).
8. J. C. Reijneveld, S. C. Ponten, H. W. Berendse and C. J. Stam, *Clin. Neurophysiol.* **118**, 2317 (2007).
9. E. Bullmore and O. Sporns, *Nat. Rev. Neurosci.* **10**, 186 (2009).
10. O. Sporns, *Networks of the Brain* (MIT Press, Cambridge, Massachusetts, 2011).
11. C. J. Stam and E. C. W. van Straaten, *NeuroImage* **62**, 1415 (2012).

182

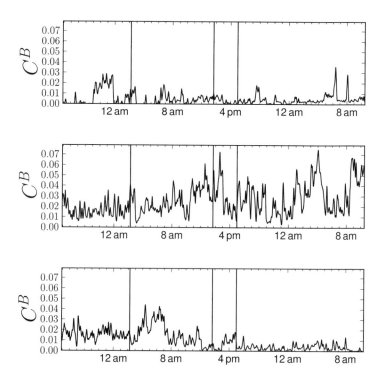

Fig. 4.   Same as Fig. 2 but for betweenness centrality.

12. A. S. Pikovsky, M. G. Rosenblum and J. Kurths, *Synchronization: A universal concept in nonlinear sciences* (Cambridge University Press, Cambridge, UK, 2001).
13. H. Kantz and T. Schreiber, *Nonlinear Time Series Analysis*, 2nd edn. (Cambridge University Press, Cambridge, UK, 2003).
14. E. Pereda, R. Quian Quiroga and J. Bhattacharya, *Prog. Neurobiol.* **77**, 1 (2005).
15. K. Hlaváčková-Schindler, M. Paluš, M. Vejmelka and J. Bhattacharya, *Phys. Rep.* **441**, 1 (2007).
16. N. Marwan, M. C. Romano, M. Thiel and J. Kurths, *Phys. Rep.* **438**, 237 (2007).
17. K. Lehnertz, S. Bialonski, M.-T. Horstmann, D. Krug, A. Rothkegel, M. Staniek and T. Wagner, *J. Neurosci. Methods* **183**, 42 (2009).
18. R. Friedrich, J. Peinke, M. Sahimi and M. R. R. Tabar, *Phys. Rep.* **506**, 87 (2011).

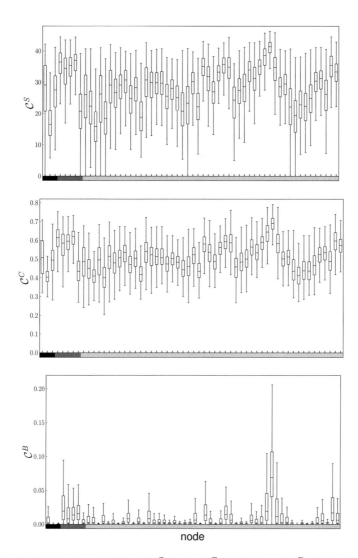

Fig. 5. Statistical characteristics of $\mathcal{C}^S$ (top) , $\mathcal{C}^C$ (middle), and $\mathcal{C}^B$ (bottom) of each node depicted as boxplot. Dashed error bars extend from the sample minimum to the sample maximum. Bottom and top of a box are the lower and upper quartile, and the vertical line in the box denotes the median. The black bar on the abscissa indicates nodes associated with the clinically defined epileptic focus, the grey bar indicates nodes associated with the immediate surrounding of the epileptic focus, and the white bar indicates distant nodes.

19. K. Lehnertz, D. Krug, M. Staniek, D. Glüsenkamp and C. E. Elger, Preictal directed interactions in epileptic brain networks, in *Epilepsy: The Intersection of Neurosciences, Biology, Mathematics, Engineering and Physics*, eds. I. Osorio, H. Zaveri, M. Frei and S. Arthurs (CRC Press, Boca Raton, FL, 2011) pp. 265–272.

20. M. Chavez, M. Valencia, V. Navarro, V. Latora and J. Martinerie, *Phys. Rev. Lett.* **104**, 118701 (2010).

21. M.-T. Horstmann, S. Bialonski, N. Noennig, H. Mai, J. Prusseit, J. Wellmer, H. Hinrichs and K. Lehnertz, *Clin. Neurophysiol.* **121**, 172 (2010).

22. G. Ansmann and K. Lehnertz, *J. Neurosci. Methods* **208**, 165 (2012).

23. E. H. Bertram, D. X. Zhang, P. Mangan, N. Fountain and D. Rempe, *Epilepsy Res.* **32**, 194 (1998).

24. A. Bragin, C. L. Wilson and J. Engel Jr, *Epilepsia* **41(Suppl.6)**, S144 (2000).

25. S. S. Spencer, *Epilepsia* **43**, 219 (2002).

26. L. Lemieux, J. Daunizeau and M. C. Walker, *Front. Syst. Neurosci.* **5**, 12 (2011).

27. A. T. Berg and I. E. Scheffer, *Epilepsia* **52**, 1058 (2011).

28. S. C. Ponten, F. Bartolomei and C. J. Stam, *Clin. Neurophysiol.* **118**, 918 (2007).

29. K. Schindler, S. Bialonski, M.-T. Horstmann, C. E. Elger and K. Lehnertz, *Chaos* **18**, 033119 (2008).

30. S. C. Ponten, L. Douw, F. Bartolomei, J. C. Reijneveld and C. J. Stam, *Exp. Neurol.* **217**, 197 (2009).

31. E. van Dellen, L. Douw, J. C. Baayen, J. J. Heimans, S. C. Ponten, W. P. Vandertop, D. N. Velis, C. J. Stam and J. C. Reijneveld, *PLoS ONE* **4**, e8081 (2009).

32. M. A. Kramer, U. T. Eden, E. D. Kolaczyk, R. Zepeda, E. N. Eskandar and S. S. Cash, *J. Neurosci.* **30**, 10076 (2010).

33. M.-T. Kuhnert, C. E. Elger and K. Lehnertz, *Chaos* **20**, 043126 (2010).

34. S. Bialonski, M. Wendler and K. Lehnertz, *PLoS ONE* **6**, e22826 (2011).

35. M. A. Kramer, U. T. Eden, K. Q. Lepage, E. D. Kolaczyk, M. T. Bianchi and S. S. Cash, *J. Neurosci.* **31**, 15757 (2011).

36. D. Gupta, P. Ossenblok and G. van Luijtelaar, *Med. Biol. Eng. Comput.* **49**, 555 (2011).

37. L. C. Freeman, *Soc. Networks* **1**, 215 (1979).

38. P. Bonacich, *Am. J. Sociol.* **92**, 1170 (1987).

39. D. Koschützki, K. Lehmann, L. Peeters, S. Richter, D. Tenfelde-Podehl and O. Zlotowski, Centrality indices, in *Network Analysis*, eds. U. Brandes and T. Erlebach, Lecture Notes in Computer Science, Vol. 3418 (Springer, Berlin, Heidelberg, 2005) pp. 16–61.

40. E. Estrada and D. J. Higham, *SIAM Rev.* **52**, 696 (2010).

41. M. Kuhnert, C. Geier, C. E. Elger and K. Lehnertz, *Chaos* **22**, 023142 (2012).

42. M. A. Kramer, E. D. Kolaczyk and H. E. Kirsch, *Epilepsy Res.* **79**, 173 (2008).

43. C. Wilke, G. Worrell and B. He, *Epilepsia* **52**, 84 (2011).

44. G. Varotto, L. Tassi, S. Franceschetti, R. Spreafico and F. Panzica, *NeuroImage* **61**, 591 (2012).
45. F. Mormann, K. Lehnertz, P. David and C. E. Elger, *Physica D* **144**, 358 (2000).
46. G. Ansmann and K. Lehnertz, *Phys. Rev. E* **84**, 026103 (2011).
47. A. Barrat, M. Barthélemy, R. Pastor-Satorras and A. Vespignani, *Proc. Natl. Acad. Sci. U.S.A.* **101**, 3747 (2004).
48. M. E. J. Newman, *Phys. Rev. E* **70**, 056131 (2004).
49. U. Brandes, *J. Math. Sociol.* **25**, 163 (2001).

PRE-SEIZURE STATES IN EPILEPTIC BRAIN NETWORKS: A SURROGATE-ASSISTED, WEIGHTED NETWORK ANALYSIS

G. ANSMANN[1,2,3,*], M.-T. KUHNERT[1,2,3], C. E. ELGER[1], and K. LEHNERTZ[1,2,3]

[1]*Department of Epileptology, University of Bonn,*
Sigmund-Freud-Straße 25, 53105 Bonn, Germany
[2]*Helmholtz Institute for Radiation and Nuclear Physics, University of Bonn,*
Nussallee 14–16, 53115 Bonn, Germany
[3]*Interdisciplinary Center for Complex Systems, University of Bonn,*
Brühler Straße 7, 53175 Bonn, Germany
*E-mail: gansmann@uni-bonn.de

In a previous study,[1] it was shown that fluctuations of characteristics of un-weighted epileptic brain networks could be attributed to daily rhythms, while relevant aspects of the epileptic process contributed only marginally. We here analyze networks derived from long-term intracranial EEG data of epilepsy patients using a weighted network approach. To identify possible confounding effects, we relate the results to those for surrogates of the respective networks. We find that 'plain' as well as surrogate-corrected network characteristics are also dominated by daily rhythms, which obfuscate possible effects of pre-seizure dynamics.

Keywords: Pre-seizure State; Daily Rhythms; Epileptic Network; Network Analysis; iEEG; Surrogate Networks

1. Introduction

In recent years network theory has been applied in various scientific fields,[2–6] amongst others to investigate functional brain networks, in which nodes usually represent brain regions and edges usually represent interactions between these brain regions.[7–10] Research over the past years indicates that both physiological and pathophysiological states of the brain are reflected by topological aspects of functional brain networks.[11–16] Recently, however, various factors that may confound the interpretation of findings from empirical networks in general and functional brain networks in particular have been identified.[1,17–23] For example, characteristics of weighted networks may not reflect the topology of a network, but mainly properties of the weight collection.[22]

In a previous study[1] unweighted functional networks constructed from long-term intracranial EEG (iEEG) recordings were analyzed. The null-model-normalized clustering coefficient and mean shortest path length were found to exhibit strong long-term fluctuations with a timescale of about one day, which dominated fluctuations with a timescale of few hours or shorter. This indicates that unweighted network characteristics are rather affected by daily rhythms and other long-term processes than relevant aspects of the epileptic process which act on timescales of a few hours or shorter. Moreover, only tendencies of a change of network characteristics were observed prior to seizures, which were inconsistent in sign over patients. Due to this, no interpretation concerning possible pre-seizure changes of the functional network was possible.

We here analyze the same data using weighted networks in order to investigate whether long-term fluctuations also confound the investigation of a possible pre-seizure state with this approach and whether new insights into pre-seizure dynamics might be gained. To identify and possibly eliminate some confounding factors, we employ surrogate networks as well as seizure-time surrogates.[24]

2. Methods

2.1. *Acquisition of weighted functional networks*

We analyze data which has already been investigated in an analysis of unweighted networks in Ref. 1. Briefly, from 13 patients undergoing presurgical evaluation, iEEG recordings were taken, each lasting between 90 h and 267 h and containing between three and nine seizures. Recordings were performed with $n = 24$ to $n = 72$ electrodes, with a sampling rate of 200 Hz, a 16 bit ADC, and a bandwidth of 0.1–70 Hz. The patients received different antiepileptic drugs, whose dose was modified during the presurgical evaluation.

The iEEG time series were split into non-overlapping windows of 20.48 s (4096 data points). In the following we describe the steps of analysis for a single time window and therefore do not denote the time dependency to ease notation. For each pair of nodes $(i, j) \in \{1, \ldots, n\}^2$, the mean phase coherence R_{ij} was estimated as a measure for phase synchronization using the Hilbert transform.[25] From the R_{ij} the $n \times n$ weight matrix W of a complete network (i.e., a network in which every edge exists) was computed:

$$W_{ij} = R_{ij}/\bar{R},$$

where $\bar{R}$ denotes the average over all mean phase coherences. For simplicity's sake, we set the diagonal elements W_{ii} to 0. Note that the W_{ij} are normalized such that the average weight of the network is 1, thus eliminating the influence of the total amount of phase synchronization.

2.2. Characterization of networks

As network characteristics we employed the mean weighted clustering coefficient

$$C := \binom{n}{3}^{-1} \sum_{i=1}^{n} \sum_{j=i+1}^{n} \sum_{k=j+1}^{n} \sqrt[3]{W_{ij}W_{jk}W_{ki}},$$

which is identical to the one proposed in Ref. 26, but without a normalization by the maximum edge weight, which may cause this quantity to dominate the clustering coefficient.[22,27]

Furthermore, we investigated the mean shortest path length L, using $d_{ij} := W_{ij}^{-1}$ as length of the edge between nodes i and j (and $d_{ij} := \infty$, if $W_{ij} = 0$):

$$L := \binom{n}{2}^{-1} \sum_{i=1}^{n} \sum_{j=1}^{i-1} \min_{l} \min_{P \in \mathcal{P}_{ij}^{l}} \sum_{k=1}^{l-1} d_{P_k P_{k+1}}, \tag{1}$$

where $\mathcal{P}_{ij}^{l} := \left\{ P \in \{1,\dots,n\}^{l} \,\middle|\, P_1 = i, P_l = j \right\}$.

To detect and eliminate confounding influences and to avoid misinterpretations, we also took into account the values of C and L for surrogate networks: For each network, we generated a collection $\mathfrak{S}$ of 4096 surrogate networks that preserve the strength sequence[22] and a collection $\mathfrak{W}$ of 4096 surrogate networks that preserve the weight collection.[28]

Using the steps of analysis as described above, we calculated the following network characteristics for each time window: C, L, $\overline{C(\mathfrak{S})}$, $\overline{C(\mathfrak{W})}$, $\overline{L(\mathfrak{S})}$, and $\overline{L(\mathfrak{W})}$ (considering C and L to be applied element-wise).

3. Results

Since number and locations of implanted electrodes varied over patients and their influence was not accounted for by the applied normalizations and surrogates, it is a priori unclear whether an application of group statistics is justified. Therefore, we here first focus on the results for an exemplary patient (patient 8 in Ref. 1) and then report on their generalizability to other patients.

3.1. *Relation to surrogate networks*

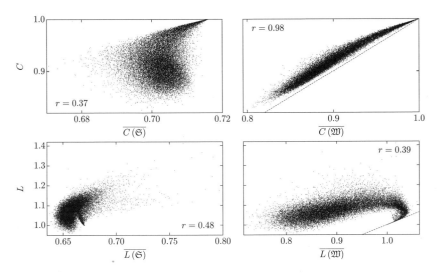

Fig. 1.   Top: Scatter plots of the time-dependent clustering coefficient C of the functional brain networks for an exemplary patient vs. its average over the respective collections of 4096 strength-preserving surrogate networks $(\overline{C\,(\mathfrak{S})}$; left) and 4096 weight-preserving surrogate networks. $(\overline{C\,(\mathfrak{W})}$; right). Bottom: Same for the mean shortest path length L. The dashed lines indicate the identity function and r denotes the Pearson correlation coefficient of the respective data.

In order to decide which surrogate-corrected network characteristics to consider in further steps of analysis, we first performed a preliminary investigation of a possible correlation of the network characteristics C and L between the actual functional brain networks and their respective surrogates.

In Fig. 1 we show scatter plots and the Pearson correlation coefficient r of time-dependent network characteristics C and L between the functional brain networks and the respective surrogates. We observed a strong correlation of the clustering coefficient C between the actual and the weight-preserving surrogate networks $\mathfrak{W}$ ($r = 0.98$, see also Fig. 2). This indicates that C mainly reflects properties of the weight collection, which confirms our previous findings for scalp EEG recordings.[22,27] Whereas in these studies we observed L to be strongly correlated to $\overline{L\,(\mathfrak{W})}$ and not correlated to $\overline{L\,(\mathfrak{S})}$, we here observed L to be moderately correlated to $\overline{L\,(\mathfrak{W})}$ ($r = 0.39$) as well as to $\overline{L\,(\mathfrak{S})}$ ($r = 0.48$, see also Fig. 2). Therefore, it remains unclear whether a surrogate correction employing $\overline{L\,(\mathfrak{S})}$ or $\overline{L\,(\mathfrak{W})}$—which may help to reduce the confounding influence of properties of the weight collection or strength sequence—is the more appropriate approach and we hence investigate both, $\left(L - \overline{L\left(\mathfrak{S}\right)}\right)/L\left(\mathfrak{S}\right)$ and $\left(L - \overline{L\left(\mathfrak{W}\right)}\right)/L\left(\mathfrak{W}\right)$ in all following steps of analysis, alongside with $\left(C - \overline{C\left(\mathfrak{W}\right)}\right)/C\left(\mathfrak{W}\right)$, C, and L.

3.2. Temporal evolutions of network characteristics

In Fig. 2 we show the temporal evolution of all these characteristics in addition to C and L for both types of surrogate networks. We did not find any of these quantities displaying any obvious prominent features consistently related to seizure onsets. However, we observed hints to long-time correlations in the order of several hours in the temporal evolutions of all quantities.

Because of this and similar observations made in Ref. 1, we investigated estimates of power spectral densities (Lomb–Scargle periodograms[29]) of C, L, $\left(C - \overline{C\left(\mathfrak{W}\right)}\right)/C\left(\mathfrak{W}\right)$, $\left(L - \overline{L\left(\mathfrak{S}\right)}\right)/L\left(\mathfrak{S}\right)$, and $\left(L - \overline{L\left(\mathfrak{W}\right)}\right)/L\left(\mathfrak{W}\right)$ (see Fig. 3). While C, L, and $\left(L - \overline{L\left(\mathfrak{S}\right)}\right)/L\left(\mathfrak{S}\right)$ displayed a dominant peak at a period between 24 h and 48 h, for $\left(C - \overline{C\left(\mathfrak{W}\right)}\right)/C\left(\mathfrak{W}\right)$ and $\left(L - \overline{L\left(\mathfrak{W}\right)}\right)/L\left(\mathfrak{W}\right)$ contributions with such periods were about the same amplitude as those from periods of a few hours. In either case, contributions with periods shorter than one hour were of considerably lower amplitude than those with larger timescales.

This suggests that a large part of temporal changes of the investigated network characteristics has to be attributed to processes acting on timescales of several hours.

3.3. Changes related to a possible pre-seizure state

We also investigated the distributions of C, L, $\left(C - \overline{C\left(\mathfrak{W}\right)}\right)/C\left(\mathfrak{W}\right)$, $\left(L - \overline{L\left(\mathfrak{S}\right)}\right)/L\left(\mathfrak{S}\right)$, and $\left(L - \overline{L\left(\mathfrak{W}\right)}\right)/L\left(\mathfrak{W}\right)$ from pre-seizure and interictal intervals (see Fig. 4). For this purpose we defined pre-seizure intervals to begin 1 h before a seizure, but not before 1 h after the previous seizure (thus omitting parts of intervals before seizures with less than 2 h distance to the previous seizure and completely omitting seizures with less than 1 h distance to the previous seizure). As interictal intervals we regarded all times with more than 1 h of distance in time from any seizure.

We observed C and L to tend to larger values and $\left(L - \overline{L\left(\mathfrak{S}\right)}\right)/L\left(\mathfrak{S}\right)$ to tend to smaller values during pre-seizure intervals. However, neither of these tendencies was prominent, and especially given the aforementioned problems due to long-term correlations, a much better statistics

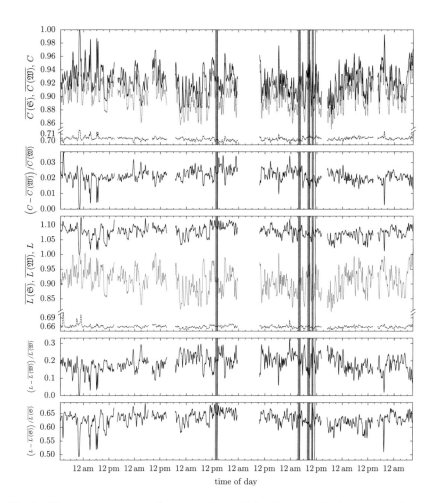

Fig. 2. Temporal evolutions of characteristics of the functional brain networks for an exemplary patient. First row: The clustering coefficient C for the actual networks (solid line) as well as for 4096 weight-preserving surrogate networks (dotted line) and for 4096 strength-preserving surrogate networks (dashed line). Second row: Normalization of C using the weight-preserving surrogate networks $\mathfrak{W}$. Third row: Same as first row for the mean shortest path length L. Fourth row: Normalization of L using the weight-preserving surrogate networks $\mathfrak{W}$. Bottom row: Normalization of L using the strength-preserving surrogate networks $\mathfrak{S}$. For better legibility all time series were smoothed using a Gaussian kernel with $\sigma = 5\,\mathrm{min}$. Solid vertical lines mark electrical seizure onsets, gray areas mark intervals taken into account as pre-seizure periods in further evaluation. Discontinuities in the time series are due to recording gaps.

192

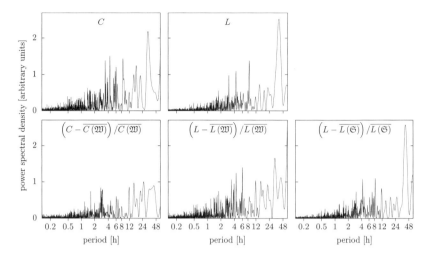

Fig. 3. Power-spectral-density estimates of selected network characteristics for an exemplary patient. Note the logarithmic period axis.

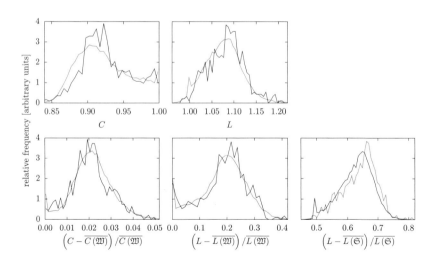

Fig. 4. Frequency distributions of selected network characteristics during interictal (dotted lines) and pre-seizure intervals (solid lines) for an exemplary patient.

(more data) would be needed to draw any meaningful conclusions. For $\left(L - \overline{L\left(\mathfrak{W}\right)}\right)/\overline{L\left(\mathfrak{W}\right)}$ and $\left(C - \overline{C\left(\mathfrak{W}\right)}\right)/\overline{C\left(\mathfrak{W}\right)}$ we did not observe any noteworthy tendencies.

If a statistical test is applied to test whether the collections of the respective characteristic from the pre-seizure and interictal intervals differ, it finds the aforementioned tendencies to be significant (see Table 1). For comparison we generated 100 seizure-time surrogates,[24] preserving only the number of seizures (and not allowing for seizures during recording gaps). For these surrogates, we also obtained significant differences of the investigated characteristics between pre-seizure and interictal intervals in most cases (see Table 1).

Table 1. Probability of a false rejection of the null hypotheses that the distributions from pre-seizure and interictal intervals are equal (Mann–Whitney–Wilcoxon test[30])

	actual data	seizure-time surrogates geometric mean[a]	median
C	$4.8 \cdot 10^{-3}$	$1.4 \cdot 10^{-8}$	$1.5 \cdot 10^{-7}$
$\left(C - \overline{C\left(\mathfrak{W}\right)}\right)/\overline{C\left(\mathfrak{W}\right)}$	$7.7 \cdot 10^{-2}$	$3.8 \cdot 10^{-6}$	$1.9 \cdot 10^{-3}$
L	$1.1 \cdot 10^{-5}$	$1.6 \cdot 10^{-6}$	$2.8 \cdot 10^{-4}$
$\left(L - \overline{L\left(\mathfrak{W}\right)}\right)/\overline{L\left(\mathfrak{W}\right)}$	$2.0 \cdot 10^{-1}$	$1.0 \cdot 10^{-8}$	$3.2 \cdot 10^{-6}$
$\left(L - \overline{L\left(\mathfrak{S}\right)}\right)/\overline{L\left(\mathfrak{S}\right)}$	$2.8 \cdot 10^{-7}$	$7.4 \cdot 10^{-6}$	$1.2 \cdot 10^{-3}$

Note: [a] For calculating the geometric mean, a few results that were zero due to numerical limitations were raised to 10^{-16}.

An explanation for these findings are the observed long-term correlations of the network characteristics: Let us regard m arbitrary pre-seizure 1 h intervals $\{I_1, \ldots, I_m\}$ and denote with L_i the collection of values of a given characteristic for times from I_i. Further, let $\Lambda := \bigcup_{i=1}^{m} L_i$ denote the collection of all values of the given characteristic from all regarded intervals and let $k = |\Lambda|$ denote the number of its elements. Finally, let Ω denote the collection of values of the given characteristics for all investigated time windows. Due to the long-term fluctuations, values in L_i are correlated to each other, since they all depend on the current state of the long-term fluctuations, which changes little during the interval I_i. E.g., the phase of a signal with a 24 h periodicity changes little during 1 h and therefore the values taken from this interval are correlated to each other. When multiple L_i are united to Λ, the aforementioned correlations remain, though their relative impact is diminished with raising m, since there is no correlation between values from different collections L_i (from different intervals).

Therefore the elements of Λ are likely to be correlated to each other more strongly than the elements of Ω. As a result of this, the expected value of $\left|\bar{\Lambda} - \bar{\Omega}\right|$ (the deviation of the mean of Λ from the mean of Ω) is larger than $\left|\bar{\Xi} - \bar{\Omega}\right|$, where Ξ denotes a collection of k randomly picked (and hence uncorrelated) values from Ω. Relatedly, a statistical test is likely to detect a spurious difference between the distributions underlying Λ and Ω if it does (as all tests known to us) not account for a priori correlations of the elements of Λ and Ω. From a slightly different perspective, the statistical test fails because it is assuming k independent samples, while the actual number of independent samples is only m.

This problem may be addressed by considering one value per pre-seizure interval only, e.g., the mean $\overline{L_i}$. As long as only few seizures are taken into account, however, an insightful statistical evaluation remains impossible. In addition, possible relevant details of the pre-seizure distributions may be missed this way.

3.4. Generalizability of results

In this section we report on whether our exemplary results hold for other patients as well as for different pre-seizure times and the alternative normalization of edge weights $W_{ij} = R_{ij} - \bar{R} + 1$ (as used in Ref. 15).

For both normalizations and all patients, we observed a strong correlation between C and $\overline{C\left(\mathfrak{W}\right)}$ ($r = 0.95 \pm 0.04$), which was higher than the correlation between C and $C\left(\mathfrak{S}\right)$ ($r = 0.46 \pm 0.28$). Similar findings were obtained for the mean shortest path length L and the alternative normalization ($r = 0.86 \pm 0.10$ between L and $\overline{L\left(\mathfrak{W}\right)}$ and $r = -0.33 \pm 0.39$ between L and $\overline{L\left(\mathfrak{S}\right)}$), which is also consistent with our previous findings for scalp EEG recordings using this normalization.[22,27] For the original normalization (see Sec. 2.1), however, we did not obtain consistent findings concerning the correlation between L for the actual and for surrogate networks but only a tendency to a correlation between L and $\overline{L\left(\mathfrak{S}\right)}$ ($r = 0.48 \pm 0.33$ between L and $\overline{L\left(\mathfrak{S}\right)}$ and $r = -0.11 \pm 0.35$ between L and $\overline{L\left(\mathfrak{W}\right)}$).

For both normalizations, all patients, and all investigated characteristics, we observed contributions on a timescale between 24 h and 48 h whose intensities were at least of the same level as those of contributions from a timescale of few hours (but higher in most cases) and higher than those of contributions from a timescale shorter than one hour.

Concerning the distinguishability of the pre-seizure interval with the applied network characteristics, we observed comparable results for all patients, i.e., at most non-prominent tendencies. The latter did, however, not have a consistent sign over patients. Comparable observations have been obtained for pre-seizure times of 15 min, 30 min, 2 h, and 4 h (with correspondingly adjusted interictal intervals and numbers of seizures taken into account).

4. Discussion

Concerning the existence of long-term fluctuations, our results are generally comparable to those for unweighted networks, as obtained by Ref. 1: All temporal evolutions of applied network characteristics exhibited long-term fluctuations with a timescale of roughly one day, which had a larger amplitude than contributions with timescales shorter than one hour. This indicates that processes acting on the former timescales, such as daily rhythms or effects of altering antiepileptic-drug doses, affect network characteristics considerably more than processes acting on the latter timescale, such as seizures or possible seizure precursors.

Our results are also comparable to the previous study in terms of the distinguishability of a possible pre-seizure state from interictal states with network characteristics: Between pre-seizure and interictal intervals, at best slight differences of network characteristics could be observed, which were not consistent in sign over patients. However, the observed differences could be fully explained by the aforementioned long-term correlations. We therefore conclude that in order to evaluate the merit of the network approach for seizure prediction, a better understanding of long-term variabilities of network characteristics is necessary, since these variablities obfuscate potential pre-seizure alterations.

Furthermore, we elaborated on how long-term correlations may severely violate the requirements of a statistical test applied to detect a possible pre-seizure state, leading to a spurious success. It is conceivable, that other investigations for a pre-seizure state are similarly affected and consequently misinterpreted, especially if only short-term data is considered, which does not allow for a detection of such long-term fluctuations.

References

1. M.-T. Kuhnert, C. E. Elger and K. Lehnertz, *Chaos* **20**, 043126 (2010).
2. M. E. J. Newman, *SIAM Rev.* **45**, 167 (2003).
3. S. Boccaletti, V. Latora, Y. Moreno, M. Chavez and D.-U. Hwang, *Phys. Rep.* **424**, 175 (2006).
4. J. F. Donges, Y. Zou, N. Marwan and J. Kurths, *Eur. Phys. J.-Spec. Top.* **174**, 157 (2009).

5. A.-L. Barabási, N. Gulbahce and J. Loscalzo, *Nat. Rev. Genet.* **12**, 56 (2011).
6. A. Bashan, R. P. Bartsch, J. W. Kantelhardt, S. Havlin and P. C. Ivanov, *Nat. Commun.* **3**, 702 (2012).
7. J. C. Reijneveld, S. C. Ponten, H. W. Berendse and C. J. Stam, *Clin. Neurophysiol.* **118**, 2317 (2007).
8. E. Bullmore and O. Sporns, *Nat. Rev. Neurosci.* **10**, 186 (2009).
9. O. Sporns, *Networks of the Brain* (MIT Press, Cambridge, Massachusetts, 2011).
10. C. J. Stam and E. C. W. van Straaten, *Clin. Neurophysiol.* **123**, 1067 (2012).
11. M. Rubinov, S. A. Knock, C. J. Stam, S. Micheloyannis, A. W. F. Harris, L. M. Williams and M. Breakspear, *Hum. Brain Mapp.* **30**, 403 (2009).
12. C. J. Stam, W. de Haan, A. Daffertshofer, B. F. Jones, I. Manshanden, A. M. van Cappellen van Walsum, T. Montez, J. P. A. Verbunt, J. C. de Munck, B. W. van Dijk, H. W. Berendse and P. Scheltens, *Brain* **132**, 213 (2009).
13. S. C. Ponten, L. Douw, F. Bartolomei, J. C. Reijneveld and C. J. Stam, *Exp. Neurol.* **217**, 197 (2009).
14. M. Chavez, M. Valencia, V. Navarro, V. Latora and J. Martinerie, *Phys. Rev. Lett.* **104**, 118701 (2010).
15. M.-T. Horstmann, S. Bialonski, N. Noennig, H. Mai, J. Prusseit, J. Wellmer, H. Hinrichs and K. Lehnertz, *Clin. Neurophysiol.* **121**, 172 (2010).
16. L. Wang, C. Yu, H. Chen, W. Qin, Y. He, F. Fan, Y. Zhang, M. Wang, K. Li, Y. Zang, T. S. Woodward and C. Zhu, *Brain* **133**, 1224 (2010).
17. L. Antiqueira, F. A. Rodrigues, B. C. M. van Wijk, L. da F. Costa and A. Daffertshofer, *NeuroImage* **53**, 439 (2010).
18. S. Bialonski, M.-T. Horstmann and K. Lehnertz, *Chaos* **20**, 013134 (2010).
19. A. Zalesky, A. Fornito, I. H. Harding, L. Cocchi, M. Yücel, C. Pantelis and E. T. Bullmore, *NeuroImage* **50**, 970 (2010).
20. S. Bialonski, M. Wendler and K. Lehnertz, *PLoS ONE* **6**, e22826 (2011).
21. F. Gerhard, G. Pipa, B. Lima, S. Neuenschwander and W. Gerstner, *Front. Comput. Neurosci.* **5**, 4 (2011).
22. G. Ansmann and K. Lehnertz, *Phys. Rev. E* **84**, 026103 (2011).
23. S. Bialonski, *arXiv* **1208.0800** (2012).
24. R. G. Andrzejak, F. Mormann, T. Kreuz, C. Rieke, A. Kraskov, C. E. Elger and K. Lehnertz, *Phys. Rev. E* **67**, 010901(R) (2003).
25. F. Mormann, K. Lehnertz, P. David and C. E. Elger, *Physica D* **144**, 358 (2000).
26. J. P. Onnela, J. Saramäki, J. Kertész and K. Kaski, *Phys. Rev. E* **71**, 065103 (2005).
27. G. Ansmann and K. Lehnertz, *J. Neurosci. Methods* **208**, 165 (2012).
28. A. Barrat, M. Barthélemy, R. Pastor-Satorras and A. Vespignani, *Proc. Natl. Acad. Sci. U.S.A.* **101**, 3747 (2004).
29. W. H. Press and G. B. Rybicki, *Astrophys J* **338**, 277 (1989).
30. H. B. Mann and D. R. Whitney, *Ann. Math. Statist.* **18**, 50 (1947).

NETWORK ANALYSIS OF GENERALIZED EPILEPTIC DISCHARGES

P. OSSENBLOK

Dept. Clinical Physics, Kempenhaeghe, P.O. Box 61
Heeze, 5590 AB, The Netherlands

P. VAN HOUDT

Dept. Research and Development, Kempenhaeghe,
Heeze, The Netherlands

A. LÜTTJOHANN

Donders Centre for Cognition, Radboud University
Nijmegen, Nijmegen, The Netherlands

G. VAN LUIJTELAAR

Donders Centre for Cognition, Radboud University
Nijmegen, Nijmegen, The Netherlands

The ultimate goal of network analysis of generalized epilepsy is to get a better understanding of the mechanisms related to the cortico-thalamo-cortical interactions responsible for the bilateral and synchronously occurring Spike-and-Wave Discharges (SWDs), which are so typically for absence seizures. The network analysis results of cortico-thalamic and thalamo-thalamic interactions in the WAG/Rij rat presented here modify the current view in showing that the thalamus is heterogeneous with respect to the dynamics in connectivity with the cortex. Some thalamic nuclei get earlier involved than others and intrathalamic dynamics are involved as well. For the MEG analysis of children with absence epilepsy presented partly the same signal analytical techniques were used as in the WAG/Rij rat studies. Evidence is discussed that these results are reminiscent to what can be observed for absence seizures of the WAG/Rij rat, namely that the pattern of bilateral synchronous generalized activity (during the waves of the SWDs) is occurring via widespread cortico-thalamo-cortical pathways, while there is a cortical source driving these generalized discharges. The methods for network analysis presented to discern the mechanisms generating the SWDs may be of diagnostic help for the clinician.

Keywords: Connectivity; absence epilepsy; spike-and-wave discharges; WAG/Rij rats; depth EEG, MEG; maximal association strength; pairwise phase consistency

Abbreviations: MEG=Magneto-Encephalo-Graphy; EEG=Electro-Encephalo-Graphy; SWDs=Spike-and-Wave Discharges; gSWDs=generalized SWDs; WAG/Rij= Wistar Albino Glaxo from Rijswijk; GAERS=Genetic Absence Epileptic Rats from Strasbourg; (r)(c)RTN= (rostral)(caudal)Reticular Thalamic Nucleus; ctx IV= layer 4 of the somatosensory cortex; ctx V= layer 5 of the somatosensory cortex; ctx VI= layer 6 of the somatosensory cortex; Po= Postero Thalamic nucleus; VPM= Ventral-Postero-Medial Thalamic nucleus; VPL=Ventral-Posteio-Lateral Thalamic nucleus; LD=Lateral-Dorsal Thalamic nucleus; ATN=Anterior Thalamic nucleus; PPC=pairwise phase consistency; EEG-fMRI=combined EEG and fMRI; CAE=Childhood Absence Epilepsy; JAE=Juvenile Absence Epilepsy; BOLD=Blood Oxygenation Level Dependent; ILAE= International League Against Epilepsy; LoC=Local Connectedness; HVHS= Hyposynchronous slowing;

Introduction

The absence seizure with as electroencephalographic hallmark the generalized 3Hz Spike-and-Wave Discharges (SWDs) with an abrupt onset and subsequent bilateral synchronization is often considered the prototypic idiopathic generalized seizure. Experimental evidence that implicates thalamic and thalamo-cortical mechanisms in the pathophysiology of generalized seizures has been offered as an explanation for the apparently "generalized" nature of these SWDs [1]. Based on studies in the feline generalized penicillin model, it was widely assumed that SWDs are generated in the thalamo-cortical circuits mediating sensory processes and consciousness, since thalamic and cortical cells show rhythmic and spike concurrent neuronal firing during cortical SWDs. Others proposed a leading role of the cortex in the initiation of SWDs without a significant role for the thalamus (for review see [2]). Studies in WAG/Rij rats and GAERS, two well validated genetic rat models of absence epilepsy, further challenged the classical theoretical point of view. Particularly, the outcome of a nonlinear association analyses of cortical and thalamic spreading of SWDs in WAG/Rij rats has led to a radical new theory for the initiation and generalization of absence seizures [3]. In this theory it is proposed that the somatosensory cortex of the WAG/Rij rats contains a focus that initiates a cascade of events which ultimately lead to the occurrence of generalized SWDs, when the cortico-thalamo-cortical network is in an appropriate state. The independent confirmation of a preferred role of specific parts of the somatosensory cortex with functional MRI (fMRI) in WAG/Rij and GAERS greatly extended the relevance of the cortical focus theory [4-6]. It has been shown, however, that an intact thalamus is necessary for the generation of full blown SWDs, since thalamic lesions affecting the lateral part of the thalamus, including the Reticular Thalamic Nucleus (RTN) were most effective [3]. Overall, these findings indicated that the functional and anatomic integrity of both thalamus and cortex is required for generalized SWDs to occur, and, even more specifically, an intact cortico-thalamo-cortical circuit is imperative for the rhytmogenesis, whereas cortical hyperexcitability is the prerequisite for the generation of the SWDs [7]. In this contribution it will be argued that according to the results presented of a Magneto-Encephalo-Graphy (MEG) study in children it seems likely that thalamo-cortical network interactions during the evolvement of generalized SWDs are imperative as well. The cortico-thalamic and intra-thalamic network analyses in genetic absence rats provides a complementary picture to the studies in patients.

1. Cortical-cortico-thalamic network analysis in a genetic model

Only a few studies have investigated the interactions between cortex and thalamus before and during SWD onset in the genetic models. Nonlinear association analysis on local field potential recordings from an epidural cortical grid and Ventro-Postero-Medial (VPM), Ventro-Postero-Lateral (VPL) and Lateral-Dorsal (LD) thalamic nucleus showed that (1) the start of SWDs was associated with an increase in association strength between an identified cortical focus and other cortical and thalamic sites, and (2) that the cortex led the thalamus during the first 500ms of a SWD [3].

SWDs arise in the subgranual layers of the somatosensory cortex and from there they quickly spread over the cortex and to the thalamus [8]. The RTN is driven/activated via cortico-thalamic pathways, the thalamo-cortical neurons are inhibited via intrathalamic pathways [9]. Sitnikova et al. [10] reported sudden and rapid increases in coupling as measured with Granger causality between frontal cortex and VPM at the onset of SWDs and a decrease at the end. Also frequency specific changes in coherence were found for local-cortical, non-local-cortical, thalamo-thalamic and cortico-thalamic networks suggesting that each circuit oscillates in its preferred frequency during SWDs [11]. However, in none of these network studies recording electrodes have targeted the focal epileptic zone in the deep layers of the somatosensory cortex together with multiple thalamic sites. This was recently done by Lüttjohann and van Luijtelaar [12] in a study in which WAG/Rij rats were equipped with multiple electrodes targeting layer IV to VI of the somatosensory-cortex, rostral RTN (rRTN) and caudal RTN (cRTN), VPM, anterior thalamic nucleus (ATN) and posterior (Po) thalamic nucleus. The latter nucleus was chosen since neurons in layer V of the somatosensory cortex have massive reciprocal connection towards the Po, a higher order thalamic nucleus that is thought to be involved in cortico-cortical communication [13].

1.1. *Dynamics of the maximal association strength*

In the study of Lüttjohann and van Luijtelaar [12] the maximal association strength between the signals from all (electrode) sensor combinations was calculated, like in the study of Meeren et al. [3], for preictal to ictal transition periods and in control periods. The dynamics of the maximal association strength showed that as early as 1.25 s prior to the ictal discharges an increase in coupling was found between cortical layer VI and Po, this was followed in time by a decrease in coupling between cRTN and Po, as illustrated in Fig. 1. This decrease reached its maximum at 750 ms prior to onset, and returned to baseline level at around 250 ms before generalized SWDs (gSWD) occurred. Next, maximal association strengths between layer V,VI and Po were found to increase. The vast majority of channel pairs showed an increase in coupling within the time windows from 250 ms prior until 125 ms following gSWDs, including layer VI and VPM (see Fig. 1). The largest increases in maximal association strength were found between all three cortical layers and Po as well as between Po and rRTN; moderate for channel pairs ctx VI-VPM, ctx IV-VPM and Po-ATN; and small for rRTN-cRTN, ATN-rRTN and ATN-cRTN. In addition, most channel pairs reached a plateau in maximal association strength at around 375 ms to 1 s after SWD onset and further remained on this level until the end of the analysis window (3 s after gSWD onset).

1.2. *Dynamics of coupling direction*

The maximal association strength between two signals is calculated as a function of the delay τ, in which one signal is shifted in time with respect to the other. In this way the delay at which the highest association strength is reached gives information on the question whether signal A predicts the future of Signal B (Signal A drives Signal B), whether Signal B predicts the future of Signal A (Signal A drives Signal B), or whether Signal A and Signal B are running equal in time (Signal A and B are driving each other and keep a bidirectional crosstalk).

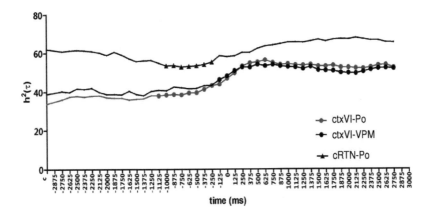

Figure 1. Maximal association strength $h^2(\tau)$ of channel pairs ctx VI-Po, ctx VI-VPM and cRTN-Po during the pre-ictal ictal transition period. Filled circles indicate significantly different values of $h^2(\tau)$ as compared to non-epileptic control periods (first data value indicated by a 'c' on the x-axis). Note that a significant increase in maximal association strength is found much earlier for channel pair ctx VI-Po as compared to ctx VI-VPM. Channel-combination cRTN-Po is the only pair for which a SWD related decrease in $h^2(\tau)$ was found. Abbreviations: c: non-epileptic control period, ctx VI: layer 6 of the somatosensory cortex, Po: Posterior thalamic nucleus, VPM: Ventral-Postero-Medial thalamic nucleus, cRTN: caudal reticular thalamic nucleus.

The dynamics of coupling direction reveal that almost all *cortico-thalamic* channel pairs for which SWD-related increases in maximal association strength have been found showed SWD-related changes in coupling direction. The cortex guided the thalamus in the majority of SWDs for these pairs and this started to occur around SWD onset and lasted only 250 to 750 ms. The only exception was channel pair ctx V-Po, where no change in coupling direction was seen despite increases in maximal association strength. Here cortex and Po kept a bidirectional crosstalk during the complete preictal to ictal transition period.

Some *intra-thalamic* channel pairs showed changes in coupling direction: the cRTN started to guide the rRTN prior to gSWD, and rRTN and ATN increased coupling direction to the Po. Many channel pairs for which no changes in maximal association strength were seen, still did show changes in coupling direction; it seemed that the Po became guided by all other thalamic nuclei except cRTN. Furthermore, the cRTN started to guide the VPM.

The same data set as used for the nonlinear association analysis was used for time-frequency and pairwise phase consistency (PPC) analysis [14]. PPC measures the stability of phase differences between two signals across trials as a function of frequency and can therefore be considered as a measure for network synchronization. Preictally, all channels showed *SWD precursor* activity in the form of an increase in power in the delta and theta frequency range, however channels differed regarding their pattern of maximal preictal power values. The earliest (2 s prior the SWD onset) and most pronounced preictal power was noticed for the deep layers of the somatosensory cortex, with ctx V showing simultaneously delta and theta precursor activity in 75% of the preictal periods. In thalamic recordings, on the other hand, maximal power values started at 0.75 s prior to SWD onset. Preictal delta and theta precursors in frontal cortex and ventral basal part of the thalamus were also described with a rather sensitive method of time frequency analyses, i.e. wavelet decomposition. Here it was found that pre-SWD cortical and thalamic EEG data consisted of delta and theta components in 80-90% of all SWDs; this co-occurrence of delta and theta was rare (7%) during control periods. The delta and theta events in pre-SWDs in the cortex preceded that in the thalamus, as one might have anticipated from a focal region [15].

PPC analysis showed that four of the 35 channel-pairs decreased PPC preictally. In 3 of these 4 cases, the cRTN was involved (Fig. 2). Most channel-pairs showed strong and abrupt increases in PPC at the transition to g SWD, for different and specific frequency bands. The differences in PPC between cortex-Po (range 8-48 Hz) and cortex VPM (12 Hz and its harmonics) is illustrated in Fig. 3. Other cortico-thalamic pairs showed different changes in PPC for different frequencies at SWD onset or during SWDs, suggesting that different cortico-thalamic channel combinations communicate differently with each other.

Intra-thalamic channel-pairs: The two intra-thalamic channel-pairs that showed a decrease in PPC preictally returned to control values around gSWD. An increase in PPC with Po at gSWD was found for all pairs except VPM. The VPM only showed increased PPC values during the ictal period with the three layers of the somatosensory cortex, but not with any other thalamic nucleus. All *cortico-cortical channel-pairs* showed abrupt increases in PPC at gSWD. Most of the changes were for a restricted frequency range. The increases in PPC were maintained until the end of the analysis window.

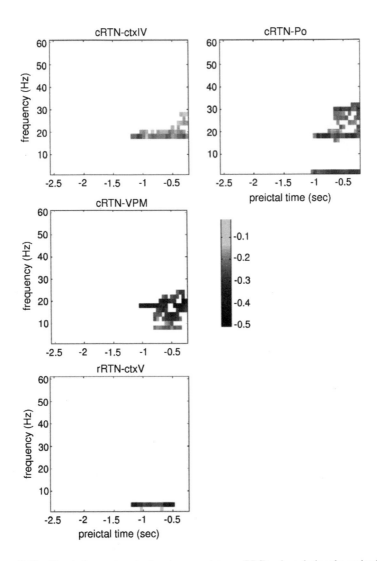

Figure 2. Significant changes in pairwise phase consistency (PPC) values during the preictal period displayed as absolute difference between control, non-epileptic PPC value and preictal PPC value (preictal PPC minus control PPC). Non-significant differences are displayed as a zero (white) difference. Note that in three of the four cases the caudal RTN decouples from a brain-structure of the somatosensory cortico-thalamic loop. Abbreviations: ctx IV: layer 4 of the somatosensory cortex, ctx V: layer 5 of the somatosensory cortex, Po: Posterior thalamic nucleus, VPM: Ventral-Postero-Medial thalamic nucleus, cRTN: caudal Reticular thalamic nucleus, rRTN: rostral Reticular thalamic nucleus.

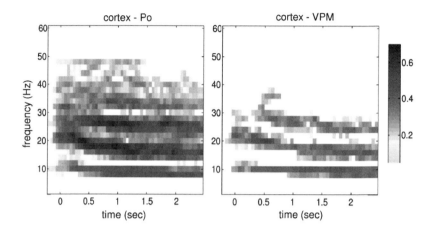

Figure 3.Changes in pairwise phase consistency (PPC) seen during SWD for channel pair ctx IV-Po and ctx V-VPM. Values are displayed as absolute difference between control, non-epileptic PPC value and ictal PPC value (ictal PPC minus control PPC). Non-significant differences are displayed as a zero (white) difference. Note the difference in the frequency-range displaying significant changes between ctx IV-Po (representatively plotted for ctx V-Po and ctx VI-Po) and ctx V-VPM (representatively plotted for ctx IV-VPM, ctx VI-VPM). Abbreviations: Po: Posterior thalamic nucleus, VPM: Ventral-Postero-Medial thalamic nucleus.

2. Cortico-Thalamo-Cortical circuit involvement in patients

A study of Williams et al. [16] showing that thalamic activity recorded from depth electrodes in patients with absence epilepsy is oscillatory and phase-locked with the SWDs seen in the scalp EEG, anticipated much of the evidence obtained in the cat penicillin model and in rat genetic models 30 years later, and suggested that both thalamic and cortical networks are involved in the expression of absence seizures. A similar conclusion has recently been reached by analyzing SWDs in patients with idiopathic generalized epilepsies by using combined EEG and fMRI (EEG-fMRI). Moeller et al. [17] investigated a homogeneous group of newly diagnosed and untreated children with childhood absence epilepsy (CAE) and showed that the 3Hz SWDs are associated with regional BOLD signal decreases in parietal areas, precuneus, and caudate nucleus along with a bilateral increase in the BOLD signal in the medial thalamus. However, when using an alternative approach of fMRI analysis showing the dynamics of BOLD signals the same authors [18] showed for an inhomogeneous group of nine patients that patient-specific BOLD signal changes were remarkably consistent in space and time across different absences of one patient but were quite different from patient to patient, despite having similar EEG pattern and clinical semiology. In addition, EEG-fMRI studies indicated that the default mode network is responsible for the impaired consciousness seen in patients during the generalized SWDs [19]. Moreover, according to a more recent study of Carney et al. [20] modifications in the parietal part of this network preceding the SWDs might play the initiating mechanism that generates the SWDs.

Although these fMRI studies are limited by their temporal resolution, their outcome appears to be quite in line with the results of the MEG studies of patients with absence epilepsy. The MEG study of Westmijse et al. [21] investigated the propagation of epileptiform activity underlying SWDs, revealing an alternating pattern of activity, with localized regional activity during the spikes and generalized activity during the slow-wave phase of the SWDs. With the analysis approach in this study the existence of significant nonlinear interactions between various brain regions could be established [22-24], using the same nonlinear association analysis (h²-estimate) as in the WAG/Rij rat studies [3, 12]. Source analysis result obtained with a beamformer, i.e SAM(g2) introduced by Robinson et al. [25], indicated significant activations underlying the spikes of the SWDs in bilateral prefrontal and parietal areas, although for four of the five patients studied with a frontal dominance [21]. Thus, both MEG and EEG-fMRI studies showed the involvement of the frontal and parietal regions. The importance of other cortical regions obtained with fMRI like the precuneus, caudate nucleus and the thalamus during absence seizures could not be confirmed with MEG. However, it is well known that MEG is less suited to establish a role of subcortical structures, is less sensitive for sources originating in the deeper (thalamic) brain structures, and does not very well represent activity from the midline where e.g. the precuneus is located [26] due to the inferior signal-to-noise ratio of MEG compared to EEG in these structures [27].

2.1. *Spatiotemporal dynamics of SWDs*

In a more recent MEG study of a large group of children with absence epilepsy (n = 27) we further developed the association analysis as presented by Westmijse et al. [21]. Our group of patients (age from 6 till 15 years) had electroclinically confirmed absences accompanied with 3 Hz SWDs, but showed different types of absence epilepsy. According to the classification of the ILAE [28] patients with absence epilepsy can be differentiated on basis of their electroclinical semiology. Patients with typical CAE, age of onset between 6 and 15, are distinguished from patients with atypical CAE whose SWDs might be more irregular while the onset and/or cessation is not as abrupt. A third group of patients are diagnosed as Juvenile Absence Epilepsy (JAE) (age of onset >10) who may show either typical or atypical absence seizures along with SWDs. Shown in Fig. 4A is a selection of four MEG signals from 1 s before the first visible onset of the SWDs (marked by a clinician) to 4 s after the onset. A nonlinear association analysis was performed for overlapping 20 ms shifted windows of 180 ms, yielding for each window k and for each pair of MEG sensors (i,j) a maximal association value h^2ij (k). Then, an average association value was computed for each sensor, called the association strength, representing the association of that MEG sensor relative to the other sensors (Fig. 4A, bottom). To be able to view at a single glance the evolvement of the changes in the association strength functions the mean association strength function was calculated over all the MEG signals (Fig. 4B). During seizure propagation a rhythmic pattern of peaks and troughs corresponding with the occurrences of SWDs in the MEG signal is related to the increasing and decreasing connectivity across time, with a maximum during the waves (red asterisk) and a minimum in an epoch centered around the maximum of the spikes (green circle). The dynamics of the SWD indicate a transition from an interictal or preictal state to an ictal state, starting at the first generalization of the SWDs, i.e. the abrupt occurrence of the bilateral synchronous distribution of these discharges, further referred to as generalized SWDs (gSWDs).

The results of a network study of Gupta et al. [29] also indicated a sharp transition (increase of the small worldness) from the preictal to the ictal state in a period starting about 1 s to 500 ms before the first visible onset of the SWDs and about 500 ms onwards, followed by a flat graph related to the rhythmic pattern of the gSWDs. Both Westmijse et al. [21] as well as Gupta et al. [29] showed that a threshold of about 95% of the association strength values sets apart the interictal from the preictal and ictal periods. Therefore in our study this threshold value has been used together with the measure of local connectedness (LoC) as network metric for the further investigation of the changes in spatial distribution of the SWDs during the evolvement of the SWDs, from the preictal to the ictal state. The LoC yields for each MEG sensor the probability that the neighboring sensors are connected [28] and is plotted color coded in a 2-dimensional projection of all MEG sensors (Fig. 4B). The LoC map obtained at, respectively, the peaks and troughs of the mean association strength function were averaged yielding the generalized pattern corresponding to the waves with typically the four regions of high LoC values located in the bilateral frontal and parietal lobes corresponding to the spikes of the gSWDs (Fig. 4B, bottom). The LoC maps shown in the upper row of Fig. 4B indicate multiple focal regions of activity at the first visible seizure activity (blue square) and widely distributed activity at the moment of the first generalization.

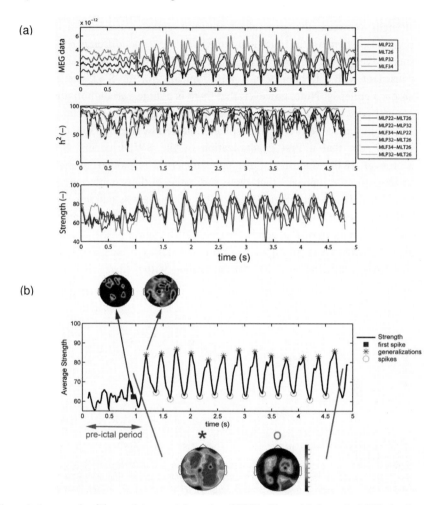

Figure 4. An example of the spatiotemporal dynamics of SWDs. Figure (a) shows the MEG signals (in fT) of four selected sensors during an SWD from 1 s before the first visible onset to 4 s after the onset (upper). The non linear association values estimated for each combination of MEG sensors ($h^2(-)$) and each analysis window (middle) and the association strength (strength (-)) calculated from the average association values per analysis window (bottom) are given in percentages. Figure (b) shows the average association strength (in percentages) over all sensors. Red asterisks indicate the maxima in the association strength, corresponding to the waves in the MEG data. During the waves, the spatial distribution is generalized. The green circles indicate the minima in the association strength, which are related to analysis windows surrounding the spikes of the SWDs. During the spikes, the spatial distribution shows focal regions (bilateral frontal and parietal) with high association values.

In Fig. 5 (left) the mean amplitude is plotted versus the mean duration of the rhythmic oscillating association strength function for each of the 27 patients studied. The amplitude is determined as the difference in average association strength between the generalizations and spikes (asterisks and circles in Figure 4), whereas the duration represents the time difference between two successive generalizations. The duration of the oscillations appear to be quite consistent with a frequency of 2-4 Hz typically for the SWDs of patients with absence epilepsy. Note, however, that there is a large variation in duration of the preictal period for the patients studied (Fig. 5, right). The preictal period starts per definition 1 s before the first spike, indicated by the blue square, and ends at the moment that a first generalization of the SWDs occurs (see Fig. 4B). Moreover, if the duration of the preictal period is plotted against the age of seizure onset it appears that there are three outliers with longer durations, typically patients older than 10 yrs of age, diagnosed as patients with JAE. It is well known that for patients with JAE the SWDs are more irregular. However, the typical pattern of a generalized spatial distribution of the LoC alternated by the four focal regions of high LoC during the spikes of the gSWDs also becomes apparent for these patients, like for the patients with CAE.

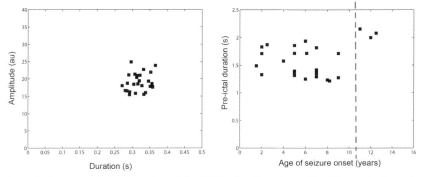

Figure 5 Summary of the dynamics of the SWDs for all patients. The left graph shows the distribution of the average amplitude vs. average duration of the oscillations in the SWDs for each patient. The right graph shows the preictal duration versus the age of seizure onset for each patient studied.

In general, it appeared that the repetitive pattern of generalized LoC maps during the waves and maps reflecting bilateral frontal and parietal regions of high LoC during the spikes is the most stable characteristic among all the patients included in this study. However, the exception are the patients who had absences provoked by hyperventilation (Fig. 6). For these patients generalization starts before the first visible onset of the SWDs, probably due to the effect of so called hyposynchronous slowing. Hyperventilation hyposynchronous slowing (HVHS) is a well described phenomenon occurring as bilateral, sometimes sharply contoured slow waves in the delta frequency range, that might complicate differential diagnosis of typical CAE, because of its sudden development and disappearance and similar frequency to SWDs [30]. Shown here are the results of a patient with JAE who had only absences when provoked by hyperventilation. However, also patients with CAE who had absences related to SWDs in unprovoked and provoked (by hyperventilation) conditions tended to show the same effect as shown in Fig. 6. Clinicians have to be aware of this phenomenon when diagnosing patients with what they call primary generalized (typical) CAE and setting these patients apart from patients with atypical CAE because there absences are so easily provoked by hyperventilation [31].

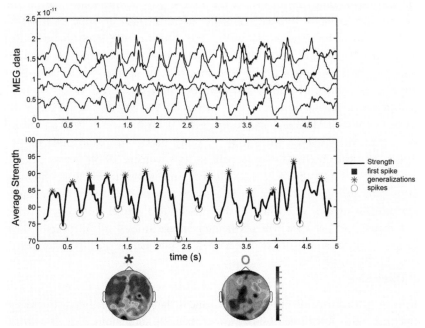

Figure 6. An example of the spatiotemporal dynamics of an SWD measured during hyperventilation. The generalization starts before the first visible onset of the SWD in the MEG data (in fT), probably due to the effect of hyposynchronous slowing. The average association values estimated for each analysis window (bottom) are given in percentages.

2.2. Cortical focus in human absence epilepsy as well?

Although the role of the cortex in absence epilepsy is not new, the fact that a focal zone was found in genetic models which mimicked SWDs and absence epilepsy rather well, increased the attention to this finding in CAE. Westmijse *et al.* [21] reported a frontal focal region at the first visible onset of the SWDs for each of the five patients studied (age ranging from 6-15 years). However, the results of our MEG study indicate that even at the early (first visible) onset of the SWDs one has to be careful to draw conclusions with regard to the driving source. For most of the patients included in our study it appeared that at the first visible onset already a more or less widely distributed spatial pattern could be discerned indicating network activations that precedes the gSWDs. This network, as shown in Fig. 4B, might reflect apart from the involvement of the bilateral frontal and parietal regions as activated during the spikes of the gSWDs dominant frontal and most often mesiofrontal activation. Gupta et al. [29] showed for a subgroup of the 27 patients presented here that the driving source is preceding the first visible onset of the SWDs. This driving source had for the homogeneous group of five patients included in the study of Gupta et al. [29] a parietal/occipital localization. However, the results of our study indicate that patient specific changes in the dynamic network during the transition from the preictal to the ictal phase of the SWDs may become apparent, like for patients with JAE. A number of studies indicated for patients with JAE involvement of (ventromedial) frontal cortex at the onset of the SWDs, based on phase synchronization of MEG signals preceding SWDs by 1.5 s [32], or in a series of twelve patients based on EEG [33]. A study of Holmes et al. [34] of five difficult to treat absence epilepsy patients (all women, 19-58 years) showed based on source analysis of 256 channel EEG recordings that both at onset and during propagation, the discharges in absence are associated with activation of only discrete regions of mainly medial frontal and orbital frontal cortex. All these results, obtained for patients ranging in age from 4 till 58 years of age, indicate a cortical source driving the SWDs, despite patient specific differences.

3. Discussion

The network analysis of cortico-thalamic and thalamo-thalamic interactions shed some new light on the role of how various thalamic subregions interact with the cortex and with each other. The data of the WAG/Rij rat study of Lüttjohann and van Luijtelaar [12] and Lüttjohann et al. [14] can be summarized by stating that there is more precursor activity in the cortex than in the thalamus. SWD related changes in local field potentials can be found more than a second prior to SWD generalization in the deep cortical layers of the somatosensory cortex. Nonlinear association analyses showed that the earliest and strongest increases in maximal association strength were seen between cortical layer V/VI and Po.

Other thalamic nuclei became later involved in SWD activity. These results are in line with the strong increases in synchrony in delta and theta activity between cortex and thalamus during the evolvement of the SWDs. In addition, at the same time point as SWD activity generalizes to the thalamus and a full blown cortico-thalamic SWD arises, the increases in maximal association strength can be seen to become accompanied by changes in coupling direction with the cortex driving the thalamus. During the first 500 ms of SWDs the cortex guided most thalamic nuclei while cortex and Po kept a bidirectional crosstalk. Most thalamic nuclei started to guide the Po until the end of the SWD. Po nucleus might be the primary thalamic counterpart to the somatosensory-cortex in the generation of SWD, instead of the VPM that was considered as the primary thalamic target for SWD activity in previous network-studies that did not take the Po into consideration [3, 10, 11]. Thus, these data also modify the picture in showing that the thalamus is heterogeneous with respect to changes in connectivity with the cortex. Some thalamic nuclei get earlier involved than others and intrathalamic dynamics of synchronization and direction of coupling emphasized a different role for the caudal and rostral RTN.

In this contribution the cortico-cortical and cortico-thalamic network involved in the initiation and spreading of SWDs based on high density EEG and MEG and fMRI studies in humans has been reviewed. EEG and MEG studies are restricted in the sense that information of subcortical networks remains enigmatic. However, the importance of the cortico-thalamo-cortical structures interconnected in a network in generating absence seizures was also confirmed by fMRI studies for both the genetic models of absence epilepsy and for children. The analysis of cortico-thalamo-cortical networks obviously has translational value for outcomes in patients with absence epilepsy. Moreover, similar signal analytical techniques were used in the animal and patient study. The association analyses provided information on the onset and propagation of absence seizures in both the WAG/Rij rats and children. The rhythmic pattern of large-scale generalization during the waves of the SWDs alternated by focal regions of high association values during the spikes appears to be the most stable characteristic of SWDs occurring in the MEG of children with absence epilepsy. Furthermore, the spatial dynamics reflected by the measure of LoC indicates that a common network is activated during the evolvement of the gSWDs, irrespective whether the patient had easy to treat (typical) CAE, difficult to treat (atypical) CAE or JAE. Here it is proposed that this repetitive pattern of bilateral synchronous generalized activity (during the waves) occurs in thalamo-cortical pathways; at each spike the thalamus is driven by the cortex and via the widespread cortico-cortical and thalamo-cortical projections the cortex is synchronously activated. Further support for the rhythmic pattern of gSWDs was provided by the connectivity study of Gupta et al. [29] indicating that a rhythmic pattern of peaks and troughs corresponding with the occurrences of SWDs in the MEG signal is related to increasing local and decreasing global connectivity across time. The network analysis as used by Gupta et al. [29] for the absence seizures, indicated a tendency to a small world network after the transition point. These results seem to be in contradiction to the findings of Ponten et al. [35] who found an increase of the local and global connectivity measures during absences compared to the preictal state. Their results were based on the synchronization likelihood [36] of 21 EEG signals. However, it has been shown that graph theoretical analysis results are highly dependent on variations of parameters like the number of sensors or length of the analysis epochs [37]. Moreover, the main interest of the study of Gupta et al. [29] was not to identify the network characteristics of the SWDs compared to the preictal period as in the study of Ponten et al. [35], but to examine the dynamics of connectivity at the transition period from the preictal to the ictal state. The results of the study of Gupta et al. [29] indeed indicated a sharp transition (increase of the small worldness) from the preictal to the ictal phase of the SWDs driven by an initial source most likely originating in the parietal/occipital cortex. The association strength approach employed in our MEG study enabled to identify both the temporal and spatial dynamics during the transition from the preictal to the ictal phase of the SWDs for a large group of absence epilepsy patients and may be of diagnostic help for the clinicians.

Acknowledgments

This study was funded by the Netherlands Organization for Scientific Research (NWO), grant number 400-04-483 to GvL and PO. We would like to thank Dr. O. Jensen for providing hospitality at the FC Donders center for NeuroImaging and the assistance of the MEG Center of VU University Medical Center.

References

1. Gloor, P., *Evlolution of the concept of the mechanism of generalized epilepsy with bilateral spike and wave discharge*, in *Modern perspective in epilepsy*, J.A. Wada, Editor. 1978, Eden Press: Montreal. p. 99-137.
2. Meeren, H., et al., *Evolving concepts on the pathophysiology of absence seizures: the cortical focus theory.* Arch Neurol, 2005. **62**(3): p. 371-6.
3. Meeren, H.K., et al., *Cortical focus drives widespread corticothalamic networks during spontaneous absence seizures in rats.* J Neurosci, 2002. **22**(4): p. 1480-95.

4. Tenney, J.R., et al., *FMRI of brain activation in a genetic rat model of absence seizures.* Epilepsia, 2004. **45**(6): p. 576-82.

5. Nersesyan, H., et al., *Dynamic fMRI and EEG recordings during spike-wave seizures and generalized tonic-clonic seizures in WAG/Rij rats.* J Cereb Blood Flow Metab, 2004. **24**(6): p. 589-99.

6. David, O., et al., *Identifying neural drivers with functional MRI: an electrophysiological validation.* PLoS Biol, 2008. **6**(12): p. 2683-97.

7. Avoli, M., *A brief history on the oscillating roles of thalamus and cortex in absence seizures.* Epilepsia, 2012. **53**(5): p. 779-89.

8. Polack, P.O., et al., *Deep layer somatosensory cortical neurons initiate spike-and-wave discharges in a genetic model of absence seizures.* J Neurosci, 2007. **27**(24): p. 6590-9.

9. Crunelli, V. and N. Leresche, *Childhood absence epilepsy: genes, channels, neurons and networks.* Nat Rev Neurosci, 2002. **3**(5): p. 371-82.

10. Sitnikova, E., et al., *Granger causality: cortico-thalamic interdependencies during absence seizures in WAG/Rij rats.* J Neurosci Methods, 2008. **170**(2): p. 245-54.

11. Sitnikova, E. and G. van Luijtelaar, *Cortical and thalamic coherence during spike-wave seizures in WAG/Rij rats.* Epilepsy Res, 2006. **71**(2-3): p. 159-80.

12. Lüttjohann, A. and G. van Luijtelaar, *The dynamics of cortico-thalamo-cortical interactions at the transition from pre-ictal to ictal LFPs in absence epilepsy.* Neurobiol Dis, 2012. **47**(1): p. 49-60.

13. Sherman, S.M., Guillery, R.W. , *Exploring the Thalamus and Its Role in Cortical Function.* 2005, Cambridge: The MIT Press.

14. Lüttjohann, A., J.M. Schoffelen, and G. van Luijtelaar, *Peri-ictal network dynamics of spike-wave discharges: Phase and spectral characteristics.* Experimental Neurology, 2012.

15. van Luijtelaar, G., E. Sitnikova, and A. Lüttjohann, *On the origin and suddenness of absences in genetic absence models.* Clin EEG Neurosci, 2011. **42**(2): p. 83-97.

16. Williams, D., *A study of thalamic and cortical rhythms in petit mal.* Brain, 1953. **76**(1): p. 50-69.

17. Moeller, F., et al., *Simultaneous EEG-fMRI in drug-naive children with newly diagnosed absence epilepsy.* Epilepsia, 2008. **49**(9): p. 1510-9.

18. Moeller, F., et al., *Absence seizures: individual patterns revealed by EEG-fMRI.* Epilepsia, 2010. **51**(10): p. 2000-10.

19. Gotman, J., et al., *Generalized epileptic discharges show thalamocortical activation and suspension of the default state of the brain.* Proc Natl Acad Sci U S A, 2005. **102**(42): p. 15236-40.

20. Carney, P.W., et al., *The core network in absence epilepsy. Differences in cortical and thalamic BOLD response.* Neurology, 2010. **75**(10): p. 904-11.

21. Westmijse, I., et al., *Onset and propagation of spike and slow wave discharges in human absence epilepsy: A MEG study.* Epilepsia, 2009. **50**(12): p. 2538-2548.

22. Lopes da Silva, F., J.P. Pijn, and P. Boeijinga, *Interdependence of EEG signals: linear vs. nonlinear associations and the significance of time delays and phase shifts.* Brain Topogr, 1989. **2**(1-2): p. 9-18.

23. Pijn, J.P.M., Vijn, P.C.M., Lopes da Silva F.H., van Emde Boas, W., Blanes, W., , *The use of signal-analysis for the location of an epileptogenic focus: a new approach* Advances in Epilptology, 1989. **17**: p. 272-276.

24. Pijn, J.P.M., *Quantitative Evaluation of EEG Signals in Epilepsy.* 1990, University of Amsterdam: Amsterdam.

25. Robinson, S.E., et al., *Localization of interictal spikes using SAM(g2) and dipole fit.* Neurol Clin Neurophysiol, 2004. **2004**: p. 74.

26. Ossenblok, P., et al., *Magnetoencephalography is more successful for screening and localizing frontal lobe epilepsy than electroencephalography.* Epilepsia, 2007. **48**(11): p. 2139-49.

27. Goldenholz, D.M., et al., *Mapping the signal-to-noise-ratios of cortical sources in magnetoencephalography and electroencephalography.* Hum Brain Mapp, 2009. **30**(4): p. 1077-86.

28. *Proposal for revised classification of epilepsies and epileptic syndromes. Commission on Classification and Terminology of the International League Against Epilepsy.* Epilepsia, 1989. **30**(4): p. 389-99.

29. Gupta, D., P. Ossenblok, and G. van Luijtelaar, *Space-time network connectivity and cortical activations preceding spike wave discharges in human absence epilepsy: a MEG study.* Med Biol Eng Comput, 2011. **49**(5): p. 555-65.

30. Epstein, M.A., et al., *Altered responsiveness during hyperventilation-induced EEG slowing: a non-epileptic phenomenon in normal children.* Epilepsia, 1994. **35**(6): p. 1204-1207.

31. Panayiotopoulos, C.P., *Typical absence seizures and related epileptic syndromes: assessment of current state and directions for future research.* Epilepsia, 2008. **49**(12): p. 2131-9.

32. Amor, F., et al., *Imaging brain synchrony at high spatio-temporal resolution: application to MEG signals during absence seizures.* Signal Processing, 2005. **85**(11): p. 2101-2111.

33. Rozas Latorre, M., et al., *Distribution and propagation of epileptiform discharges in juvenile myoclonic epilepsy.* Epilepsia, 2005. **46 (suppl 8)**: p. 268.

34. Holmes, M.D., M. Brown, and D.M. Tucker, *Are "generalized" seizures truly generalized? Evidence of localized mesial frontal and frontopolar discharges in absence.* Epilepsia, 2004. **45**(12): p. 1568-79.

35. Ponten, S.C., et al., *Indications for network regularization during absence seizures: weighted and unweighted graph theoretical analyses.* Exp Neurol, 2009. **217**(1): p. 197-204.

36. Stam, C.J. and B.W. van Dijk, *Synchronization likelihood: an unbiased measure of generalized synchronization in multivariate data sets.* Physica D: Nonlinear Phenomena, 2002. **163**(3–4): p. 236-251.

37. Rummel, C., et al., *Analyzing spatio-temporal patterns of genuine cross-correlations.* J Neurosci Methods, 2010. **191**(1): p. 94-100.

SIGNAL PROCESSING PLATFORM BASED ON CELLULAR NONLINEAR NETWORKS

J. MüLLER*, J. MüLLER, R. BECKER and R. TETZLAFF

*Fakultät Elektrotechnik und Informationstechnik,
Institut für Grundlagen der Elektrotechnik und Elektronik
Technische Universität Dresden,
01062 Dresden, Germany
* E-mail: muellerj@iee.et.tu-dresden.de
http://www.iee.et.tu-dresden.de/iee/ge*

The complexity of signals and of algorithmic methods in medical signal processing tasks imposes considerable requirements on the computing hardware. The conflicting demands for computing power and portability can currently be satisfied only by massively parallel operation. In this contribution we present the CESAR architecture of a parallel processor array utilising the underlying Cellular Nonlinear Network principle. The array is embedded into a hardware-software system forming a highly configurable signal processing platform usable both in algorithm development and in real-world applications.

Keywords: Signal processing; parallel processing; CNN; FPGA.

1. Introduction

Medical signal processing is influenced by a number of challenges dominated by the characteristics of the input signals: Multi-sensor or multivariate signals at different scales, at varying (mid-range to high) frequencies, with high levels of noise and interferences, etc. The complexity and variety of the signals often demands complex algorithmic treatment, from signal enhancement up to high-level information processing. This holds for many applications such as medical image handling, tomographic imaging, and especially for EEG/ECoG/SEEG and ECG analysis.

In the research and development of methods and algorithms, rather few restrictions are imposed on the way of producing the results. However, multiple data sets usually have to be processed (a number of recordings per patient, several patients, artificially generated data with varying characteristics), various algorithm parameters are tested, and often optimisation techniques are applied, such that high computing power is indispensable.

The restrictions change drastically with the transition to applications in a clinical environment, in healthcare, and in long-term supervision. Most of these applications require a real-time processing, implying that the *through-put* of the system is greater than the data rate of the inputs. Latency, i.e. the time delay between input events and corresponding output events, is only rarely an issue. Usually *several* processing steps, such as pre-processing, feature extraction, and classification — some of them *repeatedly* with varying parameters — have to be performed by the system. In a clinical environment some of these tasks might be accomplished by workstations or computer clusters, presumably in a remote-processing fashion. When, however, portable or wearable gadgets, or even implantable devices become necessary, requirements of size, weight, power consumption are added to that of computing power.

If we consider the traditional ways of computing, the demands for high computing power and for portability are contradictory. This conflict can be appeased by *parallel* processing — as demonstrated by the integration of up to four processing cores in recent mobile devices — and can only be solved by *massively parallel* processing with a large number of cores. Processor arrays — a very efficient structure of massively parallel cores — are inherently suited to processing of two-dimensional static or dynamic signals (such as images and videos), and of multivariate one-dimensional dynamic signals (such as EEG/ECoG streams).

In this contribution we present a digital architecture of an approved array processing principle: The Cellular Nonlinear Network (CNN). Our hardware implementation of this architecture is embedded in a hardware–software system serving as a processing platform for signals as described above.

In the following section we give a short introduction to Cellular Nonlinear Networks and to current hardware implementations, which is complemented by a presentation of our digital CNN architecture. The hardware–software system will then be discussed, followed by an example application in EEG signal processing.

2. Signal Processing using Cellular Nonlinear Networks

Vast computational tasks, like simulations of new materials' characteristics, of solid mechanics or of molecular dynamics, can be performed applying today's state-of-the-art single-core and multi-core processors. However, architectures based on the conventional way of sequential data treatment show very poor performance both in the fields of pattern recognition — where a neural structure like the human brain outperforms them easily — and in multivariate signal processing, such as EEG and ECoG/SEEG recordings.

Although *Artificial Neural Networks* are widely recognised as systems mimicking brain-like computing, they are inappropriate for an integration in silicon due to their large amount of interconnections over the whole network.[1] In order to achieve a hardware implementation exploiting the computational power of a highly parallel system *and* retaining the neural structure of interconnected simple processing elements (cells), the *Cellular Nonlinear Network* principle was proposed by Chua and Yang in 1988.[2] The CNN is strongly geared to hardware implementation, and accordingly each element of a regular grid is connected to cells in a restricted neighbourhood only (Fig. 1).

The basic elements, the cells, represent simple dynamic systems characterised by a certain state and an associated arbitrary nonlinear output function. The cells are spatially connected to the inputs and outputs of neighbouring cells, by (in the simplest case linear) coupling weights that mostly determine the dynamic behaviour of the network. The network is "programmable" since the desired input–output relation can be obtained by choosing appropriate coupling weights, threshold, and output function.

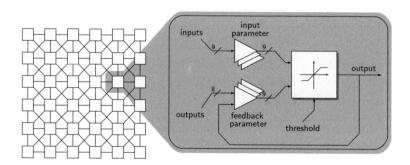

Fig. 1.   General structure of a CNN: A regular network of locally coupled cells, where each cell is connected to the outputs and inputs of its neighbours.

In space-invariant networks (all cells behave in the same manner) the parameter sets can be understood as global templates containing only 19 items for the simple case of a 3×3 neighbourhood.

As the CNN itself is a mostly mathematical description of an analogue system, some further extensions are required to build up a CNN-based computer. Thus, in 1993 the *CNN Universal Machine* (CNN–UM) was proposed — a programmable array computer based on the CNN dynamics which is equipped with memory, communication and control units, performing analogue and logic instructions.[3] Subsequently, several hardware implementations have been presented, especially for image processing purposes.

The *ACE16k* was the first suitable representative of a mixed-signal CNN–UM implementation in CMOS technology with 128×128 cells. To fully exploit the computation power of the CNN, optical sensor inputs were integrated to each cell, converting it into a programmable vision chip.[4] As a part of the standalone *Bi-i Visual System*, the CNN offered analogue image acquisition and pre-processing of more than 5 000 images per second.[5] A recent achievement of CNN-based mixed-signal vision chips is the *EyeRIS Visual System* from AnaFocus Ltd. featuring a 176×144 pixel focal-plane processor, called *Q-Eye*.[6]

Analogue and mixed-signal implementations became attractive because of their ability to couple the processing elements directly to optical sensors and due to the outstanding performance for on-chip image processing. However, they suffer from several drawbacks, namely a distinct dependency of operations on temperature and light, as well as from a very limited accuracy of calculation. The state accuracy hardly exceeds 7–8 bit when converted to digital domain. This is usually sufficient for image pre-processing tasks but not for most scientific applications such as time series analysis or the simulation of partial differential equations. Thus, digital emulations of the CNN should serve both to retain the computational speed through massively parallel processing and to enhance the system's accuracy and flexibility.

As compared to full-custom designs, implementations on field-programmable gate arrays (FPGAs) require shorter design cycles, are much more flexible, and hence are suited for research and the development of prototype systems. Emulations of the CNN–UM on FPGAs have proved to be suitable for solving numerically demanding problems, like the simulation of multi-channel retina models[7] with a performance competitive to mixed-signal full-custom designs.[8] Recently, we presented the CESAR architecture, a fully digital emulation of CNN on FPGA suitable for the implementation of CNN-based algorithms for EEG signal processing.[9,10]

3. CESAR Architecture

The underlying principle of this architecture is the analogue CNN model, which is used for digital emulation in its discretised form, to compute results in an iterative manner. The CESAR architecture is mainly composed of a cellular array of processing elements, each one directly representing one CNN cell.

The heart of each cell is formed by a pipelined multiplier, which performs both the input multiplication — to implement the linear coupling — and the state calculation. The inputs and outputs of cells in the 3×3 neighbourhood are processed accumulatively using a pipelining method. Apart from a few control signals, all interim values needed for the calculation of the next cell state are held locally at each cell, in order to use the calculation core with full capacity (Fig. 2). The accuracy of the internal state values can be freely varied, which enables the designer to choose the trade-off between accuracy and power consumption.

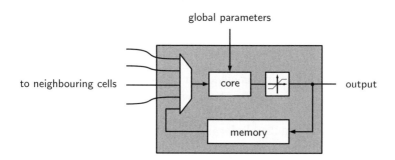

Fig. 2.   Structure of the processing element.

The cells are connected locally and form a network according to Fig. 1. This scheme is used widely and most of the existing templates have been developed especially for this structure. The local couplings of the cells are inherently present on FPGAs and can be implemented very efficiently, thus leading to high computational power. The architecture is unrestricted in network size, allowing all possible rectangular network shapes, only limited by the hardware platform for which it is configured.

To reduce the wiring effort — which can be quite complex in digital hardware implementations — a special data forwarding scheme is used.

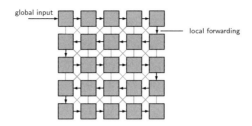

Fig. 3.   Array of processing elements with input data forwarding scheme.

Instead of feeding the input data directly from RAM to each of the hundreds of cells and hence causing an excess of wiring, the data is fed to only one corner cell of the network and from there forwarded locally to the neighbouring cells (Fig. 3). Naturally the same mechanism is used when transferring the results back to the RAM.

Given the condition of moderate data transactions, CNN algorithms can be processed at very high speed, thanks to the large degree of parallel processing. In practical applications, the CNN operations often refer to preceding results. The CNN can be programmed to either read its input values from memory or to use the result from the previous operation as the new input. This is implemented via an micro-instruction word, which in addition carries information about several network properties, like the number of iterations or the type of boundary condition. The latter informs the network how to handle cells located at the edge of the network. With the unique feature of micro-instructions, multiple sequential operations can be assigned to the network at once, hence limiting data transfers and enabling it to process real programs representing complex algorithms.

4. Hardware-Software System

As described in the previous section, CESAR is a configurable, programmable array processor. For the utilisation in the development of algorithms, or in real-world applications, some more abilities are required:

- data acquisition from the sensors or from storage, respectively
- data conditioning and pre-processing (if necessary)
- preparation of processing algorithms and mapping to CNN programs
- transfer of data and CNN programs to the CNN memories
- back-transfer of resulting data

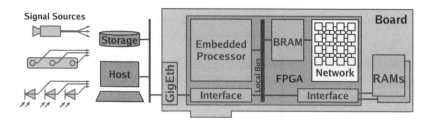

Fig. 4. Block diagram of the hardware–software system (GigEth — Gigabit Ethernet).

• post-processing, analysis, and storage of results

These tasks are accomplished by a hardware–software system, as shown in
Fig. 4, consisting of an FPGA-based embedded system, the controlling host
computer with dedicated software, and complemental storage and interface
units. The allocation of the above tasks to the components of this system,
the so-called partitioning of the processing problem, strongly depends on
the mission of the system, as will be discussed in this section.

4.1. Embedded System

The central feature of the embedded system is the *embedded processor* which
is either a dedicated physical hardware structure on the FPGA (so-called
hard core), or a generated hardware that is loaded into the FPGA fabric
during configuration (soft core). Our hardware–software system is designed
to work with both options, namely a PowerPC hard core in Xilinx Virtex-5
FPGAs, or a MicroBlaze soft core available for most modern Xilinx FPGAs.

In addition, structures like *bus connections*, *memories*, and *interfaces* to
components on the FPGA board can be installed in the configurable logic.
A block diagram of the embedded system is depicted in Fig. 5.

The *local bus* connects the embedded processor to one port (each) of
the input, state, template and operation RAMs, such that the processor
and the CNN array can access data simultaneously.

Other *memory* structures are required for storing the program code,
software stack, data buffer, temporary data, etc. They can be located within
the FPGA (so-called Block–RAM — BRAM) or on the FPGA board.
BRAMs are comparatively fast and easily accessible, but limited in size,
depending on the FPGA model. Board RAM outside the FPGA is usually calculated more generously, the access is more complex, however, and
requires additional interface logic in the FPGA. Thus the choice (or com-

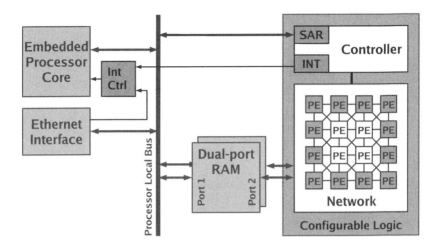

Fig. 5. Embedded system with the cellular network (SAR — Software Accessible Register, INT — Interrupt, PE — Processing Element, IntCtrl — Interrupt Controller).

bination) depends on the FPGA resources available and on the size and speed demands by the application.

The tasks of our embedded system currently comprise the reception of data over a Gigabit Ethernet interface (GigEth), their distribution to the RAMs, and the initiation of CNN operations by writing to a software-accessible register (SAR) within the CNN controller. When the CNN has finished the processing according to the micro-instructions, the controller issues an interrupt to the embedded processor. The resulting data will then be sent back over the Ethernet interface.

In a more advanced, multi-threading-based operation of the embedded system, data transfers and processing can be accomplished in parallel, allowing to receive the next chunk of data, or to send the previous results, while the CNN processes the current one. This reduces the impact of the notorious data transportation bottleneck, yet is accompanied by a higher complexity of the embedded software kernel.

4.2. Software Hierarchy and Data Flow

Since all components of the hardware–software system (host computer, embedded system, array processor) are programmable, a software hierarchy comprising all three levels has been developed accordingly. The distribution

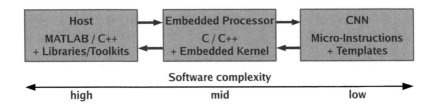

Fig. 6. Software hierarchy of the system.

(or partitioning) of the algorithm tasks to these levels strongly depends on the application field, as discussed in Section 1. Fig. 6 shows the implemented software hierarchy, with the focus on the development of algorithms.

The *host software* running on a workstation or a notebook represents the highest level in this hierarchy. All global activities and processes are controlled by the host. Data is acquired from hard disk or network storage, pre-processed according to the algorithm requirements, and converted to a common data representation processable by the CNN, using MATLAB or C++ functions. During algorithm development the same data is often processed several times, suggesting to store the pre-processed and converted data on disc. The data is then sent to and received by the FPGA board over a dedicated Ethernet port, employing operating system commands. On reception of data, the embedded system automatically starts the processing such that no further control is needed.

During development, some or all functionality of the processing array may be simulated in software instead, using the same software tools as a framework.

As described in the previous sub-section, the *embedded system* receives the data, distributes them to the memory components, orders the CNN to start, and sends the results back after completion of the processing. These mid-level activities are implemented in hardware-oriented C/C++ software, using functions of the underlying embedded kernel. Again, when the CNN processing has started, no further control of the process is required.

The *CNN program* consisting of CNN operations with their micro-instructions, as introduced in Section 3, can be regarded as a very elementary software, representing the lowest level of the hierarchy. Yet, the hardest part of processing is accomplished in the parallel kernel.

In applications requiring an autonomous operation without a host computer, higher-level software will be translated to lower levels, namely from

224

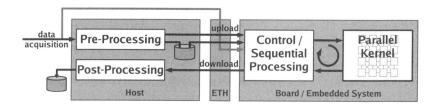

Fig. 7. Principal data flow within the hardware–software system, with a direct data input (grey line) to the embedded system (ETH — Ethernet Interface).

host level to the embedded system. This can be handled straightforwardly for C++ host software, since most of the usual library functions are also available in the embedded kernel.

Sequential pre-processing and data conversion will then be performed in the embedded system, with some constraints by the relatively slow embedded processor. Parts of these tasks that can be parallelised efficiently are also suited to a hardware implementation.

The software hierarchy can be very similarly mapped to the *data flow* in the system, as shown in Fig. 7. From this scheme it becomes quite obvious that, for an efficient operation, most of the processing has to be located in the parallel kernel, and (only secondly) in the embedded system. If the sequential part should turn out to be too slow, a trade-off between fast host processing plus data transfer and slow embedded processing has to be found.

On the other hand, for an autonomous operation all pre-/post-processing tasks are forced on the embedded system, such that a direct data input to the FPGA board becomes possible (as outlined in Fig. 7). Again, a trade-off is necessary between slow sequential procedure in the processor, and rapid parallel execution in the network. All system parameters and processing tasks can now be adapted and optimised to the particular application, making a significant reduction of the work load feasible.

5. Application in EEG Signal Processing

Despite being designed as a general-purpose computing platform, the proposed cellular array architecture is especially suited for multivariate signal processing. In this way several hundred channels of discrete time series can be handled in parallel.

225

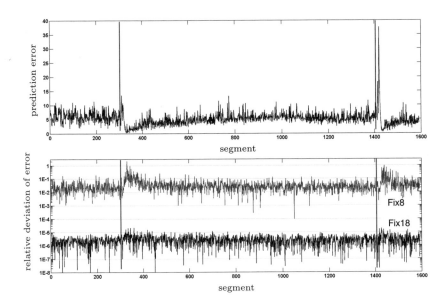

Fig. 8. Influence of data representation on the calculation accuracy in an EEG recording, with two epileptic seizures in segments 295 and 1401.

In the past, various algorithms for epileptic seizure prediction were presented[11–15] that will greatly benefit from hardware implementation on the presented system, regarding characteristics of computation time and power consumption.

An outstanding feature for EEG signal processing is the calculation accuracy, exceeding current analogue and mixed-signal implementations of the CNN–UM, while the system is matching their computing power.

In a preliminary study, we investigated the relative deviation of the EEG signal prediction error of a CNN-based spatio-temporal predictor using signal values of an intracranial EEG. In Fig. 8 the influence of data precision on the predictor quality is shown for a recording time of several hours. A reference of the prediction error calculated with a 64-bit floating-point representation is depicted in the upper diagram and the relative deviation thereof in the lower, for 8-bit (*Fix8*) and 18-bit (*Fix18*) fixed-point data, respectively. It is obvious in this example that an 8-bit accuracy is not acceptable for practical usage, as holds for many numerically demanding algorithms in multivariate time series analysis.

Apart from calculation accuracy, the system can be freely optimised for the actual number of recording channels and the considered channel combinations when investigating their interdependencies.

6. Conclusions

The proposed hardware-software system has been implemented completely and is running in a laboratory environment on various FPGA boards. The entire platform is configurable and adaptable to user requirements with a freely selectable precision of up to 18 bit due to the direct utilisation of on-chip Digital Signal Processors. It can easily be extended to arbitrary accuracies.

The system can be customised for any Xilinx FPGA of Virtex-5 series (or newer), offering massively parallel processing power outperforming state-of-the-art microprocessors.[10] An implementation on a Virtex-6 SX475 FPGA features 1225 processing elements at a power consumption of less than 10 W. We are currently adapting the cellular array to low-power components of the Xilinx Spartan series, allowing hyper-portable devices with the size of a chip card. Furthermore, an extension to more complex, non-linear weight functions between the cells is in progress.

To summarise, we presented a versatile platform suitable for any kind of signal processing that can be represented by the CNN principle. The utilisation of a cellular processor array with local couplings breaks the contradiction between computational performance and power consumption of conventional architectures. Thus, the efficient implementation of complex algorithms performing analyses on multivariate data in real-time becomes feasible on highly portable devices. In this context it seems obvious to encourage the development of novel methods based on CNN in further fields of applications.

References

1. J. Misra and I. Saha, *Neurocomputing* **74**, 239 (2010).
2. L. O. Chua and L. Yang, *IEEE Transactions on Circuits and Systems* **35**, 1257 (1988).
3. T. Roska and L. O. Chua, *IEEE Transactions on Circuits and Systems II: Analog and Digital Signal Processing* **40**, 163 (1993).
4. A. Rodríguez-Vázquez, G. Liñán-Cembrano, L. Carranza, E. Roca-Moreno, R. Carmona-Galán, F. Jiménez-Garrido, R. Domínguez-Castro and S. Meana, *Circuits and Systems I: Regular Papers, IEEE Transactions on* **51**, 851 (2004).

5. Á. Zarándy and C. Rekeczky, *Circuits and Systems Magazine, IEEE* **5**, 36 (2005).

6. Á. Rodríguez-Vázquez, R. Domínguez-Castro, F. Jiménez-Garrido, S. Morillas, J. Listán, L. Alba, C. Utrera, S. Espejo and R. Romay, The Eye-RIS CMOS Vision System, in *Analog Circuit Design*, eds. H. Casier, M. Steyaert and A. Roermund (Springer Netherlands, 2008) pp. 15–32.

7. Z. Nagy and P. Szolgay, *IEEE Transactions on Circuits and Systems I: Fundamental Theory and Applications* **50**, 774 (2003).

8. Z. Vörösházi, A. Kiss, Z. Nagy and P. Szolgay, *International Journal of Circuit Theory and Applications* **36**, 589 (2008).

9. J. Müller, J. Müller and R. Tetzlaff, A new cellular nonlinear network emulation on FPGA for EEG signal processing in epilepsy, in *Proceedings of SPIE*, 2011.

10. J. Müller, R. Becker, J. Müller and R. Tetzlaff, CESAR: Emulating Cellular Networks on FPGA, in *Cellular Nanoscale Networks and Their Applications (CNNA), 2012 13th International Workshop on*, 2012.

11. F. Gollas, C. Niederhöfer and R. Tetzlaff, *Int. J. Circuit Theory Appl.* **36**, 623 (2008).

12. D. Krug, H. Osterhage, C. E. Elger and K. Lehnertz, *Phys. Rev. E* **76**, p. 041916(Oct 2007).

13. D. Krug, C. E. Elger and K. Lehnertz, *Epilepsia* **49** (2008).

14. V. Senger, J. Müller and R. Tetzlaff, Spatio-temporal coupling of EEG signals in epilepsy, in *Proceedings of SPIE*, 2011.

15. R. Sowa, F. Morman, A. Chernihovskyi, S. Florin, C. Elger and K. Lehnertz, Estimating Synchronization in Brain Electrical Activity from Epilepsy Patients with Cellular Neural Networks, in *Proc. International Workshop on Cellular Neural Networks and Their Applications (CNNA 2004)*, 2004.

SEIZURE PREDICTION BY CELLULAR NONLINEAR NETWORKS?

V. SENGER* and R. TETZLAFF

Fakultät Elektrotechnik und Informationstechnik,
Institut für Grundlagen der Elektrotechnik
Technische Universität Dresden
*01062 Dresden * E-mail: vanessa.senger@tu-dresden.de*
www.iee.et.tu-dresden.de/iee/ge

In previous work[1] it has been shown that feature extraction algorithms based on Cellular Nonlinear Networks with nonlinear weight functions as well as discrete time Cellular Nonlinear Networks may contribute to the detection of predictive characteristics of an impending seizure. In this contribution results of two signal prediction approaches are presented – a retrospective study based on data of 15 patients with at least 4 seizures each, and first results of an approach to extract features by analyzing comparably short data segments only.

Keywords: Signal prediction, signal processing, epilepsy, EEG, CNN,

1. Introduction

Cellular Nonlinear Networks (CNN) have been an active topic of research within the seizure prediction research community. CNN have been introduced in 1988 by Chua and Yang and – by making use of their inherently massive parallel processing power – form an attractive basis for the realization of an miniaturized seizure warning device.

The local coupling of cells is defined by a so-called sphere of influence $\mathcal{N}_{ij}(r)$ of radius r in the neighborhood of each cell C_{ij}. Mostly, investigations related to seizure prediction, such as a measure based on an approximation of the correlation dimension,[2] an estimation of nonlinear interdependencies,[3–5] and of phase synchronization,[6,7] a system identification, signal prediction and level crossing approach[1,8–10] are using CNN with polynomial weight functions, following the state equation according to

$$\dot{x}_{i,j}(t) = -x_{i,j}(t) + \sum_{k,l \in \mathcal{N}_{i,j}(r)} \mathcal{P}_{k,l}(y_{k,l}(t)) + \mathcal{P}_{k,l}(u_{k,l}(t)) + z \qquad (1)$$

with

$$\mathcal{P}_{k,l}(y_{k,l}(t)) = \sum_{p=1}^{P} a_{k,l,p}[y_{k,l}(t)]^p \tag{2}$$

and

$$\mathcal{P}_{k,l}(u_{k,l}(t)) = \sum_{p=1}^{P} b_{k,l,p}[u_{k,l}(t)]^p. \tag{3}$$

In this contribution, we will present signal prediction methods based on discrete-time CNN (DT-CNN) with polynomial weight functions. An autonomous one-dimensional DT-CNN[a] can be defined according to[b]

$$x_i(t_{n+1}) = -x_i(t_n) + \sum_{j\in\mathcal{N}(i)} \sum_{p=1}^{P} a_{p,j}\,[x_j(t_n)]^p. \tag{4}$$

Results obtained by applying two CNN based signal prediction methods will be discussed. These results are based on a group of recordings of 15 patients. They have all been suffering from a focal epilepsy and each recording includes at least 4 seizures.

1.1. *Patient data*

The results presented in the following have been obtained by using recordings acquired during pre-surgical evaluations of patients suffering from focal epilepsy. For all recordings, an implantation scheme similar to Fig. 1 was used, but not all electrode channels shown here have been used for all patients – the number of electrode channels varies between 20 and 74. The duration of all recordings varies from 67.7 h to 576.4 h, with most recordings having a length between 100 h and 150 h. The number of recorded seizures varies from four to ten, with most recordings including between 4 and 6 seizures. All data was sampled with 200 Hz. Details on the number of electrode channels available for a certain patient, the duration of a recording and the number of seizures are given in Table 1.

---

[a]in the following, the index i will be used instead of i, j in order to simplifiy the notation
[b]For the sake of simplicity, the time index n will be used instead of t_n in all following equations whenever time discrete systems are considered.

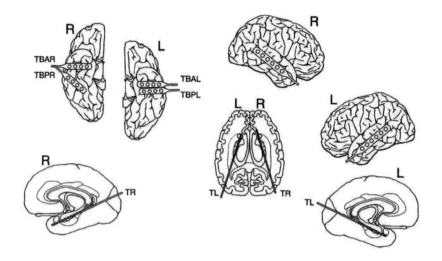

Fig. 1. Electrode implantation scheme used for patient 1 of Table 1.

2. CNN based signal prediction

Equation (4) can be transformed by introducing a time delay and assuming a signal prediction approach[c] according to

$$\hat{x}_i(n) = \sum_l \sum_{k=1}^{\kappa} \sum_{p=1}^{P} a_{l,k,p} \, x_l(n-k)^p, \qquad (5)$$

where $\hat{x}_i(n)$ denotes a value of channel i which is predicted using λ channels that may or may not include i and delayed in time by κ values each.

For data segments[d] of length N, for each segment s the coefficients $a_{l,k,p}(s)$, can be obtained by applying an optimization procedure[11] with regards to the relative root mean squared error of the data of a segment. The error can be calculated according to

$$e(s) = \sqrt{\frac{1}{N} \sum_{n=(s-1)\cdot N+1}^{s \cdot N} \frac{(\hat{x}_i(n) - x_i(n))^2}{\bar{x}_i^{\,2}}}, \qquad (6)$$

where $\bar{x}_i^{\,2}$ denotes the mean value of the squared signal segment; $\hat{x}_i(n)$ and $x_i(n)$ give the nth values of the segment of signal channel i calculated using the predictor, and the EEG signal value respectively.

---

[c]In the following, x_i denotes signal values of an EEG recording of channel i for the sake of simplicity

[d]For all values within segment s, ergodicity will be assumed throughout this contribution

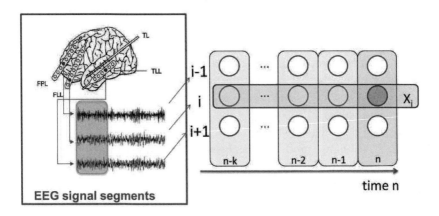

Fig. 2. Example scheme of CNN based signal prediction. $\kappa = 3$ values of 3 channels including the predicted channel are used for the prediction of a signal value x_i.

Alternatively, the coefficients $a_{l,k,p}(r)$ can be determined by introducing auto/cross-correlation functions of two time series $x_\xi(n)$ and $x_\zeta(m)$,[e]

$$\psi_{\xi,\zeta}^{p,q}(n-m) = E\{(x_\xi(n))^p, (x_\zeta)^q(m)\} \tag{7}$$

and solving the equation system

$$\mathbf{M} \cdot a = \Psi, \tag{8}$$

where the elements of the matrix $\mathbf{M}$ are submatrices

$$\mathbf{R}_{j,l}^P = \begin{pmatrix} \psi_{j,l}^{11}(0) & \cdots & \psi_{j,l}^{11}(1-\kappa) & \cdots & \psi_{j,l}^{1P}(1) & \cdots & \psi_{j,l}^{1P}(1-\kappa) \\ \vdots & \ddots & \vdots & \cdots & \vdots & \ddots & \vdots \\ \psi_{j,l}^{11}(\kappa-1) & \cdots & \psi_{j,l}^{11}(0) & \cdots & \psi_{j,l}^{1P}(\kappa-1) & \cdots & \psi_{j,l}^{1P}(0) \\ \vdots & & \vdots & & \vdots & \ddots & \\ \psi_{j,l}^{P1}(0) & \cdots & \psi_{j,l}^{P1}(1-\kappa) & \cdots & \psi_{j,l}^{PP}(0) & \cdots & \psi_{j,l}^{PP}(1-\kappa) \\ \vdots & \ddots & \vdots & \cdots & \vdots & \ddots & \vdots \\ \psi_{j,l}^{P1}(\kappa-1) & \cdots & \psi_{j,l}^{P1}(0) & \cdots & \psi_{j,l}^{PP}(\kappa-1) & \cdots & \psi_{j,l}^{PP}(0) \end{pmatrix} \tag{9}$$

of the signal. $\mathbf{M}$ has the form

$$\mathbf{M} = \begin{pmatrix} \mathbf{R}^p_{1,1} & \mathbf{R}^p_{1,2} & \cdots & \mathbf{R}^p_{1,\lambda} \\ \vdots & & \ddots & \vdots \\ \mathbf{R}^p_{\lambda,1} & \cdots & \mathbf{R}^p_{\lambda,\lambda-1} & \mathbf{R}^p_{\lambda,\lambda} \end{pmatrix}, \tag{10}$$

[e]Here, n and m denote the different time indices

$a = [a_{1,1,1} \ldots, a_{1,1,P}, \ldots, a_{1,\kappa,P}, \ldots, a_{\lambda,\kappa,P}]$ is a vector composed of the coefficients $a_{l,k,p}$ and the right hand side of Eq. (8) – $\Psi = [\psi_{i,1}^{1,1}(1), \ldots, \psi_{i,1}^{1,P}(1), \ldots, \psi_{i,1}^{1,P}(\kappa), \ldots, \psi_{i,\lambda}^{1,P}(1), \ldots, \psi_{i,\lambda}^{(1P)}(\kappa)]^T$ – consists of estimates of auto/cross correlation functions of a channel i that is predicted and other channels. All correlation functions $\psi_{j,l}^{p,q}(k_1 - k_2)$ are estimated by temporal means[12] using values $x_i(n - k_1), 1 \leq k_1 \leq \kappa$ of the channel to predict and values $x_j(n - k_2), 1 \leq j \leq \lambda, 1 \leq k_2 \leq \kappa$ of predicting channels of a certain data segment s.

The CNN signal predictor has been studied in detail in 13 by applying an optimization procedure with regards to Eq. (6) for different values of the signal prediction order κ and of the polynomial order P, as well as using coefficients derived by solving Eq. (8),[1] and order $P = 1$. Here, results obtained by applying the latter method will be presented.

2.1. *Multivariate signal prediction by CNN*

Seizure prediction methods using strategies based on EEG signal prediction and autoregressive modelling have been adressed by various authors.[14,15] A rise of the signal prediction error according to Eq. (6) prior to seizures was observed for many cases in previous studies. These included different measures– e.g. the signal prediction error and CNN coupling weights time series – and supposed preictal periods t_{pre} ranging from 10 minutes to 4 hours, Further analysis showed that the prediction error can be considered as a possible feature[1] uncovering changes of the dynamical system generating the EEG signal. In the following, results obtained by using recordings of 15 patients each including at least four seizures are given. They are based on the application of the signal prediction algorithm according to Eq. (5), by using signals of three neighboring electrode channels with $P = 1$ and $\kappa = 3$. An increase of the signal prediction error prior to a seizure has been evaluated as a possible seizure prediction feature, taking into account supposed preictal periods t_{pre} between 10 minutes and 2 hours. We use Receiver-Operating-Characteristics (ROC) analysis and the so-called Area-Under-Curve (AUC) value[16] to evaluate the seizure prediction performance.

In order to verify the significance of AUC values, we applied a surrogate analysis based on seizure onset time surrogates by using a significance level of 5%. Therefore, 19 sets of surrogate data[17] have been created for each patient. Then, AUC values have been calculated by considering the same seizure prediction horizon as for the original data that can be found in Table 1. Results have been considered significant only if all AUC values obtained for surrogate data are lower than those obtained using the original seizure times. Figure 3 shows the ROC curve and the result of the surrogate analysis for patient 9 of Table 1. We found AUC values larger than 0.65 for

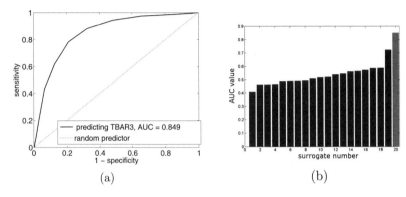

(a) (b)

Fig. 3. ROC curve (a) and AUC values for surrogate and original data (b) obtained for $e(r)$ of patient 9. Values of the channels TBAR2, TBAR3, and TBAR4 have been used in the signal prediction of channel TBAR3. $t_{pre} = 10$ min, AUC = 0.8492, maximal surrogate value $AUC_{surr} = 0.72$. AUC value of original seizure times is shown as number 20.

ten out of 15 patients. For all patients with AUC values larger than 0.65, a surrogate test validated the significance of the results. The prediction horizon of a feature is of great importance for patients; however, the preferred length of a prediction horizon varies from patient to patient.[18] A seizure prediction horizon of more than 30 minutes can be observed for only 7% of those patients with significant AUC values, making this method more suitable for patients who prefer a short seizure warning time.

The results described above underline that a feature based on signal prediction might be considered as a valuable contribution to a future implementation of a seizure warning device. However, those results are obtained in retrospective studies evaluating a large number of different electrode channel combinations using all available data, i.e. these methods cannot be applied in this form in prospective clinical studies. Therefore, we have recently proposed a modified signal prediction method.[9] In this paper, potentially appropriate features –calculated from signal prediction errors – based on the data-driven selection of a few electrode channels by analyzing comparably short data segments will be determined.

Table 1. Result of the evaluation of $e(r)$ as a possible seizure prediction feature. t_{pre} leading to best AUC values are given for all patients for which AUC values above 0.65 could be obtained

Patient number	recording duration	Number of seizures	Number of channels	AUC value	highest surr. AUC value	t_{pre}
1	94.5 h	10	48	0.71	0.69	60 min
2	106.7 h	10	53	0.74	0.72	20 min
3	576.4 h	6	20	0.70	0.65	10 min
4	141.7 h	5	20	0.72	0.63	60 min
5	67.7 h	4	22	0.68	0.63	120 min
6	115.1 h	4	32	0.56	—	—
7	113.4 h	7	22	0.70	0.65	20 min
8	151.9 h	4	46	0.51	—	—
9	209.0 h	5	42	0.85	0.72	10 min
10	187.7 h	4	62	0.85	0.55	10 min
11	135.5 h	6	22	0.44	—	—
12	257.4 h	6	20	0.60	—	—
13	137.1 h	4	76	0.68	0.48	20 min
14	154.1 h	5	78	0.54	—	—
15	140.5 h	4	74	0.65	0.58	30 min

3. Out-of-sample study of multivariate signal prediction algorithms

In this contribution we present first results of a multivariate approach of the combination of signals of channels from different regions of a brain; based on data of two patients for whom both the occurence of 10 seizures each as well as longer periods without seizures were documented.

We calculated the so-called signal prediction performance[12]

$$\epsilon_{i,l}(s) = \frac{e_i(r)}{e_{i,l}(r)} \tag{11}$$

in order to analyze the dependencies between channels from different brain regions. Here, $e_i(r)$ denotes the signal prediction error of channel i obtained in a classical univariate[19] signal prediction approach according to

$$\hat{x}(n) = \sum_{k=1}^{\kappa} a_k \cdot x(n-k), \tag{12}$$

$e_{i,l}(r)$ represents the signal prediction error[12] when signal values of channel i are predicted by those of another channel l using the multivariate approach of Eq. (5).

Data from patient 1 and 2 with 48 and 53 channels of the patient group described in Table 1 have been chosen due to the fact that for both patients10 seizures are included within the recordings. A left mesial temporal seizure origin was diagnosed for both patients.

Firstly, the CNN predictor described by Eq. (5) with $\lambda = 1$, $\kappa = 3$, and $P = 1$ was applied to predict EEG signals of each channel using those of other channels. Here, a training set with 2 seizures separated by seizure free EEG recordings of approximately 10 h have been taken from the complete recordings of both patients, each covering a period of about 100 h. The application of the proposed procedure led to time series of combinations of CNN coupling weights and signal prediction preformances $\epsilon_{i,l}(s)$ which were analyzed in order to identify pair-wise channel combinations[9] allowing an improved prediction of epileptic seizures. After the determination of the signal prediction performance given in Eq. (11) for all channel combinations, an ROC analysis was done for all 48×48 (patient 1) and 53×53 (patient 2) time series of $\epsilon_{i,l}(s)$. Here, we chose a seizure prediction horizon of 30 min. Afterwards, mean AUC values and variances were calculated for all pair-

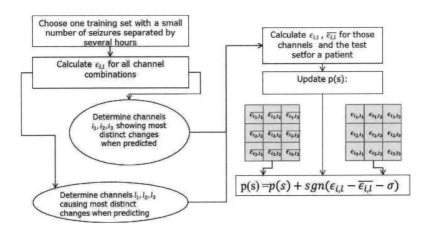

Fig. 4. Flowchart of the algorithm used to identify potentially suitable electrode channels. All combinations of signal prediction performances are calculated for a short time data segment. An ROC analysis is carried out and channels causing most distinct changes as well as showing most distinct changes are identified. Then, combinations of those channels are used to evaluate all data of a patient and a combined measure $p(s)$ is calculated.

wise channel combinations of channels predicting a certain channel. From these, three channels i_1, i_2 and i_3 having the highest mean AUC value and low variance were selected. Additionally, average AUC values for all pair-wise channel combinations of a certain channel predicting all other channels were calculated and channels l_1, l_2 and l_3 causing the most distinct changes in the prediction of signal values of any channel were selected. Then, the signal prediction performances have been determined for all 9 combinations of channels l_1, l_2, l_3 predicting channels i_1, i_2, i_3 for the test set as shown in Fig. 4.

Since slow oscillations of the signal prediction performance with a period of several hours can be observed for all patients and channel combinations so far, we introduced a mean signal prediction performance according to

$$\bar{\epsilon}_{i,l}(s) = \frac{1}{h_m} \cdot \sum_{n=0}^{h_m} \epsilon_{i,l}(s-n), \tag{13}$$

with a mean length h_m of 30 min. An increased dependency of the signal prediction on different regions of the brain directly prior to a seizure would lead to more pronounced changes of $\epsilon_{i,l}$ and a rise above the mean signal prediction performance $\bar{\epsilon}_{i,l}$. In a last step, by using all 9 possible features, the evaluation measure $p(s)$ according to

$$p(s) = \sum_i \sum_l sgn(\epsilon_{i,l} - \bar{\epsilon}_{i,l} - \sigma) \tag{14}$$

was calculated. Here, a step-value σ was introduced in order to smooth very small fluctuations of the signal prediction performances. For the results presented here a value of $\sigma = 0.033$ was used and an ROC analysis was carried out, now taking into account the test set for each patient. Results were compared to the performance of time series of $\epsilon_{i,l}(s)$ determined before. Table 2 shows AUC values of all selected channel combinations – both of the short time analysis and of all data available for patient 1, evaluating a rise of the signal prediction performance $\epsilon_{i,l}$ prior to a seizure as a possible feature, and taking into account a preictal period of $t_{pre} = 30$ min. All AUC values drop significantly when considering the test set. However, an increased significance of the AUC value of $p(s)$ can be obtained as compared to the results shown in Table 2. Here, it should be emphasized that the seizure prediction horizon as well as the interval h_m used in calculating the mean signal prediction performance $\bar{\epsilon}_{i,l}$ according to Eq. (13) were not adjusted to the patient but chosen based on assumptions made before the analysis. ROC-curves of $p(s)$ and of 2 signal prediction performances $\epsilon_{i,l}(s)$, evaluated for the test set of 100 h of patient 1 are shown in Fig. 5.

Likewise,channel combinations were selected and the evaluation procedure was applied to data of patient 2. Results of the AUC analysis for the selected channel combinations are shown in Table 3. Again, no adjustment of the parameters to the patient was carried out. When taking into account

237

Table 2. AUC values of patient 1, ROC analysis carried out
for a short training set of approximately 10 h with two seizures
and for the test set. Evaluating a rise of the signal prediction
performance, preictal period $t_{pre} = 30$ min.

test set

pred. signal	signal from predicting electrode		
from electrode	$l_1 = TBPR1$	$l_2 = TLR02$	$l_3 = TL01$
$i_1 = TR02$	0.8133	0.8173	0.8151
$i_2 = TR01$	0.8080	0.8067	0.8122
$i_3 = TR05$	0.7959	0.7923	0.7889

training set

pred. signal	signal from predicting electrode		
from electrode	$l_1 = TBPR1$	$l_2 = TLR02$	$l_3 = TL01$
$i_1 = TR02$	0.6167	0.6195	0.6050
$i_2 = TR01$	0.5581	0.5596	0.5555
$i_3 = TR05$	0.6319	0.6244	0.6155

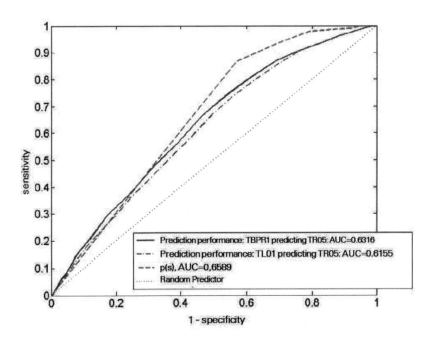

Fig. 5. ROC curves and AUC values of $\epsilon_{TR05,TBPR1}$, AUC = 0.616, $\epsilon_{TR05,TR02}$, AUC = 0.6319 and $p(s)$, AUC = 0.6589 for patient 1. A slightly increased AUC value can be observed for $p(s)$

only the test set of about 10 h, again, AUC values of 0.8 could be obtained for all 9 electrode combinations. However, when taking into account the test set for the patient, these AUC values drop below 0.6, practically equal to a random predictor. With $p(s)$, the combination of them led to an AUC value of 0.654, exceeding those of a random predictor as shown in Fig. 6. Since optimal electrode channels chosen by the method presented here are located in different regions of the brain, the dependencies of such channels may possibly indicate network phenomena also observed by other groups.[20]

4. Discussion

In this contribution, we present results of a CNN based signal prediction approach as a possible feature extraction method for seizure prediction using long-term recordings of 15 patients suffering from temporal lobe epilepsy. We find promising results for 66.7% of all patients with AUC values up to 0.85. AUC values of surrogate data are clearly separable from those of real seizure times for all patients with AUC values above 0.65. Apart from the results presented here, various other studies focus on the application of CNN based methods ranging from nonlinear interdependencies[3] and synchronization measures[5,6] to an approximation of the correlation dimension.[10] Most of those studies also show promising results which could be a basis for a future implementation of a miniaturized seizure warning device.

We presented first results of an approach dedicated to be applied and verified for data sets of two patients by identifying features based on a small subset of the available data. The proposed method can be regarded

Table 3.   AUC values of patient 2, ROC analysis carried out for a training set of app. 10 h with two seizures and for the test set available. Evaluating a rise of the signal prediction performance, preictal period $t_{pre} = 30$ min.

training set			
pred. signal	signal from predicting electrode		
from electrode	$l_1 = TL03$	$l_2 = LR02$	$l_3 = BPR01$
$i_1 = TR02$	0.8250	0.8266	0.8242
$i_2 = TR01$	0.8201	0.8161	0.8175
$i_3 = TR03$	0.8041	0.8031	0.8030

test set			
pred. signal	signal from predicting electrode		
from electrode	$l_1 = TL03$	$l_2 = LR02$	$l_3 = BPR01$
$i_1 = TR02$	0.5966	0.5962	0.5961
$i_2 = TR01$	0.5850	0.5851	0.5846
$i_3 = TR03$	0.5799	0.5793	0.5794

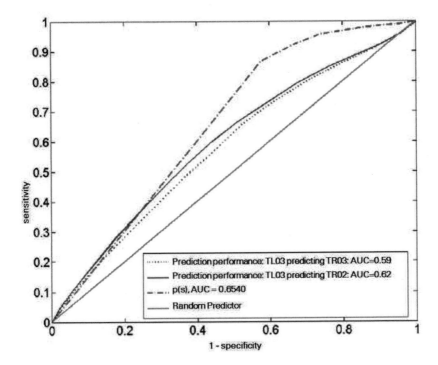

Fig. 6. ROC curves and AUC values for $\epsilon_{TR03,TL03}$, AUC $= 0.5799$, $\epsilon_{TR02,TL03}$, $AUC = 0.5966$ and $p(s)$, AUC $= 0.6540$ for patient 2. The AUC value obtained for $p(s)$ exceeds those of all $\epsilon_{i,l}$ and the random predictor.

as a first step in the development of CNN based signal prediction methods which are more appropriate for applications in clinical practice. They should be further developed and evaluated, e.g. by applying it to data of a larger group of patients and secondly by evaluating how many seizures would be needed to be considered in the suggested data-driven selection method. A third step possibly leading to an improvement of the method would be to focus on the proposed evaluation measure – the mean horizon used in the calculation of the mean signal prediction performance as well as the step value used for determining $p(r)$ have been chosen prior to the calculations. A detailed analysis of the seizure free period included within the short data segment chosen as test data could lead to an improved and more individualized evaluation measure. First results presented here indicate that the combination of the feature calculated using recordings from different areas of the brain can lead to increased AUC values as compared to univariate prediction.

Acknowledgment

This work was obtained using ressources of the high performance computation center Dresden (ZIH). We would like to thank Klaus Lehnertz from
the Department of Epileptology, University Hospital in Bonn, Germany for
providing the EEG data.

References

1. F. Gollas and R. Tetzlaff, Spatio-temporal analysis of brain electrical activity
   in epilepsy based on Cellular Nonlinear Networks., in *Proceedings of SPIE
   Europe, Microtechnologies for the new millennium*, 2009.
2. R. Kunz, R. Tetzlaff and D. Wolf, Brain electrical activity in epilepsy: Characterization of the spatio-temporal dynamics with Cellular Neural Networks
   based on a correlation dimension analysis, in *Proceedings of the ISCAS*, 2000.
3. D. Krug, H. Osterhage, C. E. Elger and K. Lehnertz, *Physical review. E* **76**,
   p. 041916 (2007).
4. H. Dickten, C. E. Elger and K. Lehnertz, Measuring directed interactions us-
   ingCellular Neural Networks (CNN) with complex topologies., in *This Issue*,
   2011.
5. D. Krug, C. E. Elger and K. Lehnertz, A CNN-based synchronization analysis for epileptic seizure prediction: Inter- and intraindividual generalization
   properties, in *Proceedings of the 2008 11th International Workshop on Cellular Neural Networks and their Applications.*, eds. D. Vilarino, D. Ferrer and
   V. Sanchez2008.
6. A. Chernihovskyi, C. E. Elger and K. Lehnertz, *EURASIP Journal on Advances in Signal Processing* , p. 582412 (2009).
7. R. Sowa, A. Chernihovskyi, F. Mormann and K. Lehnertz, *Phys. Rev. E* **71**,
   p. 061926 (2005).
8. F. Gollas and R. Tetzlaff, Analysis of EEG-signals in epilepsy: Spatio-
   temporal models, in *Proceedings of the 11th International Workshop on Cellular Nonlinear Networks and their Applications (CNNA 2008)*, eds. D. Vilarino, D. Ferrer and V. Sanchez (Santiago de Compostela, Spain, 2008).
9. V. Senger and R. Tetzlaff, Multichannel prediction analysis in epilepsy, in
   *Proc. of the 20th Conference on Nonlinear Dynamics and Electronic Systems,
   (NDES 2012)*, 2012.
10. R. Kunz and R. Tetzlaff, *Journal of Circuits, Systems and Computation* **12**,
    825(December 2003).
11. C. Niederhöfer, F. Gollas and R. Tetzlaff, EEG analysis by multi layer Cellu-
    lar Nonlinear Networks (CNN), in *Proceedings of the 2006 IEEE Conference
    on Biomedical Circuits and Systems (BioCAS 2006)*, 2006.
12. V. Senger, J. Müller and R. Tetzlaff, Spatio-temporal coupling of EEG signals
    in epilepsy., in *Proceedings of SPIE*,

13. C. Niederhöfer, F. Gollas and R. Tetzlaff, Dynamics of eeg-signals in epilepsy: Spatio temporal analysis by Cellular Neural Networks, in *Proceedings of the 18th European Conference on Circuit Theory and Design (ECCTD 2007)*, 27–30 Aug. 2007.

14. C. Niederhöfer and R. Tetzlaff, Prediction of epileptic seizures using multi-layer delay-type discrete time cellular nonlinear networks (DTCNN) - long-term studies, in *Proceedings of SPIE's Microtechnologies for a New Millenium*, (Sevilla, Spain, 2005).

15. L. Chisci, A. Mavino, G. Perferi, M. Sciandrone, C. Anile, G. Colicchio and F. Fuggetta, *IEEE Trans Biomed Eng* **57**, 1124 (2010).

16. T. Fawcett, *Pattern Recognition Letters* **27**, 861 (2006).

17. R. Andrzejak, F. Mormann, T. Kreuz, C. Rieke, A. Kraskov, C. E. Elger and K. Lehnertz, *Phys Rev E* **67**, p. 010901 (2003).

18. A. Schulze-Bonhage, F. Sales, K. Wagner, R. Teotonio, A. Carius, A. Schelle and M. Ihle, *Epilepsy & Behavior* **18**, 388 (2010).

19. S. Haykin, *Adaptive Filter Theory* (Prentice Hall International, New Jersey, 1996).

20. K. Lehnertz, S. Bialonski, M.-T. Horstmann, D. Krug, A. Rothkegel, M. Staniek and T. Wagner, *Journal of Neuroscience Methods* **183**, 42 (2009).

MEASURING DIRECTED INTERACTIONS USING CELLULAR NEURAL NETWORKS WITH COMPLEX CONNECTION TOPOLOGIES

H. DICKTEN[1,2,3,*], C. E. ELGER[1], K. LEHNERTZ[1,2,3]

[1]*Department of Epileptology, University of Bonn,*
Sigmund-Freud-Straße 25, 53105 Bonn, Germany
[2]*Helmholtz-Institute for Radiation and Nuclear Physics, University of Bonn,*
Nussallee 14–16, 53115 Bonn, Germany
[3]*Interdisciplinary Center for Complex Systems, University of Bonn,*
Brühler Straße 7, 53175 Bonn, Germany
[*]*E-mail: hdickten@uni-bonn.de*

We advance our approach of analyzing the dynamics of interacting complex systems with the nonlinear dynamics of interacting nonlinear elements. We replace the widely used lattice-like connection topology of cellular neural networks (CNN) by complex topologies that include both short- and long-ranged connections. With an exemplary time-resolved analysis of asymmetric nonlinear interdependences between the seizure generating area and its immediate surrounding we provide first evidence for complex CNN connection topologies to allow for a faster network optimization together with an improved approximation accuracy of directed interactions.

Keywords: CNN; Directed Interactions; Nonlinear Interdependence; iEEG; Complex Networks; Time Series Analysis; Seizure Prediction Device

1. Introduction

Synchronization phenomena play an important role in nearly all fields of science, including physics, chemistry, economy, and the neurosciences.[1,2] The human epileptic brain can be regarded as a prominent example in which different forms of synchronization can be observed. Estimators for synchronization[3,4] are highly attractive to characterize interactions between brain areas involved in ictogenesis.

Promising computational platforms for approximating these estimators are, among other approaches,[5] Cellular Neural (or Nonlinear) Networks (CNN) as they are capable of universal computation and offer massive computing power while minimizing space and energy consumption and are already available as analogue integrated circuits.[6-9] Recent studies have shown that the approach of analyzing the dynamics of interacting complex systems with the nonlinear dynamics of interacting nonlinear elements can also be extended to the concepts of phase synchronization[10] and generalized synchronization.[11] With the latter concept symmetric and asymmetric nonlinear interdependence measures can be defined that allow one to characterize strength and direction of interactions.[11-15]

We investigated whether a CNN-based characterization of directed interactions can further be improved by modifying the canonical Chua–Yang CNN.[16] This CNN consists of a regular (lattice-like) arrangement of cells which we replace by complex topologies.[17,18] We evaluate approximation accuracies through the analysis of directed interactions in long-term, multi-channel, intracranial electroencephalographic (iEEG) recordings from an epilepsy patient.

2. Methods

2.1. *Nonlinear Interdependencies*

Let A and B denote two dynamical systems and let $a_n, n = 1, \ldots, N$ and $b_n, n = 1, \ldots, N$ denote time series of some observable of the respective system. With

$$\vec{a}_n = \left(a_n, \ldots a_{n-(d_e-1)\tau}\right) \quad \text{and} \quad \vec{b}_n = \left(b_n, \ldots, b_{n-(d_e-1)\tau}\right) \tag{1}$$

we denote the reconstructed delay vectors in state space[19,20] with an appropriate chosen time delay τ and embedding dimension d_e. Given some reference point in state space, the mean-squared Euclidean distance to its k nearest neighbors reads:

$$R_n^{(k)}(A) = \frac{1}{k} \sum_{j=1}^{k} \left(\vec{a}_n - \vec{a}_{r_{n,j}}\right)^2, \tag{2}$$

where $r_{n,j}, j = 1, \ldots, k$ denote the time indices of the k nearest neighbors of $\vec{a}_n$. With $s_{n,j}, j = 1, \ldots, k$ as time indices of the k nearest neighbors of $\vec{b}_n$, $R_n^{(k)}(B)$ is defined analogously. In addition, the B-*conditioned* mean-squared Euclidean distance in the state space of system A is derived by replacing the nearest neighbors of $\vec{a}_n$ by the equal-time partners of the nearest neighbors of $\vec{b}_n$:

$$R_n^{(k)}(A|B) = \frac{1}{k} \sum_{j=1}^{k} \left(\vec{a}_n - \vec{a}_{s_{n,j}}\right)^2. \tag{3}$$

$R_n^{(k)}(B|A)$ is defined in complete analogy, and the nonlinear interdependence $S^{(k)}$ then reads[12]

$$S^{(k)}(A|B) = \frac{1}{M} \sum_{n=1}^{M} \frac{R_n^{(k)}(A)}{R_n^{(k)}(A|B)}, \qquad (4)$$

where M denotes the total number of state space vectors. Strength and direction of interactions can be characterized via a symmetric and asymmetric measure:

$$
\begin{aligned}
S_{\text{symm}}^{(k)} &= \frac{S^{(k)}(A|B) + S^{(k)}(B|A)}{2} \\
S_{\text{asymm}}^{(k)} &= \frac{S^{(k)}(A|B) - S^{(k)}(B|A)}{2}.
\end{aligned}
\qquad (5)
$$

2.2. Cellular Neural Networks (CNN)

Artificial Neural Networks (ANNs) are computational tools inspired by the brain that have found extensive utilization in complex real-world problems.[21] An ANN consists of simple artificial *cells* or *processing units* which are connected via *edges*, but there exists no single formal definition of what an ANN exactly is. ANNs feature characteristics such as high parallelism, intrinsic nonlinearity, as well as fault and noise tolerance. More importantly, ANNs can be trained using a set of given examples and offer the ability to generalize.[22,23]

A Cellular Neural Network (CNN) is a subset of ANN where—in contrast to a Hopfield network[24]—only local connections between cells are allowed.[16] Hence the number of edges increases only linearly with the number of cells of the network.

2.2.1. Dynamics of a CNN

Following Ref. 25, a CNN is a spatial arrangement of locally connected cells, where each cell is a dynamical system which has an input u, bias z, output $y(t)$ and state $x(t)$ evolving according to some state equation (cf. Fig. 1).

Let us first consider a CNN which consists of a two-dimensional $\mathcal{M} \times \mathcal{N}$ translation-invariant lattice of cells with nonlinear interactions. The corresponding state equation for cell (i,j) ($i \in [1, \mathcal{M}]$ and $j \in [1, \mathcal{N}]$) reads

$$\dot{x}_{ij}(t) = -x_{ij}(t) + \sum_{lm \in \mathcal{I}_{ij}} \mathcal{A}_{lm}\big(y_{lm}(t)\big) + \sum_{lm \in \mathcal{I}_{ij}} \mathcal{B}_{lm}\big(u_{lm}\big) + z, \qquad (6)$$

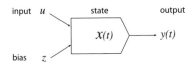

Fig. 1. Representation of a single cell of a CNN. Each cell is a dynamical system with state $x(t)$ evolving according to some state equation.

where $\mathcal{I}_{ij}$ denotes the *sphere of influence* of cell (i, j), and $l, m \in \mathcal{I}_{ij}$. $\mathcal{A}_{lm}$ and $\mathcal{B}_{lm}$ denote the feedback and feed-forward template functions, respectively. In order to present the time series $a_n, b_n, N = 4096$ to the network, we used a line wise alignment, i.e., the rightmost cell in a row is connected to the leftmost cell in the following row. Time series a_n was assigned to the input u and time series b_n to the initial state $x(0)$ of the CNN. Together with the chosen boundary condition this alignment preserves the temporal order of the time series. Nevertheless it may introduce correlations between uncorrelated data points within the time series.

Following Ref. 11, we here define the canonical Chua–Yang CNNcan as a quadratic network arrangement ($\mathcal{M} \times \mathcal{N} = 64$) with a minimum possible 3×3 sphere of influence as well as polynomial-type template functions of order three (cf. Fig. 2 left). In order to investigate whether complex connection topologies allow for an improved CNN-based characterization of directed interactions, we additionally consider two modified versions of CNNcan:

With CNNlr we define a topology, in which some short- and long-ranged connections between cell (i, j) and cells of its sphere of influence are introduced. The distance of the long-ranged connections corresponds to the time of the first maximum of the autocorrelation function of time series a_n and b_n, respectively (normalized by the sampling interval), thus minimizing the aforementioned effect of connecting possibly uncorrelated data. Short-ranged connections exist between cells (i, j) and $(i, j - 1)$ and between cells (i, j) and $(i, j + 1)$ (cf. Fig. 2 middle). Eventually we fully relax the canonical topology by choosing connections between cell (i, j) and eight other cells (that comprise the sphere of influence) at random (CNNran; cf. Fig. 2 right). Each sphere of influence remained translation-invariant and consisted of nine (eight to other cells and one to itself) connections to ensure comparability between different topologies.

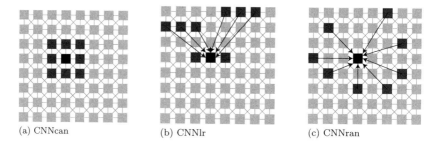

(a) CNNcan   (b) CNNlr   (c) CNNran

Fig. 2. CNN with the canonical (a) and with complex connection topologies (b and c). In (b) long-ranged connections are chosen according to the time of the first maximum of the autocorrelation function for each time series separately. In (c) short- and long-ranged connections are chosen at random.

2.2.2. *Optimization and Validation*

In the following, we denote with U, $X(t)$, and $Y(t)$ the inputs, states and outputs of all CNN cells. In order to optimize the networks we used an evolutionary algorithm[26,27] with the following parameters: population size: 50, number of survivors: 10, number of immigrants: 10, maximum number of iteration steps: 300.

We performed an in-sample optimization of our CNN using $V = 20$ representative pairs of time series of 20.48 s duration (in total ≈ 7 min EEG) each along with the corresponding value of the nonlinear interdependence measure calculated according to Eq. (5) (denoted as $S^{\text{ref.}}$ in the following) with $\tau = 5, d_e = 10$, and $k = 6$. Half of the values represented weakly dependent time series ($S^{\text{ref. low}}_{\text{asymm.}} \in [-0.04, -0.02]$), and the other half stronger dependent time series ($S^{\text{ref. high}}_{\text{asymm.}} \in [0.04, 0.06]$), respectively.[28] To check for possible over-optimization of our CNN, we performed an additional out-of-sample validation using a similar setup as before but with another set of 20 pairs of time series along with the corresponding values of the nonlinear interdependence.

The approximated asymmetric nonlinear interdependence measure $S^{(k)}_{\text{asymm}}$ was obtained by the rescaled mean output of all cells:

$$S^{\text{CNN}}_{\text{asymm.}} = \left(\frac{S^{\text{ref. high}}_{\text{asymm.}} - S^{\text{ref. low}}_{\text{asymm.}}}{\mathcal{M}\mathcal{N}} \sum_{i,j=0}^{\mathcal{M},\mathcal{N}} \frac{y_{i,j}(\tau_{\text{trans}}) + 1}{2} \right) + S^{\text{ref. low}}_{\text{asymm.}} \qquad (7)$$

After choosing random initial values for the components of templates $\mathcal{A}$ and $\mathcal{B}$ and for the global cell bias z the global error was minimized:

$$E_g = \frac{1}{V} \sum_{v=0}^{V-1} \left(\frac{1}{4\mathcal{M}\mathcal{N}} \sum_{i,j=0}^{\mathcal{M},\mathcal{N}} \left(y_{i,j,v}(\tau_{\text{trans}}) - Y_v^{\text{ref}} \right)^2 \right) \tag{8}$$

where τ_{trans} denotes some fixed transition time.[29,30] All calculations were performed using our distributed computing system,[31] and network simulations were performed with Conedy.[32]

3. CNN-based iEEG Analysis

We analyzed directed interactions in multi-channel iEEG recordings from an epilepsy patient who underwent presurgical evaluation of a left-sided mesial temporal lobe epilepsy. After selective amygdalo-hippocampectomy the patient is completely seizure-free. The patient had signed informed consent that the clinical data might be used and published for research purposes. The study protocol had previously been approved by the ethics committee of the University of Bonn. iEEG was measured from bilaterally implanted intrahippocampal depth electrodes. iEEG data were sampled at 200 Hz using a 16 bit analog-to-digital converter and filtered within a frequency band of 0.5–85 Hz.

In the following we report our findings of estimating directed interactions between the seizure generating area and its immediate surrounding in a time-resolved manner (moving window analysis; non-overlapping windows of 20.48 s duration). We here restrict ourselves to an interictal recording lasting for about 25 hours.

First of all we note that short- and long-term fluctuations of nonlinear interdependencies between brain regions could well be approximated even with CNN with complex connection topologies. This observation does not only extend previous findings[11] but it also indicates that the use of complex topologies leads to a faster optimization and validation of the CNN (cf. upper parts of Fig. 3–5). More importantly, when comparing performance data of the three investigated CNN, approximation accuracy increased from 87.5 % (CNNcan) to 90.1 % (CNNran) to 92.7 % (CNNlr) (cf. lower parts of Fig. 3–5).

4. Conclusion

We have investigated whether a CNN-based approximation of directed interactions between the dynamics of different areas of the human epileptic brain can be improved by replacing the lattice-like arrangement of CNN

248

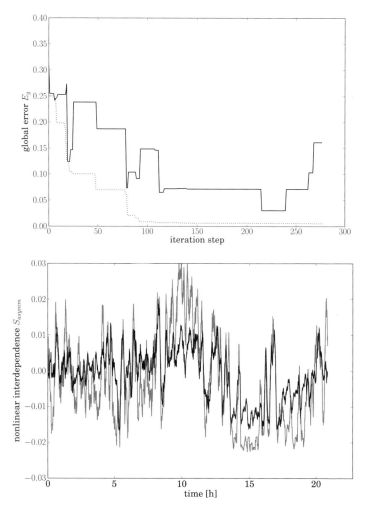

Fig. 3. Exemplary findings obtained with CNNcan. Top: Global error E_g (cf. Eq. (8)) depending on the number of iteration steps during in-sample optimization (dotted line) and during out-of-sample validation (solid line). Bottom: Temporal evolution of analytically calculated (black line) and approximated nonlinear interdependence S_{asymm} (gray line) between the seizure generating area and its immediate surrounding. Profiles are smoothed using a 15-point ($\approx 5\,\mathrm{min}$) moving-average filter for better visualization. The CNN-approximation was performed with the templates $\mathcal{A}$ and $\mathcal{B}$ and the global cell bias z obtained in iteration step 80.

cells by complex connection topologies. Findings obtained from an exemplary analysis of directed interactions in intracranial electroencephalo-

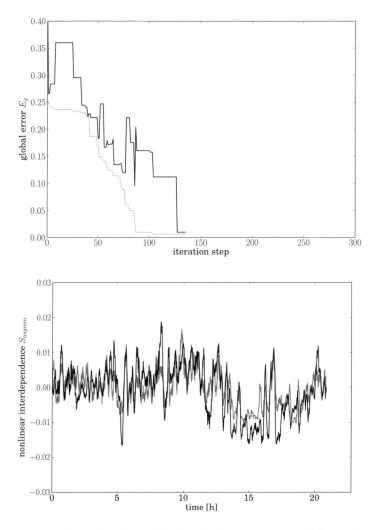

Fig. 4. Same as Fig. 3 but for CNNlr. The CNN-approximation of the nonlinear interdependence S_{asymm} was performed with the templates $\mathcal{A}$ and $\mathcal{B}$ and the global cell bias z obtained in iteration step 58.

graphic recordings from an epilepsy patient indicate that complex connection topologies allow for a faster optimization of CNN together with an improved approximation accuracy of nonlinear interdependence. Our preliminary though promising findings need to be validated on the data from a larger group of patients.

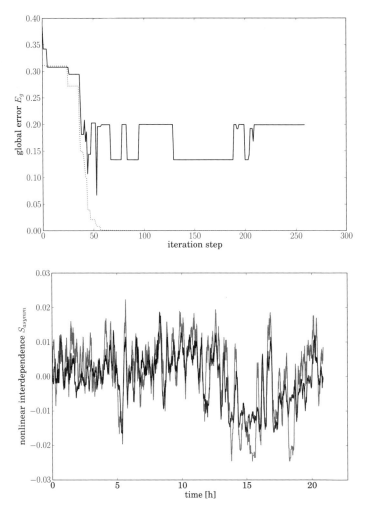

Fig. 5. Same as Fig. 3 but for CNNran. The CNN-approximation of the nonlinear interdependence S_{asymm} was performed with the templates $\mathcal{A}$ and $\mathcal{B}$ and the global cell bias z obtained in iteration step 40.

Although our findings are, at present, restricted to simulated or digital realizations of CNN, their powerful computational capacity and generalization capability combined with small size and low power consumption of hardware realizations render these networks highly attractive for the development of miniaturized seizure prediction devices.

Acknowledgments

This work was supported by the Deutsche Forschungsgemeinschaft (Grand No. LE660/2-4).

References

1. A. S. Pikovsky, M. G. Rosenblum and J. Kurths, *Synchronization: A universal concept in nonlinear sciences* (Cambridge University Press, Cambridge, UK, 2001).
2. S. Boccaletti, J. Kurths, G. Osipov, D. L. Valladares and C. S. Zhou, *Phys. Rep.* **366**, 1 (2002).
3. K. Lehnertz, S. Bialonski, M.-T. Horstmann, D. Krug, A. Rothkegel, M. Staniek and T. Wagner, *J. Neurosci. Methods* **183**, 42 (2009).
4. K. Lehnertz, *Physiol. Meas.* **32**, 1715 (2011).
5. K. Abdelhalim, V. Smolyakov and R. Genov, *IEEE Trans. Biomed. Circuits Syst.* **5**, 430 (2011).
6. L. O. Chua and T. Roska, *Cellular neural networks and visual computing* (Cambridge University Press, Cambridge UK, 2002).
7. A. Chernihovskyi, F. Mormann, M. Müller, C. E. Elger, G. Baier and K. Lehnertz, *J. Clin. Neurophysiol.* **22**, 314 (2005).
8. R. Tetzlaff, T. Niederhofer and P. Fischer, *Int. J. Circ. Theor. Appl.* **34**, 89 (2006).
9. T. Roska, *Int. J. Circ. Theor. Appl.* **36(5-6)**, 523 (2008).
10. R. Sowa, A. Chernihovskyi, F. Mormann and K. Lehnertz, *Phys. Rev. E* **71**, 061926 (2005).
11. D. Krug, H. Osterhage, C. E. Elger and K. Lehnertz, *Phys. Rev. E* **76**, 041916 (2007).
12. J. Arnhold, P. Grassberger, K. Lehnertz and C. E. Elger, *Physica D* **134**, 419 (1999).
13. D. Chicharro and R. G. Andrzejak, *Phys. Rev. E* **80**, 026217 (2009).
14. R. G. Andrzejak, D. Chicharro, K. Lehnertz and F. Mormann, *Phys. Rev. E* **83**, 046203 (2011).
15. K. Lehnertz, D. Krug, M. Staniek, D. Glüsenkamp and C. E. Elger, Preictal directed interactions in epileptic brain networks, in *Epilepsy: The Intersection of Neurosciences, Biology, Mathematics, Engineering and Physics*, eds. I. Osorio, H. Zaveri, M. Frei and S. Arthurs (CRC Press, Boca Raton, FL, 2011) pp. 265–272.
16. L. O. Chua and L. Yang, *IEEE Trans. Circuits Syst.* **35**, 1257 (1988).
17. D. J. Watts and S. H. Strogatz, *Nature* **393**, 440 (1998).
18. K. Tsuruta, Z. Yang, Y. Nishio and A. Ushida, *IEIC Technical Report* **103**, 67 (2003).
19. H. Whitney, *Ann. Math.* **37**, 645 (1936).
20. F. Takens, Detecting strange attractors in turbulence, in *Dynamical Systems and Turbulence (Warwick 1980)*, eds. D. A. Rand and L.-S. Young, Lecture Notes in Mathematics, Vol. 898 (Springer-Verlag, Berlin, 1981) pp. 366–381.

21. K. Priddy and P. Keller, *Artificial neural networks: an introduction* (SPIE Press, Bellingham, WA, 2005).
22. T. L. H. Watkin, A. Rau and M. Biehl, *Rev. Mod. Phys.* **65**, 499 (1993).
23. S. Haykin, *Neural Networks - A Comprehensive Foundation*, 10 edn. (Tom Robbins, London, UK, 1999).
24. J. Hopfield, *Proc. Natl. Acad. Sci. U.S.A.* **79**, 2554 (1982).
25. L. O. Chua, *CNN: A paradigm for complexity* (Singapore: World Scientific, 1998).
26. J. H. Holland, *Adaptation in natural and artificial systems* (The University of Michigan Press, Ann Arbor, USA, 1975).
27. R. Kunz, A. Loncar and R. Tetzlaff, SCNN 2000, Part I and II, in *Proceedings of the 6th IEEE International Workshop on Cellular Neural Networks and Their Applications*, ed. L. Fortuna (IEEE Press, Piscataway, NJ, 2000).
28. D. Krug, C. E. Elger and K. Lehnertz, A CNN-based synchronization analysis for epileptic seizure prediction: Inter- and intraindividual generalization properties, in *11th International Workshop on Cellular Neural Networks and Their Applications, 2008.*, eds. D. Vilarino, D. Ferrer and V. Brea Sanchez (IEEE Press, Piscataway, NJ, 2008).
29. R. Kunz, R. Tetzlaff and D. Wolf, Brain electrical activity in epilepsy: Characterization of the spatio-temporal dynamics with cellular neural networks based on a correlation dimension analysis, in *Proceedings of the IEEE International Symposium on Circuits and Systems*, eds. J. Vandevalle and M. Hassler (IEEE Press, Piscataway, NJ, 2000).
30. D. Krug, A. Chernihovsky, H. Osterhage, C. E. Elger and K. Lehnertz, Estimating generalized synchronization in brain electrical activity from epilepsy patients with cellular nonlinear networks, in *Proc. 10th IEEE International Workshop on Cellular Neural Networks and their Applications*, eds. V. Tavsanoglu and S. Arik (IEEE Press, Piscataway, NJ, 2006).
31. A. Müller, H. Osterhage, R. Sowa, R. G. Andrzejak, F. Mormann and K. Lehnertz, *J. Neurosci. Methods* **152**, 190 (2006).
32. A. Rothkegel and K. Lehnertz, *Chaos* **22**, 013125 (2012).

SEIZURE PREDICTION USING OPTICAL MEASUREMENTS OF BLOOD FLOW AND OXYGENATION

M. ZHAO, H. MA AND T. H. SCHWARTZ

Department of Neurological Surgery, Weill Medical College of Cornell University,
New York Presbyterian Hospital, New York, New York 10021
Correspondence should be addressed to: Theodore H. Schwartz, MD Department of
Neurological Surgery, Weill Medical College of Cornell University, 525 East 68th Street,
Box 99, New York, NY 10065 E-mail: schwarh@med.cornell.edu

The ability to predict seizure occurrence is extremely important to trigger abortive therapies and to warn patients and their caregivers. Optical imaging of hemodynamic parameters such as blood flow, blood volume and tissue and hemoglobin oxygenation has already been shown to successfully localize epileptic events with high spatial and temporal resolution. Recent studies have now found pre-ictal optical changes in both human and animal seizures. Such optical measurements of blood flow and oxygenation may become increasingly important for predicting as well as localizing epileptic events.

Key Words: seizure, optical imaging, predication, neurovascular coupling, vasoconstriction

1. Introduction

1.1. *Seizure prediction*

Epilepsy is a clinical term referring to a disease that affects between 1 and 2% of the population of the United States involving recurrent seizures. Seizures can be sudden and occur without warning, which can cause significant injuries. The possibility of identifying events, whether they be behavioral, electrographic or hemodynamic, that reliably occur before epileptic seizures would have a dramatic impact on our ability to warn patients and their families of an upcoming event, thereby giving patients the ability to remove themselves from harm's way. Attempts have been made to forecast epileptic seizures using a variety of methodologies such as electroencephalogram (EEG) [1], functional magnetic resonance imaging (fMRI) [2, 3], single-photon emission computer tomography (SPECT) [4], among others[5]. Such, pre-ictal signals could also provide information for 'closed-loop' abortive therapies such as cortical stimulation [6], focal drug perfusion [7, 8], cooling [9], and optical inhibition [10-12]. Additionally, seizure prediction mechanisms can offer insights into epileptogenesis [13].

Traditional analysis of EEG signals has not shown any obvious or consistent pre-ictal changes [14, 15]. Complex non-linear mathematic algorithms for electrographic data can be used to predict seizure with increasing reliability [16, 17]. Recently, our laboratory reported a ~20s focal hemodynamic change before seizure onset in human lesional neocortical case. In addition, we have shown pre-ictal vessel constriction as early as 5 s prior to seizure onset in an animal model using a two-photon microscope [18, 19]. Elaboration of these findings, among others, and their significance will be the main subject of this chapter.

1.2. Neurovascular coupling and epilepsy

Neurovascular coupling concerns the relationship between neuronal activity, metabolism, tissue oxygenation, and blood flow. Adequate coupling is critical to supply the energy demands of the brain during normal physiological function as well as pathological conditions. Seizures create a large focal increase in metabolism and result in a dramatic increase in cerebral blood flow (CBF) to the ictal focus to provide adequate oxygenation. Whether or not CBF is adequate to meet the demands of an epileptic event has been a long-standing debate.

Optical imaging of intrinsic signals (ORIS) is a technique for measuring hemodynamic changes in the brain, based on enhanced light absorption of active neural tissue, which is caused by focal increases in cerebral blood flow (CBF), deoxygenation of hemoglobin and enhanced scattering of light [20, 21]. At wavelengths such as 570 nm, an isosbestic wavelength of hemoglobin, ORIS provides a direct measure of total hemoglobin (Hbt). Hbt is equivalent to cerebral blood volume (CBV) if the hematocrit remains constant, and CBV is proportional to CBF. At 610 nm, deoxygenated hemoglobin (Hbr) absorbs light more strongly than oxygenated hemoglobin (HbO_2) and it is possible to directly quantify both Hbr and Hbt with the appropriate calculation [22]. At 800 nm, or near infrared wavelengths, the optical signal is largely derived from light scattering related to cell swelling as well as intra- and extracellular fluid shifts, which provide an indirect representation of neuronal activity, less influenced by the changes in cerebral blood volume and hemoglobin oxygenation that dominate the intrinsic signal at lower wavelengths.

Several studies have shown that ORIS can be used to map the onset and spread of epileptic events via their hemodynamic sequellae with very high spatial and temporal resolution, as well as high spatial sampling [25, 34-40]. Epileptic events initiate a large focal increase in metabolism and cerebral blood flow (CBF) at the seizure focus. In contrast, decreases in CBF have been demonstrated surrounding the focus, the etiology of which is unknown. The relationship between these events and neuronal activity and metabolism are also unknown. Studies using techniques with limited spatial and temporal resolution such as fMRI, PET, SPECT and autoradiography have shown that the relative increase in CBF more than meets the increase in metabolism leading to an increase in blood oxygenation. But studies using higher temporal resolution techniques such as near infra-red spectroscopy (NIRS) and ORIS showed that CBF is inadequate to meet the metabolic demands of the epileptic tissue leading to a decrease in both tissue and hemoglobin oxygenation (see review [23])

2.   Optical measurement and seizure prediction

2.1.   *Optical imaging of pre-ictal changes*

The idea of pre-ictal vascular reactivity predicting the seizure onset was proposed (mistakenly at the time) as early as 1933 by Gibbs [24]. More recently, studies have found increases in cerebral perfusion 20 min before focal and generalized spike-and-wave events using transcranial Doppler [25]. Fortuitously, we recorded ORIS from human cortex intraoperatively in a patient with recurrent focal seizures arising from a cavernous malformation [18]. We found that focal changes in cerebrovascular hemodynamics preceded the seizure onset by ~20 s, and occurred focally over the known location of the lesion and the seizure onsets (Fig. 1). Three spontaneous seizures were successfully recorded, two at 610 nm and one at 570 nm, providing data on Hbr and CBV. Each seizure was accompanied by a dramatic, focal change in the intrinsic signal.   At 610 nm, a significant increase light reflectance began 23.74 ± 8.67 s prior to the electrographic onset of the seizure (Fig. 1 D and F). The spatial maps of the two seizures recorded at 610 nm were remarkably similar. At 570 nm, a significant decrease in light reflectance began 15.0 s prior to the electrographic onset of the seizure (Fig. 1 E), again restricted to the known epileptic gyrus consistent with a focal drop in CBV. Prior to the onset of the seizures, the signal inverted to a significant increase in light reflectance (increase in CBV), which reached maximum amplitude of 46.2%, peaking 58.1 s after the onset of the seizure. Again the signal was restricted to the known epileptic gyrus consistent with a focal drop in CBV. Prior to the onset of the seizures, the signal inverted to a significant increase in light reflectance (increase in CBV), which reached maximum amplitude of 46.2%, peaking 58.1 s after the onset of the seizure. This pre-ictal finding from spontaneous human epilepsy suggests that optical measurements may be useful to predict the seizure onset and location prior to any electrographic changes.

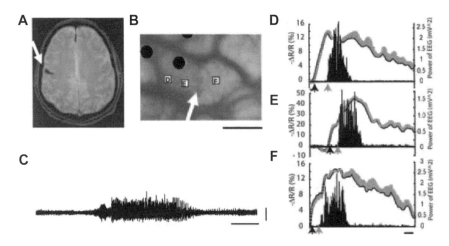

Figure 1. Pre-ictal changes of optical signal in human epilepsy. (A) Gradient echo axial MRI scan demonstrates a small cavernous malformation the right motor strip. (B) Surface of the brain under glass footplate. The black circles highlight the location of the recording electrodes. The rectangles demonstrate three regions of interest (ROIs), which contained the pixel values with the most statistically significant changes for each of the three seizures. The label on the rectangle corresponds to the graphs within this figure. (C) ECoG recording of a typical seizure. Scale bars: 20 seconds and 1 millivolt. The time course of (D and F) oximetry and (E) perfusion related intrinsic optical signal calculated as $-\Delta R/R$ (%) during each seizure from each ROI in (B) is graphed along with the power of the ECoG. Error bars represent SD of pixel values from each ROI. The onset of statistically significant optical signal changes is indicated with a black arrow and the onset of significant change in the power of the ECoG is indicated with a gray arrow. Scale bar: 1 cm. (see detail in [18])

Despite the discovery of pre-ictal optical signal in human spontaneous epilepsy, many of our animal studies in pharmacologically-induced recurrent focal neocortical seizures using 4-aminopyridine injection (4-AP) did not find any pre-ictal changes in intrinsic optical imaging, autofluorescence flavoprotein metabolism or direct tissue measurements [19, 26-29]. In another study, however, we divided these 4-AP seizures into two groups based on their electrographic onset pattern. While some seizures began with a large population spike, followed by low-voltage fast activity (LVFA), others began with LVFA without an initial spike. Of the 67 seizures, 47 began with an initial spike and 20 began without the initial spike. Using ORIS to record CBV, when an initiating spike occurred, increases were identified 0.653 ± 0.482 s after the initial spike. However, for the 20 seizures that did not begin with an initial spike but a LVFA recruiting rhythm, CBV increases occurred 1.525 ± 1.218 s before the first significant change in the LFP [30]. Thus, pre-ictal increase in CBV can depend on pattern of seizure onset (Fig. 2).

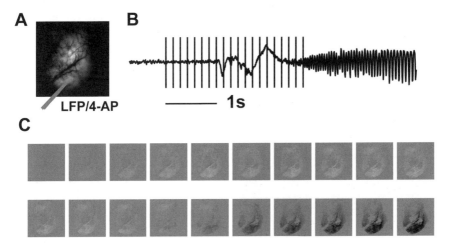

Figure 2. Pre-ictal decrease in CBV precede seizure onset. (A) Image of cortical surface to demonstrate location of 4-AP and LFP electrode (gray bar). (B) LFP recording of one seizure. The black lines showed the frame markers in (C). CBV images at selected time points (B) with respect to seizure onset show pre-ictal decrease in CBV then increase in CBV after seizure onset (light indicates the decrease of CBV and the dark indicates the increase of CBV.

2.2. Pre-ictal surround vasoconstriction

To determine the etiology of the pre-ictal vascular signals, we recently measured changes of arteriolar diameter during acute 4-AP seizures using 2-photon imaging and found pre-ictal vasoconstriction in cortex surrounding an ictal focus [19]. In vivo images of cortical vasculature were used to measure vessel diameter (Fig. 3A). High-magnification movies of individual arterioles allowed for tracking diameter changes during seizure activity near (Fig. 3B-C) and far (Fig. 3D-E) from the seizure focus (Fig. 3 A-E). We found that arterioles dilated in response to the seizure in the focus, with a decreasing amount of dilation with increasing distance from the 4-AP injection site ($n = 4$ rats, 71 vessels, 45 seizures, 143 measurements). Plotting the temporal profile of vasodilation compared with vasoconstriction (Fig. 3F and G), we determined that vasodilation in the focus occurred 0.5 ± 0.1 s after seizure onset, whereas vasoconstriction in the surround occurred 5.3 ± 0.5 s before seizure onset. Note that all vasoconstriction was observed to occur before seizure onset.

In previous studies, we had demonstrated an inverted ORIS signal in the surround consistent with a decrease in CBV [29]. It was not clear form these studies whether the surrounding decrease in CBF or CBV was caused by a passive shunting of blood into the ictal focus or by active shunting of blood due

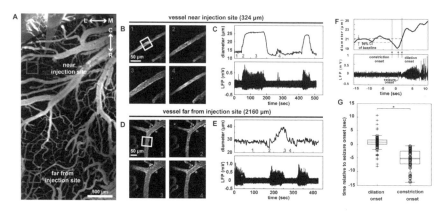

Figure 3. Seizures induce spatially-dependent vascular changes. (A) 2-photon image of fluorescently-labeled surface vasculature (Gray arrow, implanted electrode. boxed areas, near and far regions from the seizure focus highlighted in parts B–E). L↔M, lateral-medial axis; C↔R, caudal-rostral axis. Scale bar: 500µm. (B) Example of a representative vessel adjacent to the injection site in the focus demonstrates vascular dilation concurrent with seizure onset and evolution. (C) Plot of vessel diameter (above) in the white box in (B) during ictal events (below). Note vascular dilation with each event. Numbered timestamps in (C) top correspond to images in (B). (D) 2-photon images in located vessel > 2 mm from the injection site reveals a transient constriction of arterioles at the onset of the seizure. (E) Plot of vessel diameter (above) in the white box in (D) during ictal events (below). Note vascular constriction at the onset of each event, followed by dilation. Numbered timestamps in (E) top correspond to images in (D). (F) Representative example of vascular diameter (top panel) and simultaneous LFP recording (bottom panel) of seizure onset demonstrate pre-ictal vasoconstriction and post-ictal vasodilation. A 99% confidence interval about the mean diameter is shown in (F). Arrows indicate constriction (first arrow), seizure onset (second arrow), and dilation (third arrow). (G) Boxplot of dilation and constriction onset times relative to seizure onset. Gray and black lines represent mean and median respectively. Circles are individual data points and cross hairs are statistical outliers. *: p < 1.0E-7. (n= 4 rats, 71 vessels, 45 total seizures, 143 total measurements). [19]

to vasoconstriction on the surrounding brain tissue. Using the 2-photon microscope to look directly at the arterioles, we demonstrated active pre-ictal vasoconstriction, indicating that ictal onset may be preceded by vasoconstriction in small arterioles surrounding an ictal focus. The etiology of pre-ictal surround vasoconstriction is unclear. One possibility is the active shunting of oxygenated blood to the imminent seizure focus. Another possibility is that the vasoconstriction is reaction to pre-ictal surround inhibition in the 'ictal penumbra' [31, 32].

3. Discussion

The principal findings of pre-ictal optical changes in both human and animal seizures provides converging evidences for the existence of anticipatory changes in cerebral blood flow and hemoglobin oxygenation. Although the etiology of those changes is currently unknown, ORIS can be used as a method to detect these early events.

Whether these vascular events are truly pre-ictal or rather represent subtle underlying neuronal or glial events is also unclear and will require more sensitive measurements of both signals. For example, fast ripples (very high frequency activity) and microseizures have been recorded in human epilepsy using high-resolution ECoG techniques [33-38], which were not applied in the above studies. Ictal change in the ECoG or the LFP are a reflection of synchronous dendritic activity in large groups of neurons. ORIS recordings mostly arise from sub-threshold activity in an area 5-10 times larger than the area of spiking cells. Hence, subtle pre-ictal activity may not be recorded by the ECoG or LFP electrode but clearly recorded by optical methods. Additionally, pre-ictal signals may not be elicited by neurons but rather astrocyte- or pericyte-medicated signaling or local potassium and local neurotransmitter/neuropeptide release [39-43]. Hemodynamic changes may also be influenced by glia, which are not directly recorded with standard electrophysiological methods.

What is the significance of the pre-ictal optical signal? The ultimate goal of optical seizure prediction is not only to warn of an impending seizure but also to prevent seizure from occurring. New novel epilepsy therapies such as cortical stimulation, local short-acting, powerful drug application, and focal cooling have been investigated to stop seizures [6-9, 44]. All of these methodologies would be more efficacious if those closed-loop intervention systems can predict the onset of seizures. In this model, an optode could be implanted over an epileptic focus to record blood flow. Pre-ictal blood flow changes would trigger an abortive therapy such as focal cooling or drug injection. An alternative use for optical mapping, for which there are already prototypes available, would be chronically implanted optode-electrode combinations to localize the seizure focus in preparation for surgical intervention. Likewise, transcranial optical monitoring at the bedside could be used to map seizures to localize foci in preparation for surgery or an implant.

Currently, most of those systems use recording electrodes to provide ongoing feedback of cortical physiology. Number and location of electrodes may be important to provide a sufficiently early detection of an ongoing seizure. Complex mathematical algorithms applied to electrographic data for seizure prediction have recently garnered much attention [16]. The pre-ictal optical signals we describe here may provide an alternative method. Additionally, the optical method is an non-invasive measurement, which can avoid the brain damage caused by implanted electrodes [45]. New neuroimaging and neuro-modulatory techniques such as 'optogenetics', which combines optical and genetic techniques, have emerged as a popular tool to probe and control neuronal function with light [46-50]. Recently, optical suppression of epilepsy has been studied by using optogenetic techniques and caged compounds [10, 11]. The combination of optical pre-ictal detection and optical control would be a novel optical device to terminate seizures.

In summary, we have found clear pre-ictal optical signals from both human epilepsy and acute pharmacologically induced seizures in animal models. Optical measurements of blood flow and oxygenation may be extremely useful tools for predicting and localizing seizure onset, which can have a myriad of uses in warning patients and triggering abortive therapies.

Acknowledgments

This work was supported by the NINDS RO1 NS49482 (T.H.S), CURE Taking Flight Award (H.M.), the Clinical and Translational Science Center (CTSC) Grant UL1 RR 024996 Pilot Grant (M.Z), and the Cornell University Ithaca-WCMC seed grant (M.Z.).

References

1. J. R. Williamson, D. W. Bliss, D. W. Browne and J. T. Narayanan. *Epilepsy Behav.*. 25(2): 230-238 (2012)
2. U. J. Chaudhary, J. S. Duncan and L. Lemieux. *Hum. Brain Mapp.* 34(2): 447-466 (2013)
3. P. Federico, D. F. Abbott, R. S. Briellmann, A. S. Harvey and G. D. Jackson. *Brain.* 128(8): 1811-1817 (2005)
4. E. L. So and T. J. O'Brien, *Chapter 27 - Peri-ictal single-photon emission computed tomography: principles and applications in epilepsy evaluation*, in

Handbook of Clinical Neurology, H. Stefan and W.H. Theodore, Editors., Elsevier, Amsterdam, Netherland. 107: pp 425-436 (2012)

5. F. Mormann, R. G. Andrzejak, C. E. Elger and K. Lehnertz. *Brain*. 130(2): 314-333 (2007)

6. E. H. Kossoff, E. K. Ritzl, J. M. Politsky, A. M. Murro, J. R. Smith, R. B. Duckrow, D. D. Spencer and G. K. Bergey. *Epilepsia*. 45(12): 1560-1567 (2004)

7. H. G. Eder, A. Stein and R. S. Fisher. *Epilepsy Res*. 29(1): 17-24 (1997)

8. A. G. Stein, H. G. Eder, D. E. Blum, A. Drachev and R. S. Fisher. *Epilepsy Res*. 39(2): 103-114 (2000)

9. J. M. Burton, G. A. Peebles, D. K. Binder, S. M. Rothman and M. D. Smyth. *Epilepsia*. 46(12): 1881-1887 (2005)

10. X. F. Yang, B. F. Schmidt, D. L. Rode and S. M. Rothman. *Epilepsia*. 51(1): 127-35 (2010)

11. J. Tonnesen, A. T. Sorensen, K. Deisseroth, C. Lundberg and M. Kokaia. *Proc Natl Acad Sci U S A*. 106(29): 12162-7 (2009)

12. M. Ledri, L. Nikitidou, F. Erdelyi, G. Szabo, D. Kirik, K. Deisseroth and M. Kokaia. *Eur. J. Neurosci*. 36(1): 1971-1983 (2012)

13. M. Gavaret, A. McGonigal, J.-M. Badier and P. Chauvel, *Chapter 41 Physiology of frontal lobe seizures: pre-ictal, ictal and inter-ictal relationships*. in *Supplements to Clinical Neurophysiology* M. Hallett, L. H. Phillips D. L. Schomer, J. M. Massey Editors., Elsevier, Amsterdam, Netherland. 57: pp 400-7 (2004),

14. Z. Rogowski, I. Gath and E. Bental. *Biol. Cybern*. 42(1): 9-15 (1981)

15. A. Katz, D. A. Marks, G. McCarthy and S. S. Spencer. *Electroencephalogr. Clin.Neurophysiol*. 79(2): 153-156 (1991)

16. B. Litt and J. Echauz. *Lancet Neurol*. 1(1): 22-30 (2002)

17. H. Feldwisch-Drentrup, M. Staniek, A. Schulze-Bonhage, J. Timmer, H. Dickten, C. E. Elger, B. Schelter and K. Lehnertz. *Fron. Compu. Neurosci*. 5.(2011)

18. M. Zhao, M. Suh, H. Ma, C. Perry, A. Geneslaw and T. H. Schwartz. *Epilepsia*. 48(11): 2059-67 (2007)

19. M. Zhao, J. Nguyen, H. Ma, N. Nishimura, C. B. Schaffer and T. H. Schwartz. *J. Neurosci*. 31(37): 13292-13300 (2011)

20. R. D. Frostig, E. E. Lieke, D. Y. Ts'o and A. Grinvald. *Proc Natl Acad Sci U S A*. 87(16): 6082-6 (1990)

21. D. Malonek and A. Grinvald. *Science*. 272(5261): 551-4 (1996)

22. S. A. Sheth, M. Nemoto, M. Guiou, M. Walker, N. Pouratian, N. Hageman and A. W. Toga. *J. Neurosci*. 24(3): 634-41 (2004)

23. T. H. Schwartz, S. B. Hong, A. P. Bagshaw, P. Chauvel and C.-G. Bénar. *Epilepsy Res*. 97(3): 252-266 (2011)

24. F. A. Gibbs. *Arch Neurol Psychiatry*. 30(5): 1003-1010.(1933)

25. B. Diehl, S. Knecht, M. Deppe, C. Young and S. R. Stodieck. *Epilepsia*. 39(12): 1284-9 (1998)

26. S. Bahar, M. Suh, M. Zhao and T. H. Schwartz. *Neuroreport.* 17(5): 499-503 (2006)

27. M. Suh, H. Ma, M. Zhao, S. Sharif and T. H. Schwartz. *Mol. Neurobiol.* 33(3): 181-97 (2006)

28. H. Ma, M. Zhao, M. Suh and T. H. Schwartz. *J. Neurophysiol.* 101(5): 2550-62 (2009)

29. M. Zhao, H. Ma, M. Suh and T. H. Schwartz. *J. Neurosci.* 29(9): 2814-23 (2009)

30. H. Ma, M. Zhao and T. H. Schwartz. *Cerebral. Cortex.* Published online ahead of print on April 11, 2012 (2012)

31. C. A. Schevon, S. A. Weiss, G. McKhann, Jr., R. R. Goodman, R. Yuste, R. G. Emerson and A. J. Trevelyan. *Nat. Commun.* 3: 1060 (2012)

32. A. J. Trevelyan and C. A. Schevon. *Neuropharmacology.* Published online ahead of print on June 18 2012 (2012)

33. A. Bragin, I. Mody, C. L. Wilson and J. Engel, Jr. *J. Neurosci.* 22(5): 2012-21 (2002)

34. R. J. Staba, L. Frighetto, E. J. Behnke, G. W. Mathern, T. Fields, A. Bragin, J. Ogren, I. Fried, C. L. Wilson and J. Engel, Jr. *Epilepsia.* 48(11): 2130-8 (2007)

35. P. Jiruska, G. T. Finnerty, A. D. Powell, N. Lofti, R. Cmejla and J. G. R. Jefferys. *Brain.* 133(5): 1380-1390 (2010)

36. C. A. Schevon, S. K. Ng, J. Cappell, R. R. Goodman, G. J. McKhann, A. Waziri, A. Branner, A. Sosunov, C. E. Schroeder and R. G. Emerson. *J. Clin. Neurophysiol.* 25(6): 321-330 (2008)

37. C. A. Schevon, R. R. Goodman, G. J. McKhann and R. G. Emerson. *J. Clin. Neurophysiol* . 27(6): 406-411 (2010)

38. M. Stead, M. Bower, B. H. Brinkmann, K. Lee, W. R. Marsh, F. B. Meyer, B. Litt, J. Van Gompel and G. A. Worrell. *Brain.* 133(9): 2789-2797 (2010)

39. E. Hamel. *J. Appl. Physiol.* 100(3): 1059-64 (2006)

40. E. Hamel, B. W. Day, J. H. Miller, M. K. Jung, P. T. Northcote, A. K. Ghosh, D. P. Curran, M. Cushman, K. C. Nicolaou, I. Paterson and E. J. Sorensen. *Mol. Pharmacol.* 70(5): 1555-64 (2006)

41. C. M. Peppiatt, C. Howarth, P. Mobbs and D. Attwell. *Nature.* 443(7112): 700-4 (2006)

42. X. Wang, N. Lou, Q. Xu, G.-F. Tian, W. G. Peng, X. Han, J. Kang, T. Takano and M. Nedergaard. *Nat. Neurosci.* 9(6): 816-823 (2006)

43. J. A. Filosa, A. D. Bonev, S. V. Straub, A. L. Meredith, M. K. Wilkerson, R. W. Aldrich and M. T. Nelson. *Nat. Neurosci.* 9(11): 1397-1403 (2006)

44. G. K. Motamedi, P. Salazar, E. L. Smith, R. P. Lesser, W. R. S. Webber, P. I. Ortinski, S. Vicini and M. A. Rogawski. *Epilepsy Res.* 70(2-3): 200-210 (2006)

45. M. P. Cox, M. Hongtao, M. E. Bahlke, J. H. Beck, T. H. Schwartz and I. Kymissis. *Electro. Devices, IEEE Transactions on.* 57(1): 174-177 (2010)

46. D. Boison. *Neuroscientist.* 11(1): 25-36 (2005)

47. A. R. Adamantidis, F. Zhang, A. M. Aravanis, K. Deisseroth and L. de Lecea. *Nature*. 450(7168): 420-424 (2007)
48. D. Boison. *Trends. Pharmacol. Sci.* 27(12): 652-658 (2006)
49. F. Zhang, L.-P. Wang, M. Brauner, J. F. Liewald, K. Kay, N. Watzke, P. G. Wood, E. Bamberg, G. Nagel, A. Gottschalk and K. Deisseroth. *Nature*. 446(7136): 633-639 (2007)
50. L. Zayat, M. G. Noval, J. Campi, C. I. Calero, D. J. Calvo and R. Etchenique. *Chembiochem*. 8(17): 2035-8 (2007)

OBSERVING THE SLEEP-WAKE REGULATORY SYSTEM TO IMPROVE PREDICTION OF SEIZURES

M. SEDIGH-SARVESTANI[1] and B. J. GLUCKMAN[1,2*]

1. Center for Neural Engineering, Department of Engineering Science and Mechanics
2. Departments of Physics, Neurosurgery, and Bioengineering
The Pennsylvania State University
University Park, PA 16802, USA
* E-mail: BruceGluckman@psu.edu

We describe our ongoing efforts to understand the dynamics of the sleep-wake regulatory system to improve seizure prediction. Although mathematical models of its dynamics have been developed, the activity of this system is difficult to observe directly. Therefore we have developed a data assimilation framework that combines sparse measurements of the sleep-wake regulatory system together with a mathematical model of its dynamics to estimate the unmeasured variables. This toolset will allow us to understand the interaction between modulators of the state-of-vigilance and seizure susceptibility and may provide meaningful indicators of an impending seizure.

Keywords: Sleep and Seizure; State-of-vigilance; Data assimilation.

1. Introduction and Motivation

We, along with our colleagues at the Center for Neural Engineering at Pennsylvania State University, have been seeking novel engineering solutions to identify,[1] observe,[2,3] predict and also prevent[4] the dynamics that lead to epileptic seizures. The objectives of clinically meaningful seizure prediction extend beyond statistically significant prediction of an impending event in a local region of the brain. They include understanding the whole-brain mechanisms that result in transitions of a network from its usual stable or non-seizing state to the seizure. Within this approach, successful prediction of seizures stems from first understanding and second detecting preseizure dynamics and the whole-brain mechanisms that modulate the likelihood of a transition into seizure.

One of the best established modulators of the preseizure state is the state-of-vigilance (SOV) or sleep-state. SOV has been shown to play a role in seizure susceptibility in several experimental animal models of epilepsy.[5–8] In humans, observations of correlations between SOV and seizure frequency predate the advent of the electroencephalogram.[9] In neurology literature and practice, the relationship between SOV and seizures is well accepted and used to diagnose epilepsy syndromes.[10]

Long-term observation of the SOV and seizure relationship is difficult in humans. In animal models of epilepsy, long-term experiments predesigned for adequate statistical power are possible given current signal acquisition technology. However, only a handful of such studies exist.[11–13] The relationship between SOV and seizure onset remains to be adequately explored in even the most prevalent animal models of epilepsy.

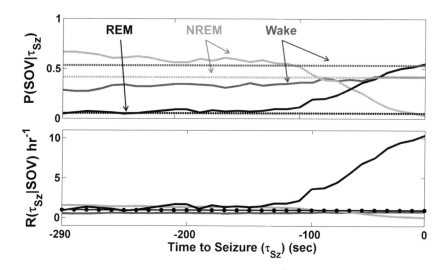

Fig. 1. Preseizure State-of-vigilance (SOV) for 7 days of continuous recording including 165 seizures from one animal. Seizures were induced with a focal injection of tetanus toxin in the ventral hippocampus.[14] SOV was scored in 10 second windows. (Top) Probability of each SOV vs. time to seizure onset (τ_{Sz}) is shown in solid lines where black indicates REM, light gray indicates NREM and dark gray indicates Wake. Dashed lines represent fraction of each SOV during the recording period. Nearly half of all seizures arise from REM, although only 5% of time is spent in this state. (Bottom) The rate of seizure onset conditioned on SOV was calculated from the posterior probability by multiplying by the SOV measurement rate.The rate of seizure onset conditioned on REM rises significantly higher than the average rate of seizure shown in dotted- black (0.98 hr^{-1}), or the rate conditioned on any other SOV, 120-130 seconds prior to seizure onset.

We conducted a series of experiments on the relationship between SOV and seizure-onset in the rat tetanus toxin model of mesial temporal lobe epilepsy.[14] Sample results for one rat are shown in Fig. 1. We scored the SOV, in continuous 10 second windows for the duration of the recordings, including the 300 second preseizure window. We determined $P(SOV|\tau_{Sz})$ the fraction contributed by each SOV in each window prior to seizure, as shown in Fig. 1(top) for wakefulness (Wake), rapid-eye-movement sleep (REM), and non-REM sleep (NREM). Nearly half of all seizures occur following REM. The fraction of preseizure windows in REM begins to increase 120-130 seconds before seizure onset. This increase is concurrent with a decrease in the fraction of windows in NREM over the same period. We also calculated $P(SOV)$, shown in dashed horizontal lines in Fig. 1(top), and observed that REM occurs only about 5% of the time whereas NREM occurs about 50% of the time.

To better compare the correlation between SOV and seizure onset, we used Bayes rule to calculate the SOV-conditioned probability of seizure-onset in the preseizure window: $P(\tau_{Sz}|SOV) = \frac{P(SOV|\tau_{Sz})P(\tau_{Sz})}{P(SOV)}$. Here $P(\tau_{Sz})$ is the probability of observing a seizure within τ_{Sz} seconds. We then calculated the rate of seizure onset by multiplying this probability by the SOV measurement rate of 360 hr^{-1} (360, 10- second windows per hour): $R(\tau_{Sz}|SOV) = P(\tau_{Sz}|SOV) * 360$. As we show in Fig. 1(bottom), the rate of seizure conditioned on REM is several times higher than the unconditioned average rate of seizure (shown in dashed black) and than the rate of seizure conditioned on any other SOV. This observation suggests that we can use SOV information for prediction: observation of REM should increase anticipation of seizure and observation of NREM should decrease it. Regardless of the particular SOV that most often precedes a seizure, the relationship between SOV and seizure onset can be utilized in this way to improve seizure prediction efforts in animal experiments.

In our experiments, SOV information results in notable improvement of prediction accuracy but does not allow us to predict all seizures. Although nearly half of all seizures arise from REM, only 20% of REM bouts lead to seizure and we have no way to distinguish preseizure REM bouts based on our observations. To fully utilize our observations of a strong correlation between SOV and seizure onset we would need to go beyond the statistics and understand the underlying mechanisms that cause seizures to preferentially arise from a particular SOV. To accomplish this task, we need to develop methods to observe the relevant brain processes that regulate SOV and potentially modulate seizure susceptibility. This includes the neuronal, neurotransmitter and hormonal, glial, and vascular dynamics that together define the activity of sleep and seizure regulatory networks.

We have implemented a research program that aims to improve seizure prediction by better understanding the mechanisms of sleep regulation. The aim is to develop tools that allow us to observe the dynamics of the sleep-wake regulatory system (SWRS) so as to understand how this network modulates seizure susceptibility. These observation tools would also be applicable to other neurological disorders such as depression and schizophrenia in which sleep plays a role. To meet this aim, we have developed a framework that utilizes detailed mathematical models of the SWRS along with sparse observations of relevant neural activity to 'observe' the remaining unmeasured components. The core objective of our framework is to accurately reconstruct and predict SWRS dynamics from a small set of measurements. A second objective is to develop methods that determine the optimal sets of biological measurements from the available set of potentially costly measurements.

In the remainder of this chapter we describe our research program. We begin with an overview of the SWRS and the mathematical models that describe the interactions within this system. We then introduce our data assimilation framework based on the unscented Kalman filter (UKF) and outline the core methods that we have developed thus far. These include methods to optimize the UKF parameters, methods to determine the optimal variables for measurement and methods to estimate model parameters. We conclude with a discussion of implementation of this framework to the experimental animal, the next step in our program.

2. Sleep-Wake Regulatory System Physiology

Sleep-wake cyles arise primarily due to the interaction of cell groups in the brainstem and hypothalamus.[15] GABAergic ventrolateral preoptic nucleus (VLPO) neurons in the hypothalamus promote NREM. Monoaminergic cell groups in the brainstem such as the noradrenergic locus coeruleus (LC) and the serotonergic dorsal raphe (DR) neurons, promote wake behavior. Mutual inhibition between these two groups forms a flip-flop switch as each group promotes its own activity by inhibiting the other's. The transitions between NREM and REM are thought to arise from interactions between cholinergic cell-groups in the brainstem, including the laterodorsal tegmentum (LDT) and pedunculopontine tegmentum (PPT), and the monoaminergic cell-groups LC and DR. In addition, neurotransmitters such as orexin and adenosine have been implicated in further regulation of the sleep network.

These dynamics are further modified by the 24-hour circadian drive, regulated by the suprachiasmatic nucleus (SCN) in the hypothalamus. The SCN has indirect projections to the VLPO which results in inhibition of sleep during subjective day.[16] The SCN clock, which arises from subcellular genetic cycles, can be modulated by afferent cortical inputs in response to a variety of external cues, most importantly light. Light input from melonopsin expressing ganglion cells in the retina entrains the SCN and can shift the circadian phase.[17,18]

Different hypotheses have been proposed to explain the SOV-seizure relationship observed in various animal and human expressions of epilepsy, although further study is needed to elucidate this relationship. Genetic abnormalities resulting in acetylcholine disturbances in the ascending arousal system, discovered in a population of patients with nocturnal frontal lobe epilepsy, suggests a genetic basis for the sleep-seizure link in some syndromes.[19] Retrograde trace studies have shown that a number of central nervous system sites innervate the SCN in the rat[20] thus implying a neuro-anatomical pathway for the observed effect of SOV on seizure states. Finally, several systemic neurotransmitters such as adenosine whose concentrations change in response to SOV and SCN-related oscillations are believed to play a role in seizure generation.[21]

In the past decade, several investigators have developed mathematical models of sleep dynamics.[22–26] Ideally, we would like to use these models to predict sleep-wake behavior. We therefore need to differentiate between various models by validating each model against the detailed neural dynamics that occur in real brains. Although decades of research into the brain's sleep regulatory system give us insight into the activity and connection of several different brain regions, we can measure only a few relevant variables in a real biological system. Therefore alternate methods are needed.

3. Data Assimilation Framework

Any alternate 'observation' method must meet a series of criteria. Most importantly, it must be able to reconstruct estimates of unmeasured variables. There must also be a method to determine the optimal variables for measurement. The optimal variable is that which strikes a balance between accuracy of the reconstructed estimates and cost of measurement. We propose that data assimilation can serve this purpose by directly linking the neurophysiology of sleep, embedded into mathematical models, together with available measurements of a real and noisy biological system.

Data assimilation is the process by which measurements are incorporated into a mathematical model of a real system.The degree of incorporation depends on the estimated uncertainty of both the measurements and the model. Measurement uncertainty can usually be calculated from the measurement process but estimating model uncertainty is challenging. We therefore require a method of model uncertainty optimization. In addition there is no *ab inito* link between the biological system and the model parameters. Therefore we require a method for estimating model parameters. Finally, because neither measurements nor the model will be perfect representations of the biological system, a successful data assimilation framework must be able to handle sparse and noisy measurements as well as inadequate models.

We have developed a data assimilation framework capable of reconstructing the unmeasured variables of the sleep-wake regulatory system which performs within these criteria. This framework includes three aspects: The UKF for estimating unmeasured variables using sparse measurements together with a filter model; an intuitive method for determining which variables can be used as measurements to optimally reconstruct remaining unmeasured variables, which we also use to optimize model uncertainty; and a method to estimate unknown fixed and slowly moving model parameters from sparse measurements. We will give a brief introduction to our framework in this section and invite the interested reader to Sedigh-Sarvestani et al.[3] for an in-depth discussion of the methods and results.

3.1. *Reconstructing Unmeasured Variables*

For illustration of our data assimilation framework in this chapter we use the Diniz Behn model of sleep.[24] We have also used other mathematical models[22,23] within this framework. Ten variables in this model represent the firing rate and output neurotransmitter of the NREM-active VLPO cell group, the Wake-active DR cell group, the Wake-active LC cell group, the REM-active LDT/PPT cell group and the Wake/REM active LDT/PPT cell group. Modeled off of the physiology described above, these cell groups mutually inhibit each other and give rise to sleep-wake cycles. Another variable represents the homeostatic sleep drive and modulates the firing threshold of the VLPO cell group.

We generate data by integrating the model. We then apply an observation function to this generated data by selecting one or a few of the variables, to which we add noise, as our limited observed data set. This data set, with or without the correct parameters used to generate it, is then passed

270

onto the data assimilation framework. The UKF[27,28] is used to reconstruct the unobserved variables and a parameter estimation method[28] is used to estimate the underlying parameter set. To validate our results, we compare the reconstructed estimates and parameters with the fully observed original data set.

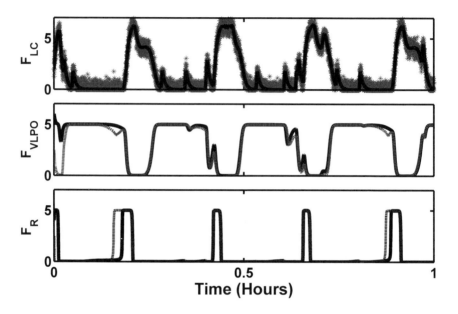

Fig. 2. Reconstruction of Diniz Behn model dynamics. Noisy measurements of the firing rate of Wake-active LC (F_{LC}) (gray asterisks), were passed to the unscented Kalman filter framework to track and reconstruct all other variables of the model. Shown are the reconstructions (gray) and true values (black) for the firing rate of NREM-active VLPO (F_{VLPO}), the REM-active LDT/PPT (F_R). Other variables of the model are also reconstructed well.

An example of this procedure is shown in Fig. 2, where 1 hour of sleep-wake data was generated from the Diniz Behn model. The limited observation function produced a noisy version of variable (F_{LC})-the firing rate of the wake-active LC region. This 'measurement' is shown in gray asterisks. The remaining 11 variables of the model were unmeasured and reconstructed by the UKF. The reconstruction (gray) and unmeasured true (black) value of the NREM-active firing rate variable F_{VLPO} and the REM-active firing rate variable F_R are shown.

The UKF reconstructs the unobserved variables using a prediction-correction scheme where model-generated predictions are used to constrain the dynamics and a correction factor is used to assimilate the observation. When the model state is far from the observations, as occurs when model initial conditions are chosen arbitrarily, the correction factor increases and outweighs the model prediction. This prediction-correction scheme causes the model state to be gradually dragged toward the observation. However, once the model state nears the observations in state-space, the model predicted state estimates are no longer outweighed by the observation and the reconstruction stays close to the true value. See the textbook by Schiff[29] for equations, examples, and detailed discussion of the UKF.

In this example the UKF assimilates observations of F_{LC} and reconstructs NREM-active F_{VLPO}, which is inhibited by F_{LC} in a flip-flip fashion, well. F_R, firing rate of the REM-active cell group in the LDT/PPT is reconstructed less well than F_{VLPO}. This relative accuracy in reconstruction stems from different partial observability of these variables from F_{LC} as discussed in the next section. In summary, by observing F_{LC} as can be done easily with a microelectrode in the LC, the UKF can reconstruct the remaining model variables reasonably well.

3.2. *Choosing Optimal Variables for Measurement*

Some of the cell groups included in the Diniz Behn model are easier to reach and measure in the rat brain than others. Similarly, off-the-shelf electrochemical sensors are available for some, but not all, of the neurotransmitters included in this model. But not all observable variables serve equally well to reconstruct unmeasured states. The reconstruction fidelity of any particular variable depends on qualities that are inherent to the model dynamics such as observability. Observability is a structural property of a model defined as the ability to recover the model state through the observation of one or more of its outputs.[30] In most biological models, not all variables can be used as observables to reconstruct the full dynamics. Nonetheless, information regarding the partial observability of each variable can be used to choose the optimal variable for measurement in the UKF framework. The optimal variable is that which reconstructs the state space well and whose measurement is practical and efficient given current technology.

Analytical methods to determine observability for nonlinear systems generally determine in a binary fashion whether or not a variable or set of variables can be used to reconstruct the remaining state space. Letellier et al.[31,32] proposed a simple algebraic solution to rank all variables of a system according to their relative partial observability, and demonstrated it on relatively low-dimensional (3 or 4-dimensional) physical models. This method did not not work well for the high-dimensional biological models presented here. Therefore, we developed an empirical metric to rank the partial observability of each variable based on the reconstruction error as detailed below.

We use the mean square difference between the reconstructed $(\hat{x}_i)$ and true (x_i) values for each variable to quantify the accuracy of state reconstruction. We normalize this error by the variance of each variable's dynamics to form ε_i^2, a normalized mean square error for the ith variable. We use the inverse of $1 + \varepsilon_i^2$, which is bounded between [0,1] as a metric of reconstruction fidelity which we have termed the empirical observability coefficient (EOC). The EOC also relates to the partial observability of variable i, given observation of variable j:

$$\varepsilon_i^2 = \frac{\langle (x_i - \hat{x}_i)^2 \rangle}{var(x_i)}$$

$$EOC_{i,j} = \frac{1}{1 + \varepsilon_{i|j}^2}$$

(1)

In Fig. 3, we show the EOC for each variable (down the columns) as a function of observation variable (across rows), in matrix format for the Diniz Behn model of sleep. In this color coded plot, white indicates good reconstruction, and black indicates poor reconstruction.

Given observation of F_{LC}, the firing rate of the wake-active LC group, the best reconstructed variable is $F_{W/R}$, the firing rate of the Wake/REM-active cell group in the LDT/PPT. Several other variables are reconstructed well according to high values down the column marked F_{LC}. The worst reconstructed variables are F_R and its synaptic output $C_{A(R)}$, the concentration of acetylcholine. We interpret this to mean that F_R is relatively *less observable* from F_{LC} than is $F_{W/R}$. Thus, the EOC can be used to determine which reconstructed variables to 'trust' given a certain observation and which variables to measure to insure accurate reconstruction of particular variables.

We investigated pairings of two or more variables with respect to their relative partial observability. We found that for the Diniz Behn model, the EOC of variable i given measurements of variables j and k is always at least as good as the individual EOC: $EOC_{i,(j,k)} \geq max\{EOC_{i,j}, EOC_{i,k}\}$. For this model, we also observed that good reconstruction of all variables

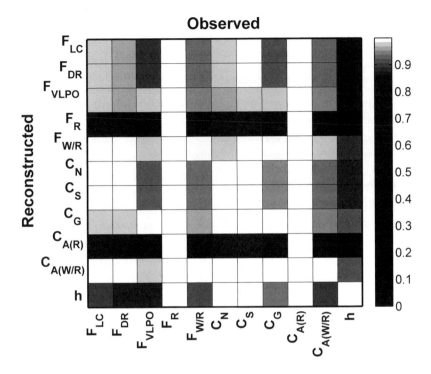

Fig. 3. **Empirical Observability Coefficient (EOC) Matrix.** *EOC* for the Diniz Behn model. $EOC_{i,j}$ is an empirical measure of how well variable i is reconstructed from measurement of variable j. $EOC_{i,j} \in [0,1]$ with perfect reconstruction being 1. From the *EOC* matrix, we observe that F_R (row) is poorly observed - poorly reconstructed - from most variables, although its measurement (column) yields good reconstruction of all other variables.

requires some measurement of both Wake and REM dynamics. These states are readily observed from real biological systems through external physiological measurements such as power bands in the EEG, muscle tone, and movement. For the subsequent computations, we assimilate noisy measurements of both Wake-active F_{LC} and REM-active F_R dynamics.

Because the *EOC* is a measure of reconstruction fidelity, we demonstrate that we can optimize framework parameters using the *EOC* matrix as the optimization metric. An important UKF parameter is the model covariance inflation matrix, which gets added to the model uncertainty matrix and affects how much the UKF weighs model predictions vs. measurements. Quantitative methods to optimize this parameter to improve reconstruction fidelity have been proposed but are not clearly defined for general use. In

274

Sedigh-Sarvestani et al.,[3] we describe an intuitive approach to use the *EOC* to optimize this parameter.

3.3. *Estimating Model Parameters*

We have implemented a version of a multiple-shooting method[28] for parameter estimation. To ensure that parameter dynamics are estimated well, parameter estimation is carried out iteratively with UKF state reconstruction over short-windows. Estimation is performed by minimizing the distance between UKF reconstructed traces from the previous iteration and short model-generated trajectories that originate on these reconstructed traces. The set of trajectories that remains closest to the reconstructed trajectories define the next parameter update. The test trajectories are generated from models wherein the parameter of interest is slightly larger or smaller than the current estimate. In this way, the optimal parameter value is eventually reached over several iterations of variable and parameter reconstruction.

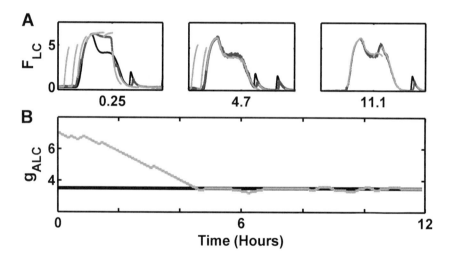

Fig. 4. The parameter g_{ALC} is estimated iteratively in short windows. Updated parameters are used for the UKF filter in the next short window. A) Trajectories for the short model-generated (light gray), reconstructed (dark gray) and true (black) F_{LC} dynamics during different time-points in the convergence of g_{ALC}. B) Convergence of the estimate of g_{ALC} (light gray) to its true value (black). As the parameter approaches its true value, the short trajectories of F_{LC} become closer to the reconstructed dynamics and the reconstructed dynamics become closer to the true dynamics.

For illustration purposes we generated data with fixed parameters and assimilated noisy measurements of F_{LC} and F_R to reconstruct the dynamics. Initially, all model parameters in the UKF were set to the same values used to generate the true data set, except g_{ALC}, the parameter that couples acetylcholine output from F_R and $F_{W/R}$ into F_{LC} dynamics. To this we supplied an arbitrary initial value.

As seen in Fig. 4B, our estimation of g_{ALC} converges to the true value. In Fig. 4A, we plot trajectories for the short model-generated (light gray), reconstructed (dark gray), and true (black) F_{LC} dynamics for different periods of the convergence of g_{ALC}. Note that initially, for g_{ALC} significantly different than the true value, the short trajectories diverge quickly from the reconstructed values, and the reconstructed values of F_{LC} are different from the true ones. When g_{ALC} approaches the true value, both the short model-generated and reconstructed trajectories approach the true dynamics.

The iterative estimation of parameters over small windows is crucial in the estimation of slowly varying parameters. Using the approach outlined above we have successfully tracked a slowly varying parameter with 24-hour circadian periodicity.[3]

3.4. *Inadequate Models and Inadequate Measurements*

The dual nature of the UKF in incorporating both measurements and model-predictions allows for much flexibility if the uncertainty in either quantity becomes large. The uncertainty of the model prediction is continuously updated with each measurement. This affects how much or little model-predictions are weighed in the next reconstruction step. Measurement uncertainty is usually taken to be a constant over the reconstruction period. Given temporal information about the noise in the measurement, the UKF could dynamically guide its estimates to trust or ignore the measured values. For instance, during Wake, measurements of the Wake-active LC neurons are likely to be more robust than during NREM or REM, states during which this groups of cells is mostly inactive. Using such a scheme, the UKF could handle inadequacies in measurement.

The UKF is also robust in handling model inadequacies to some degree, a fortunate fact given that our most sophisticated models of neuronal networks will likely fail to capture all relevant dynamics. As discussed above, and shown in Sedigh-Sarvestani et al.,[3] the UKF is able to capture dynamics such as 24-hour periodicity, that are not included in the UKF filter model. In addition, estimation of parameters uniquely for each biological

276

system will help to make a robust mathematical model more 'adequate'.

4. Future Work: Translation to the Experimental Animal

We have developed a framework capable of estimating unmeasured variables and parameters and have validated our methods with simulation studies. Implementation of this toolset in the experimental animal requires a few further steps. First, prior to making any measurements, off-line analytical study of the observability and identifiability properties of the SWRS model must be carried out if possible. Identifiability analysis for parameters is similar to observability analysis for variables, where the aim is to determine which set of parameters can be uniquely identified from observing the state of the system. Identifiability analysis will help to determine the order of parameters to estimate and which parameters, if any, can be pulled together to reduce model complexity. Second, once we have determined the the optimal observables, we will make corresponding measurements in the rat brain. Third, we will use these observations to reconstruct variables and estimate both model and UKF parameters off-line. Finally, we will use these parameter values along with a smaller subset of observables to reconstruct and predict SWRS dynamics in real time. These predictions will be used to validate and improve the mathematical models.

The last step of our program will be to incorporate this toolset in the epileptic animal. This will allow us to observe the components of the SWRS that modulate seizure susceptibility and to determine which set of variables and parameters serve as useful features for seizure prediction. We will also be able to utilize these experiments to determine how the epileptic brain modulates SOV dynamics.

References

1. M. Sedigh-Sarvestani, G. I. Thuku, S. Sundaram, S. L. Weinstein, S. J. Schiff and B. J. Gluckman, *Unpublished Results* (2013).
2. S. Sunderam, N. Chernyy, N. Peixoto, J. P. Mason, S. L. Weinstein, S. J. Schiff and B. J. Gluckman, *J. Neurosci. Methods* **163**, 373 (2007).
3. M. Sedigh-Sarvestani, S. J. Schiff and B. J. Gluckman, *PLoS Comput. Biol.* **8**, p. e1002788 (2012).
4. S. Sunderam, N. Chernyy, N. Peixoto, J. P. Mason, S. L. Weinstein, S. J. Schiff and B. J. Gluckman, *J. Neural Eng.* **6**, p. 046009 (2009).
5. J. W. Miller, G. M. Turner and B. C. Gray, *Epilepsy Res* **18**, 195 (1994).
6. M. N. Shouse, P. R. Farber and R. J. Staba, *Clin Neurophysiol* **111 Suppl**, S9 (2000).

7. L. V. Colom, A. García-Hernández, M. T. Castañeda, M. G. Perez-Cordova and E. R. Garrido-Sanabria, *J. Neurophysiol.* **95**, 3645 (2006).
8. V. F. Kitchigina and M. V. Butuzova, *Exp Neurol* **216**, 449 (2009).
9. S. R. Sinha, *J. Clin. Neurophysiol.* **28**, 103 (2011).
10. T. Loddenkemper, S. W. Lockley, J. Kaleyias and S. V. Kothare, *J. Clin. Neurophysiol.* **28**, 146 (2011).
11. A. Coenen, W. Drinkenburg, B. Peeters, J. Vossen and E. van Luijtelaar, *Neurosci. Biobehav. Rev.* **15**, 259 (1991).
12. M. Quigg, M. Straume, M. Menaker and E. H. Bertram, *Ann. Neurol.* **43**, 748 (1998).
13. G. Matos, S. Tufik, F. A. Scorza, E. A. Cavalheiro and M. L. Andersen, *Prog. Neurobiol.* **95**, 396 (2011).
14. J. Jefferys and M. Walker, *Tetanus toxin model of focal epilepsy*, in *Models of Seizures and Epilepsy*, eds. A. Pitkanen, P. Shwartzkroin and S. Moshe (Elsevier, 360 Park Ave, New York, NY, USA, 2006).
15. C. B. Saper, T. Scammel and J. Lu, *Nature* **437**, 1257 (2005).
16. S. Deurveilher and K. Semba, *Neuroscience* **130**, 165 (2005).
17. S. Panda, T. Sato, A. Castrucci, M. Rollag, W. DeGrip, J. Hogenesh, I. Prevenico and S. Kay, *Science* **298**, p. 22132216 (2002).
18. S. Hattar, H.-W. Liao, M. Takao, D. M. Berson and K.-W. Yau, *Science* **295**, 1065 (2002).
19. L. Ferini-Strambi, V. Sansoni and R. Combi, *Neurologist* **18**, 343 (2012).
20. K. Krout, J. Kawano, T. Mettenleiter and A. Loewy, *Neuroscience* **110**, 73 (2002).
21. D. Boison, *Open Neurosci. J.* **4**, 93 (2010).
22. Y. Tamakawa, A. Karashima, Y. Koyoma, N. Katayama and M. Nakao, *J. Neurophysiol.* **95**, 2055 (2006).
23. C. D. Behn, E. Brown, T. Scammel and N. Kopell, *J. Neurophysiol.* **97**, 3828 (2010).
24. C. G. Diniz Behn and V. Booth, *J Neurophysiol* **103**, 1937 (2010).
25. J. Phillips and P. Robinson, *J. Biol. Rhythms* **22**, 167 (2007).
26. M. Rempe, J. Best and D. Terman, *J. Math. Biol.* **60**, 615 (2010).
27. S. J. Julier and J. K. Uhlmann, *P SPIE* **3068**, 182 (1997).
28. H. U. Voss and J. Timmer, *Int. J. Bifurcation Chaos Appl. Sci. Eng.* **14**, 1905 (2004).
29. S. J. Schiff, *Neural Control Engineering* (MIT Press, 55 Hayward Street, Cambridge, MA, USA, 2012).
30. R. E. Kalman, *Proc. IFAC 1st International Congress* **1**, 481 (1960).
31. C. Letellier, L. A. Aguirre and J. Maquet, *Phys. Rev. E* **71**, p. 066213 (2005).
32. C. Letellier and L. Aguirre, *Phys. Rev. E* **79**, p. 066210 (2009).

THE WORLD'S LARGEST EPILEPSY DATABASE: CONTENT AND STRUCTURE

M. IHLE*, B. SCHELTER[+], J. TIMMER[+] and A. SCHULZE-BONHAGE*

*Epilepsy Unit, University Hospital of Freiburg, Germany
[+]FDM, University of Freiburg, Germany

The evaluation, standardization, and reproducibility of studies in the field of seizure prediction has always been hampered by the lack of access to high-quality long-term electroencephalography (EEG) data. In this article we present the European Epilepsy database EPILEPSIAE with long-term EEG recordings of 275 patients, annotated by EEG experts and supplemented with extensive meta-data. Since the first 60 datasets have been made available in 2012, we illustrate the content and structure of the database that will affect current standards in the field of prediction and facilitate reproducibility and comparison of studies. Beyond seizure prediction, it may also be of considerable benefit for studies focusing on seizure detection, basic neurophysiology, and related topics including computational neuroscience.

Keywords: Epilepsy, EEG, Seizures, Annotations, Relational Database

1. Introduction

More than 0.5 percent of the world's population suffers from epilepsy with patients being severely restricted in daily life due to the unforeseen seizures being characteristic for this neurologic disorder. Since seizure control cannot be achieved by drugs or surgery for a considerable percentage of patients, it is crucial to find alternative treatment methods. A reliable prediction of seizure onsets would enable closed-loop interventions[1] and allow seizure prevention by timely targeted seizure-suppressive medication[2] or electrical stimulation.[3,4]

Hence, much effort has been invested to identify reliable precursors of seizures in electroencephalography (EEG).[5,6] Thereby, mathematical analysis of the complex changes in neural activity preceding seizures has shown more promise than mere visual inspection. But early studies often focused on sensitivity by including only selected pre-ictal data for a small number of seizures with predictors suffering from poor specificity when applied to interictal data.

With research groups becoming increasingly aware of the shortcomings mentioned above some publicly accessible databases were installed. The first such database was compiled by the epilepsy center in Bonn[a] containing 5 datasets of about 40 minutes of discontinuous EEG.

A more comprehensive database was provided by Flint Hills Scientific, LLC. This *Flint Hills ECoG Database* comprises 1419 hours of continuous, intracranial long-term ECoG recordings from 10 patients and contains 59 clinically manifest and approximately 1174 subclinical seizures. Additionally, the database contains meta-information on seizure onsets and electrode locations. Unfortunately, the database is no longer publicly available.

The *Freiburg EEG database*[b] contains 21 patients with 24 hours of interictal EEG without seizure activity and a total of 89 seizures with at least 50 min preictal data. In total the database comprehends 509 hour of EEG. Electrode positions are indicated on implantation schemes.

The *CHB-MIT Scalp EEG Database*[c] was compiled at the Boston Children's Hospital containing more than 800 hours of scalp EEG recordings from 23 pediatric subjects with intractable seizures and a total of 198 seizures.

Although being a first step in the right direction,[7] those databases still contained only small amounts of data and provided little annotations and meta-data. A recent study showed that the sensitivity of previously published prediction algorithms was negatively correlated with both recording duration and number of seizures contained.[8] An ideal study should be based on continuous long-term data used for optimizing the prediction system and a second data set from the same patient for evaluating its performance in a quasi-prospective manner. Hence, high-quality long-term EEG recordings of many patients containing sufficient interictal data is required. To facilitate reproducibility, publicly available databases are of great benefit.

2. The EPILEPSIAE project database

To overcome this limitations, the EU funded in 2008 the EPILEPSIAE project[d] in its 7th Framework Program with six partners from hospitals, academic institutions and industry in France, Germany, Italy, and Portugal (www.epilepsiae.eu). In the course of this project, the largest epilepsy

---

[a]http://epileptologie-bonn.de/cms/front_content.php?idcat=193
[b]http://epilepsy.uni-freiburg.de/freiburg-seizure-prediction-project/eeg-database
[c]http://www.physionet.org/pn6/chbmit/
[d]Grant 211713, website: http://www.epilepsiae.eu/

database worldwide with more than 40.000 hours of EEG and 2500 seizures has been compiled, exceeding earlier databases by more than an order of magnitude.

One of the main advantages of the EPILEPSIAE database, setting it apart from all previous EEG databases, is its extensive collection of meta-data supplementing the EEG and its standardized EEG annotation scheme. Based on both video analysis and EEG screening, for each patient all clinical manifest seizures and selected subclinical seizures as well as characteristic interictal patterns have been annotated by experienced EEG experts.

In 2012 this database has been made available to the public (http://epilepsy-database.eu/), allowing researchers worldwide to conduct high-quality studies not only in the field of seizure prediction, but also seizure detection, basic neurophysiology, and other fields.

2.1. *Database content*

The database contains data acquired during pre-surgical evaluations of 275 epilepsy patients at the epilepsy centers of the University Hospital Freiburg, Germany, the University Hospital of Coimbra, Portugal, and the Hospital de la Pitie-Salpetriere in Paris, France. Thereby, the database comprehends data of different modalities: 1) binary files containing the EEG recorded during the long-term monitoring of the patient, as well as MR-Imaging data for most patients, and 2) a relational database containing supplementary meta-data.

The usage of a relational database enables users to comfortably query the meta-data by the standard database query language SQL and therefore allows for selection of homogeneous patient groups. The scope of the database and the variety of possible queries the database offers to researchers is illustrated in a first report[9] presenting some basic characteristics of the patient datasets contained in the database. In this paper the distribution of seizures during the course of recordings, with respect to time of the day, to circadian rhythm and to the state of vigilance has been examined, as well as the duration of ictal and interictal periods, differences between clinical and EEG based seizure onsets, and spatial propagation of seizures.

Each of the 275 patient datasets had to meet certain conditions for being included into the database and annotation had to fulfill standards defined by the consortium of collaborating epilepsy centers.

Thus, recordings of the patients have an average duration of 165 hours with a maximum of 500 hours, and the number of seizures per patient

```
start_ts=2004-02-18 11:32:25.000
num_samples=921600
sample_freq=256
conversion_factor=0.165000
num_channels=29
elec_names=[FP1,FP2,F3,F4,C3,C4,P3,P4,O1,O2,F7,F8,T3,T4,T5,T6,FZ,CZ,PZ,
SP1,SP2,RS,T1,T2,EOG1,EOG2,EMG,ECG,PHO]
pat_id=23902
adm_id=239102
rec_id=23900102
duration_in_sec=3600
sample_bytes=2
```

Fig. 1. A typical .head file with supplementary information for a binary EEG file.

ranges from 3 to 94.

2.2. The binary EEG file format

The long-term EEG recordings are segmented into blocks of usually one hour length, each of them stored in a .data-file with a simple binary format supplemented by an additional header file containing information about channels, sampling frequency, number of samples, as well as start, duration of the block (see Fig. 1).

The .data-file itself simply consists of a sequence of samples. Thereby, each sample contains the sampled values for each channel multiplexed as 2 or 4-byte-integers into it (see Table 1). There is a constant conversion factor with that the real microvolt values can be calculated from the stored integer representations. Storing an integer representation of a sampled value is more space efficient in comparison to floats containing the sampled microvolt value.

Table 1. Logical alignment of bytes in a .data file with a 2-byte itemsize and 30 channels.

	channel 1	channel 2	...	channel 30
sample 1	bytes 1&2	bytes 3&4	...	bytes 59 & 60
sample 2	bytes 61&62	bytes 63&64	...	bytes 119&120
sample 3	bytes 121 & 122	bytes 123 & 124	...	bytes 179 & 180
...	...	...	...	...

The rationale behind the data format is the ease of use for the target audience, the seizure prediction and detection research community. It allows to easily use numerical computing environments like MATLAB, where a `.data`-file can simply be mapped into a matrix:

$$data = \mathbf{fread}(\ fid,\ [channels * \text{samples}],\ dtype\ );$$

Thereby, fid is the file descriptor of the file retrieved by the `fopen` command, and *channels*, *samples*, and *dtype* can be retrieved either the `.head`-file or from the database.

The drawback of this storage approach is the need for data conversion before being able to view the EEG files in most of the EEG system viewers, although conversion to the common EDF file format[10] is quite simple since it basically consists of a header part and several sequences of channel-multiplexed samples with a duration of up to one second. EDF is probably the most prevalent of the non system-specific file formats.

Typical sizes for such an one-hour recording block are 54 MB (30 channels, sampled at 250 Hz) to 900 MB (122 channels, sampled with 1024 Hz). Since the recording duration of a patient often exceeds 150 hours, the storage requirements for one patient may sum up to 200 GB. Typical patient datasets with surface EEG sampled at 250Hz have a size of 5 to 10 Gb, while datasets with invasive EEG sum up to 300 GB and more.

2.3. *The relational database*

A unique feature with respect to the previously available databases is the supplemented relational database with meta-data about patients as well as recordings, electrodes and EEG annotations like seizures.

Since this meta-data is stored in a relational database it can be fully queried by the SQL query language. With SQL, client applications may be built for viewing and querying the database, e.g. the web-based client that is provided for customers of the database for viewing the datasets without the need for a local database installation (see Fig. 2). Users have to be familiar with the database schema for being able to formulate and perform such queries.

2.3.1. *Database schema*

The general structure of the database schema is summarized in Fig. 3. It shows a hierarchical structure with the patient table at the top, directly referenced by the admission table, the root of the clinical meta-data. Beneath, the recording table forms the root of meta-data related to EEG recordings and annotations.

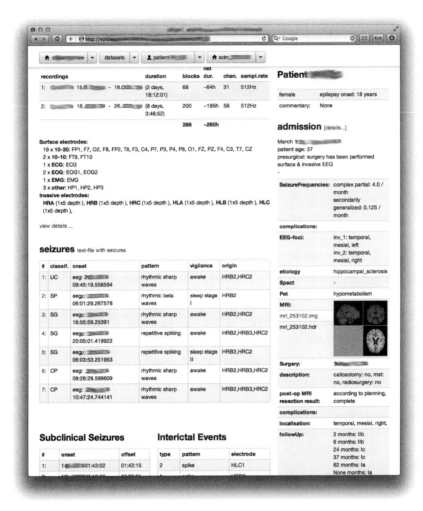

Fig. 2. Patient overview in the web-client provided for customers of the European Epilepsy Database (Dates have been blurred).

The patient table contains general information about patients, not tied to a particular evaluation period during a hospital admission. Since the database is pseudonymized only the patient's gender and epilepsy onset age are available as personal information. The table also has a field containing a code to publicly identify the patient in publications (*patientcode*).

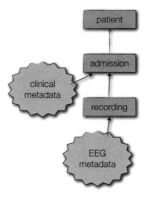

Fig. 3. The hierarchcal structure of the database schema.

2.3.2. Hospital admissions and clinical meta-data

An admission of a patient in a hospital, usually for evaluating if a surgery would be a suitable treatment, is represented by the `admission` table. The table itself contains general information like the admissions date, hospital and type of EEG (surface or invasive), as well as the final decision about a potential surgery.

The relevant information for this decision, collected during the patient's evaluation is spread across several separate tables, directly or indirectly referencing the admission table. This clinical meta-data encompass potential epilepsy causes (in the `etiology` table), findings from PET, SPECT and MR images if performed (including files in case of MRI), medication for each day including dosage, frequency of seizures before the admission extracted from seizure diaries, results from neuropsychological tests of cognitive capabilities, potential complications, and localisation (lobe and lateralisation) of EEG foci.

In case of performed surgeries, it also contains information about the surgery, its localisation (lobe and lateralisation), potential complications, histology and outcome.

2.3.3. EEG recordings and annotations

During such an pre-surgical evaluation, the EEG of the patient is recorded continuously, at least in principle. In practice, the recording may be interrupted and restarted for various reasons like a change in the electrode setup, e.g. the addition of supplementary surface electrodes for an invasive recording, technical problems of the recording system (crash, electrode impedance tests), or due to examinations like a stimulation of the patient. Whether a new recording is started after a crash or the old one is continued with a gap depends on the EEG system software.

EEG systems usually split recordings into several blocks for storage on hard disk. Thereby, some cause system immanent gaps between two blocks, some cause these only in the case of a failure.

In the database the idea behind the recording table is an episode of the patient's long-term EEG recoding with identical parameters like the contained electrodes or the sampling rate. Besides these parameters the *recording*-table contains timestamps for the beginning and the end, the net duration, the number of blocks and channels, as well as some characteristics of the recorded EEG like the background rhythm or the localisation (lobe and lateralisation) of potentially obtained EEG slowings. Thereby, one or several recordings may be related to one admission. Whether subsequent recordings all have different parameters depends on the EEG system.

Each recording block is represented by an entry in the block table containing the block specific meta-data: besides the block number and the reference to the respective recording, it contains timestamps of the beginning and the end, the duration of the block, the gap to the previous block and the size of sample values in bytes. It also redundantly contains the number of channels and samples. Lastly, it holds the conversion factor that is needed to calculate the measured potential amplitudes out of the stored raw integer value for each sample. The information is basically the same found in the `.head` files introduced in section 2.2.

Additionally, the block table holds a reference to the files table that provides information about the storage of the block in the file system. Since records in this table refer to files on the hard disk, the tables attributes correspond to properties of the respective file: besides fields containing the name, the path, the length and the file creation time, the md5-checksum of the file is stored in the checksum field. It also contains a format field which is set to 'raw' for EEG files since this table is also used for other binary files, such as MR images.

2.3.4. *Recording channels & Electrodes*

While the electrode table only contains the number of channels, detailed information about the recording channels is contained in the separate table `electrode_usage` with attributes *position* and *name* resembling the number and the name of the channel in the recording. This information is identical to the channel description in the .head-files. The `function`-field of this table may indicate if a channel is suitable as reference or acts as ground electrode. But this is rarely used since ground electrodes are not visible as separate channels in the hitherto used EEG systems.

Besides the reference to the recording table, it also has references to the tables `electrode` and `electrode_array`. Underlying these tables are the ideas of distinct physical electrode contacts, respectively the arrangement of such physical contacts into associated groups, e.g. all electrodes of the 10-20 electrode reference system, all ECG electrodes, or all 64 contacts of an invasive 8x8-grid electrode.

In our schema, the electrode table corresponds to individual electrode contacts. It provides the fields for the electrode name, in both the official ILAE nomenclature (*name*) and a potentially deviating internal name used in the EEG system (*moniker*). Additionally, it has a field indicating possible artifacts and a reference to a focus defined in the EEG focus table (currently unused). In order to reduce the number of joins in queries, we use a common table for surface and invasive electrodes, with the Boolean attribute *invasive* indicating invasive electrodes. Hence, the table has three attributes that are only used for invasive electrodes, each of them holding one dimension of the 3D coordinates of the electrode localisation in the brain. Coordinates are either given in the Montreal Neurologic Institute (MNI) coordinate system[11] or the equally widespread Talairach coordinates,[12] depending on the hospital. Lastly, it contains a reference to the table `electrode_array`.

Arrays have a name, a type, a configuration and, in case they are invasive, an implantation date. The name usually derives from the location of the array, e.g., TLA in case of the first strip electrode in the left temporal lobe or '10-20' for the standard surface electrodes of the 10-20 system. The type is a reference to the electrode array type domain table that contains a list of the possible invasive electrodes like grids, depth electrodes or electrode groups like surface or ECG electrodes. Additionally, this table has a field indicating if the array is invasive or not. Lastly, the configuration may have additional information about the array, e.g., '8x8' in case of a 64-channel grid electrode.

2.3.5. *Annotated EEG events*

The EEG contained in the database is completely manually reviewed, and three different types of EEG events have been annotated according to a common basis on definition and interpretation at different levels of detail:

Table 2.   Examplary Annotation of a seizure according to the database annotation protocol.

timestamp	annotation
2004-03-23 06:00:59	@SP/NREM I
2004-03-23 06:01:29	EEG-ON: beta: HRB2
2004-03-23 06:01:39	Prop 1: HRB1, HRB3
2004-03-23 06:02:11	CLIN-ON
2004-03-23 06:02:47	Prop 2: HRC3
2004-03-23 06:02:47	EEG-OFF
2004-03-23 06:02:47	CLIN-OFF

clinical manifest seizures, subclinical seizures and interictal events.

Such EEG annotations are markers set by the epilepsy experts during the review for EEG events, consisting of timestamp and textual content. We have developed a protocol defining a standard for syntax (see Fig. 4) and semantics of such annotation markers that can be deployed in the clinical workflow to ease the integration of datasets into the database, albeit annotations according to this protocol exceed the requirements for clinical use. Table 2 shows exemplary annotations of a seizure.

Clinical manifest seizures are clearly the most important of the considered EEG events and therefore annotated at the greatest level of detail. Thereby, the parsed textual content as well as the marker timestamps are used to fill the various fields of the tables `seizure` and `propagation`: The fields *classification*, indicating a simple, complex partial, or secondarily generalized type of seizure, and *vigilance* with the patients state of vigilance determined 10 seconds before seizure onset, are directly taken from the @-marker (see Table 2).

The onset and offset times for both the seizures clinical and the EEG manifestations are directly taken from the timestamps of the respective markers (Table 2) and written to the fields *eeg_onset, eeg_offset, clin_onset, clin_offset*. Thereby, the clinical onset/offset is determined by video surveillance, which is not included in the database due to data privacy requirements, and may not be available in case of missing video. The EEG onset/offset is determined by EEG and may not be available in case of severe artifacts. Not available annotations are indicated by *NA* markers.

If applicable, the first change in the EEG and the first clinical sign of a seizure are annotated with *EEG-?* and *CLIN-?* markers and again, the timestamp of these markers is written to the fields *first_eeg_change* and *first_clin_sign*.

288

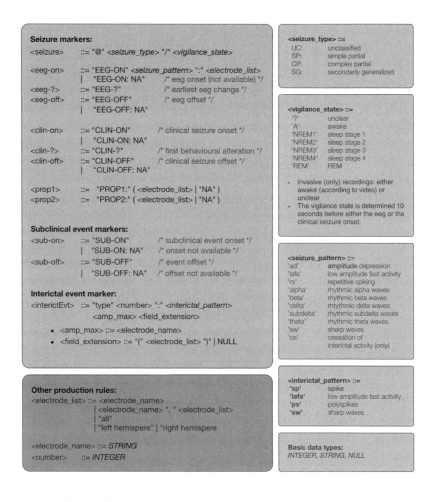

Seizure markers:

\<seizure\>	::= "@" \<seizure_type\> "/" \<vigilance_state\>	
\<eeg-on\>	::= "EEG-ON" \<seizure_pattern\> ":" \<electrode_list\>	
	| "EEG-ON: NA"	/* eeg onset (not available) */
\<eeg-?\>	::= "EEG-?"	/* earliest eeg change */
\<eeg-off\>	::= "EEG-OFF"	/* eeg offset */
	| "EEG-OFF: NA"	
\<clin-on\>	::= "CLIN-ON"	/* clinical seizure onset */
	| "CLIN-ON: NA"	
\<clin-?\>	::= "CLIN-?"	/* first behavioural alteration */
\<clin-off\>	::= "CLIN-OFF"	/* clinical seizure offset */
	| "CLIN-OFF: NA"	
\<prop1\>	::= "PROP1:" (\<electrode_list\> | "NA")	
\<prop2\>	::= "PROP2:" (\<electrode_list\> | "NA")	

Subclinical event markers:

\<sub-on\>	::= "SUB-ON"	/* subclinical event onset */
	| "SUB-ON: NA"	/* onset not available */
\<sub-off\>	::= "SUB-OFF"	/* event offset */
	| "SUB-OFF: NA"	/* offset not available */

Interictal event marker:

\<interictEvt\> ::= "type" \<number\> ":" \<interictal_pattern\>
    \<amp_max\> \<field_extension\>

- \<amp_max\> ::= \<electrode_name\>
- \<field_extension\> ::= "(" \<electrode_list\> ")" | NULL

Other production rules:

\<electrode_list\> ::= \<electrode_name\>
    | \<electrode_name\> ", " \<electrode_list\>
    | "all"
    | "left hemispere" | "right hemispere"

\<electrode_name\> ::= STRING
\<number\> ::= INTEGER

\<seizure_type\> ::=

UC:	unclassified
SP:	simple partial
CP:	complex partial
SG:	secondarily generalized

\<vigilance_state\> ::=

'?'	unclear
'A'	awake
'NREM1'	sleep stage 1
'NREM2'	sleep stage 2
'NREM3'	sleep stage 3
'NREM4'	sleep stage 4
'REM'	REM

- invasive (only) recordings: either awake (according to video) or unclear
- The vigilance state is determined 10 seconds before either the eeg or the clinical seizure onset.

\<seizure_pattern\> ::=

'ad'	amplitude depression
'lafa'	low amplitude fast activity
'rs'	repetitive spiking
'alpha'	rhythmic alpha waves
'beta'	rhythmic beta waves
'delta'	rhtythmic delta waves
'subdelta'	rhythmic subdelta waves
'theta'	rhythmic theta waves
'sw'	sharp waves
'ce'	cessation of interictal activity (only)

\<interictal_pattern\> ::=

'sp'	spike
'lafa'	low amplitude fast activity
'ps'	polyspikes
'sw'	sharp waves

Basic data types:
INTEGER, STRING, NULL

Fig. 4.   Syntax of markers in the database annotation protocol.

Additionally the *EEG-ON* marker defines a token for the seizure pattern and a list of electrodes names at which the seizure originates. While the seizure pattern is simply written to the *pattern* field as reference to the domain table `seizure_pattern`, for each electrode in the origin list a new record in the `propagation` table is created with references to the according records in the `electrode` and `seizure` tables and the *origin* field set to *true*.

In addition to the seizure origin electrodes the protocol defines two further sets of electrodes involved in propagation phases: the electrodes involved in the seizure within the first ten seconds after seizure onset, and electrodes being involved later (see the *prop* markers in table 2). Again, for each such electrode a new record in the `propagation` table is created, but here, either the field *early* or *late* is set depending on the propagation phase.

Directly related to a seizure is the semiology table holding detailed information about the seizures semiology, i.e., the clinically observed signs of the seizure. Among them are ictal and post-ictal, subjective symptoms, motor, vegetative signs and aspects like language capabilities and reactivity.

For subclinical events, electrographic ictal patterns without clinical manifestation, only the beginning and the end is annotated in the EEG. Hence, the table `subclinicalEvent` contains only the fields *onset* and *offset* with the timestamps of the according markers besides the references to the respective recording and block. Because subclinical events may possibly allow further insights into the seizure generating processes, it was decided to mark at least ten subclinical events per day for each patient. While a complete analysis of all subclinical events is not possible, database users may thereby study at least some of the subclinical events that occurred.

Interictal events, i.e., abnormal EEG activity in the phase between two seizures, cannot be annotated in full extent as well in long-term recordings. So it was decided to mark some characteristic events exemplarily for each of the patients types of interictal events. Here, a type is determined by the pattern of the event and the electrode where the event has its maximum amplitude. Like with subclinical patterns, this information can be used to analyze EEG changes related to these events.

3. Discussion

Up to now, the seizure prediction research was hampered since only few research groups had access to EEG data. Data used were often short and/or non-continuous, and underlying groups of patients were often small. This led to overfitting and little statistical reliability of the results obtained. Moreover, due to missing standards, studies were hardly comparable and reproducibility was not always ensured. To conduct high-quality prediction studies, standardized long-term EEG recordings of many patients containing interictal data are required. Therefore, data may be split into a continuous long-term dataset used for optimizing the prediction system and a second dataset for evaluating its performance in a quasi-prospective manner.

In the course of the EU-funded EPILEPSIAE project, the largest epilepsy database worldwide has been compiled.[13] Consisting of datasets of 275 patients and comprising more than 2,500 seizures, it exceeds earlier databases by more than one order of magnitude. In addition to the standardized annotated recordings of the EEG and ECG of the patients, it contains extensive meta-data on technical and clinical details of the recordings and clinical information about patients. The first 60 of the 275 datasets have been made publicly available in 2012 (conditions listed at epilepsy-database.eu), and the remaining datasets will be available in the future. It solves the problem of public availability of well-annotated continuous long-term EEG/ECG data. And it will allow for annotation standards and facilitate reproducibility and comparison of prediction studies as well as studies focusing on seizure detection, basic neurophysiology, and other fields. The data included were limited to those from patients who were undergoing pre-surgical monitoring, as these patients are pharmaco-resistant and were of particular relevance for applications of seizure prediction as targeted in the EU project EPILEPSIAE. Certainly this criterion as well as the required seizure frequency led to a strong selection bias, and data are not representative of all patients with focal epilepsy. In principle, the database is open to a future extension to other EEG data from patients with a variety of syndromes and investigated for other diagnostic reasons.

References

1. W. Stacey and B. Litt, *Nat Clin Pract Neurol* **4**, 190 (2008).
2. A. G. Stein, H. G. Eder, D. E. Blum, A. Drachev and R. S. Fisher, *Epilepsy Res* **39**, 103 (2000).
3. W. H. Theodore and R. S. Fisher, *Lancet Neurol.* **3**, 111 (2004).
4. I. Osorio, M. G. Frei, S. Sunderam, J. Giftakis, N. C. Bhavaraju, S. F. Schaffner and S. B. Wilkinson, *Ann Neurol.* **57**, 258 (2005).
5. F. Mormann, R. Andrzejak, C. Elger and K. Lehnertz, *Brain* **130**, 314 (2007).
6. B. Schelter, J. Timmer and A. Schulze-Bonhage (eds.), *Seizure prediction in epilepsy: from basic mechanisms to clinical applications* (Wiley-VCH, Berlin, Germany, 2008).
7. C. Gierschner and A. Schulze-Bonhage, *Considerations on Database Requirements for Seizure Prediction*, in *Seizure Prediction in Epilepsy*, (Wiley-VCH, Berlin, Germany, 2008), ch. 20.
8. A. Schulze-Bonhage, H. Feldwisch-Drentrup and M. Ihle, *Epilepsy Behav.* **22**, S88 (2011).
9. J. Klatt, H. Feldwisch-Drentrup, M. Ihle, V. Navarro, M. Neufang, C. Teixeira, C. Adam, M. Valderrama, C. Alvarado-Rojas, A. Witon, M. Le Van Quyen, F. Sales, A. Dourado, J. Timmer, A. Schulze-Bonhage and B. Schelter, *Epilepsia* **53**, 1669 (2012).

10. B. Kemp, A. Vrri, A. C. Rosa, K. D. Nielsen and J. Gade, *Electroencephalogr Clin Neurophysiol* **82**, 391 (1992).

11. A. Evans, D. Collins, S. Mills, E. Brown, R. Kelly and T. Peters, 3D statistical neuroanatomical models from 305 MRI volumes, in *Nuclear Science Symposium and Medical Imaging Conference, 1993., 1993 IEEE Conference Record.*, oct-6 nov 1993.

12. J. Talairach and P. Tournoux, *Co-planar stereotaxic atlas of the human brain* (Thieme, Stuttgart, Germany, 1988).

13. M. Ihle, H. Feldwisch-Drentrup, C. A. Teixeira, A. Witon, B. Schelter, J. Timmer and A. Schulze-Bonhage, *Comput Methods Programs Biomed* **106**, 127 (2012).